Progress in Drug Research

Vol. 55

Edited by Ernst Jucker, Basel

Authors
Q. May Wang and Beverly A. Heinz
Jay A. Glasel
Gerlie C. de los Reyes, Robert T. Koda and
Eric J. Lien
Angelo Vedani and Max Dobler
Paul A. Keifer
Laurane G. Mendelsohn
Satya P. Gupta

Springer Basel AG

Editor

Dr. E. Jucker
Steinweg 28
CH-4107 Ettingen
Switzerland
e-mail: jucker.pdr@bluewin.ch

Visit our PDR homepage: http://www.birkhauser.ch/books/biosc/pdr

© 2000 Springer Basel AG
Originally published by Birkhäuser Verlag, Basel, Switzerland in 2000
Cover design and layout: Gröflin Graphic Design, Basel
ISBN 978-3-0348-9544-6   ISBN 978-3-0348-8385-6 (eBook)
DOI 10.1007/978-3-0348-8385-6

9 8 7 6 5 4 3 2 1

Contents

Foreword by the Editor

Volume 55 of *Progress in Drug Resarch* contains seven articles with the latest information on important and actual fields of drug research. In addition, this volume contains several indices which facilitate the use of these monographs. Over the 41 years of its existence, PDR covered practically all important fields of drug research and also serve as an encyclopedic source of information.

The articles in volume 55 deal with the prevention and treatment of hepatitis C virus infections, with NMR spectroscopy and its role in solving important problems in the field of drug discovery, with the roles of opioid peptides and narcotics on the growth of a variety of cells, including those of the immune system. Osteoarthritis is one of the most prevalent problems detected in elderly people. Until recently, anti-inflammatory drugs have been used in standard treatments. In the last few years, however, it was discovered that glucosamine sulfate and chondroitin sulfate and their derivatives are effective and safer alternatives to alleviate symptoms of osteoarthritis. Here, the findings are comprehensively reviewed. Another article deals with the newly synthesised non-steroid androgen agonists which may have tissue-selective effects on prostatic cancer and, hopefully, demonstrate useful therapeutic effects. The last contribution is devoted to the quantitative structure-activity relationships (QSAR) of cardiotonic agents.

All these reviews contain comprehensive bibliographies, thus enabling the interested reader to access the original literature.

Since the founding of PDR in 1958/59, drug research has undergone drastic changes. The original purpose of this series of monographs, however, remained unchanged: dissemination of information about the actual trends and directions of drug research and its consequences for the therapy of life treatening diseases. The editor is anxious to maintain the high standard of these monographs and is greatly assisted by the authors who are willing to undertake the hard work of writing comprehensive review articles for the benefit of the ill and of those who are involved with drug research. I would like to thank all authors for their excellent contibutions. My gratitude goes also to the members of the Board of Advisors for their advice and for suggesting current topics. The reviewers have greatly helped improve these monographs, and I am grateful to them as well.

Last but not least, I would like to express my deep gratitude to the staff of Birkhäuser Publishers Inc. Daniela Brunner gave me most valuable assistance. She greatly influenced the presentation of the scientific facts and did not hesitate to critisize some of my – probably old-fashioned – attitudes. Ruedi Jappert, Bernd Luchner, Eduard Mazenauer and Gregor Messmer invested their vast experience and knowledge in the layout and the actual production of the book. My very special thanks go to Mr. Hans-Peter Thür, Birkhäuser Publishing's CEO. Over the many decades of close cooperation, I did and still do enjoy Mr. Thür's full support linked with his encouragement to continue – after so many years – with the editorship of PDR.

Basel, September 2000   Dr. E. Jucker

Progress in Drug Research, Vol. 55 (E. Jucker, Ed.)
©2000 Birkhäuser Verlag, Basel (Switzerland)

Recent advances in prevention and treatment of hepatitis C virus infections

By Q. May Wang and
Beverly A. Heinz

Infectious Diseases Research, Lilly
Research Laboratories, Eli Lilly and
Company, Indianapolis, IN 46285,
USA

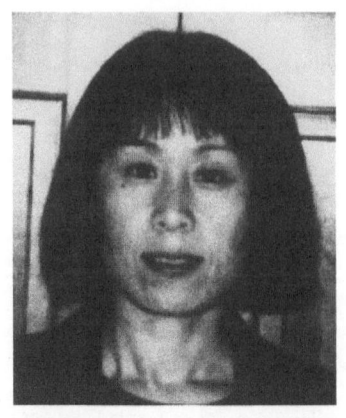

Q. May Wang

received her B.S. and M.S. degrees with a major in Biology from Shandong University, China. She earned her Ph.D. in Biochemistry from Purdue University, Indiana and then had post-doctoral training at Indiana University School of Medicine. Dr. Wang joined Lilly Research Laboratories as a Senior Biochemist in 1995.

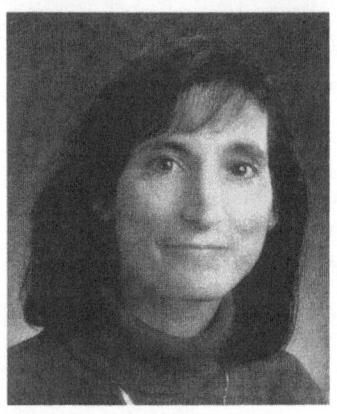

Beverly A. Heinz

earned a B.S. in Biology from Rensselaer Polytechnic Institute in Troy, New York, and her M.S. and Ph.D. degrees from the Department of Bacteriology at the University of Wisconsin-Madison. She then completed four years of post-doctoral training at the Institute for Molecular Virology at UW-Madison. In 1990, Dr. Heinz joined Lilly Research Laboratories as a Senior Virologist working in the field of antiviral drug discovery.

Summary

Hepatitis C virus (HCV) is the leading cause of chronic hepatitis in humans. As members of the flavivirus family, HCVs are a group of small single-stranded, positive-sense RNA viruses. Upon translation of the genome, a polyprotein precursor is synthesized and further processed by both cellular and viral proteases to generate functional viral proteins. Treatment options are currently limited to the administration of α-interferon alone or in combination with ribavirin. Unfortunately, these approaches are characterized by relatively poor efficacy and an unfavorable side-effect profile. Therefore, intensive effort is directed at the discovery of novel molecules to treat this disease. These new approaches include the development of prophylactic and therapeutic vaccines, the identification of interferons with improved pharmacokinetic characteristics, and the discovery of novel drugs designed to inhibit the function of three major viral proteins: protease, helicase and polymerase. Finally, the HCV RNA genome itself, particularly the IRES element, is being actively exploited as an antiviral target using antisense molecules and catalytic ribozymes. This review summarizes the most recent findings in each of these areas. Although not intended to be comprehensive, it should serve as a first resource for those individuals who desire updated information in this rapidly changing field.

Contents

Keywords
Hepatitis, hepatitis C virus, interferon, ribavirin, antiviral inhibitors, IRES, protease inhibitors.

Glossary of abbreviations
ALT, aminotransferase levels; CTL, cytotoxic T lymphocyte; HCC, hepatocellular carcinoma; HCV, hepatitis C virus; IFN, interferon; IMPDH, inosine monophosphate dehydrogenase; IRES, internal ribosome entry site; NS, nonstructural; NTR, non-translated region; ORF, open reading frame; PTB, polypyrimidine tract binding; SAR: structure-activity relationship.

1   Introduction

Hepatitis C virus (HCV) was first identified in 1989 as the etiologic agent of non-A, non-B hepatitis [1] and is currently recognized as the leading cause of chronic liver disease worldwide. In contrast to hepatitis B virus infection, in which only about 5% of adult infections become chronic, more than 80% of HCV-infected patients develop chronic hepatitis. Moreover, 20–50% of those persistently infected with HCV will develop liver cirrhosis and hepatocellular carcinoma (HCC) [2]. It is estimated that there are 10,000 deaths in the USA per year due to chronic liver failure or HCC [3]. In addition, HCV disease is responsible for 25–50% of all liver transplants in US centers, and the recurrence of HCV infection following liver transplantation is universal [4]. Typically, HCV disease emerges after a 10–20 year period during which symptoms, if they exist at all, are mild and non-specific. Although the prevalence varies greatly among different countries, it has been estimated that up to 170 million people (3% of the world's population), are infected with HCV [5]. A recent study in the USA found that 65% of all HCV-infected persons are 30 to 49 years old [6].

The modes of HCV transmission include blood transfusion, occupational exposure and injection drug abuse. In addition, there are a large number of cases that continue to be attributed to unknown risk factors; these most likely result from incidental parenteral exposure to contaminated objects, such as sharing razors or toothbrushes. The frequency of sexual transmission of HCV appears to be low, except in cases of co-infection with HIV [7]. Current views on the epidemiology of HCV were recently summarized [8].

1.1   Pathogenesis

HCV disease typically begins with an acute infection which resembles other forms of acute viral hepatitis, beginning with malaise, nausea and right upper quadrant pain. Although the mean incubation period to onset of symptoms is ~7 weeks, HCV RNA is detectable in serum within 1–2 weeks. After several weeks, serum alanine aminotransferase (ALT) levels increase. Only about a third of patients will develop jaundice or other symptoms; the majority of infections are subclinical.

In at least 85% of cases, the HCV infection becomes chronic (for review see [9]). Symptoms seen in these patients, such as nausea, anorexia and dark urine, are generally mild and nonspecific, and serum ALT levels tend to fluctuate between elevated and normal. The major serious complication of chronic HCV infection, which can take from 1 to 30 years to develop, is cirrhosis. The development of cirrhosis is characterized by the symptoms of end-stage liver disease, including severe fatigue, muscle weakness and jaundice. Cirrhosis caused by HCV infection is currently the most frequent cause of liver transplantation in the USA and western Europe. In addition, chronic HCV infection is a major cause of hepatocellular carcinoma, a disease for which treatments are inadequate. The molecular relationship between HCV infection and hepatocarcinogenesis was recently reviewed [10]. Finally, several nonhepatic manifestations of HCV infection are known as well, including arthritis, glomerulonephritis, essential mixed cryoglobulinemia, and porphyria cutanea tarda [11].

The pathogenesis of HCV infection is believed to have a basis in immunological injury, involving both humoral and cellular factors (reviewed in [12]). In these models, liver cell damage is caused by soluble cytotoxic mediators and the activation of inflammatory cells. A role for apoptosis has been proposed as well (summarized in [13]). Unfortunately, research in these areas is hampered by the lack of a cell culture virus replication system and a small animal model for infection.

1.2   Infectious agent

The HCV virion is composed of a lipid bilayer with two species of membrane glycoprotein (E1 and E2) surrounding a nucleocapsid. The genome, as shown in Figure 1, consists of one piece of single-stranded, positive-sense RNA containing approximately 9500 nucleotides encoding a single open reading frame (ORF). The plus-strand RNA is replicated *via* a negative-stranded intermediate. Although HCV cannot yet be replicated reliably in cell culture, transcripts encoding the plus-sense RNA have been shown to be infectious in the chimpanzee animal model [14, 15]. The overall genome sequence and organization of HCV, as well as its apparent method of replication, most closely resemble the family *Flaviviridae*. This family of viruses contains the classic flaviviruses, such as the yellow fever and dengue fever

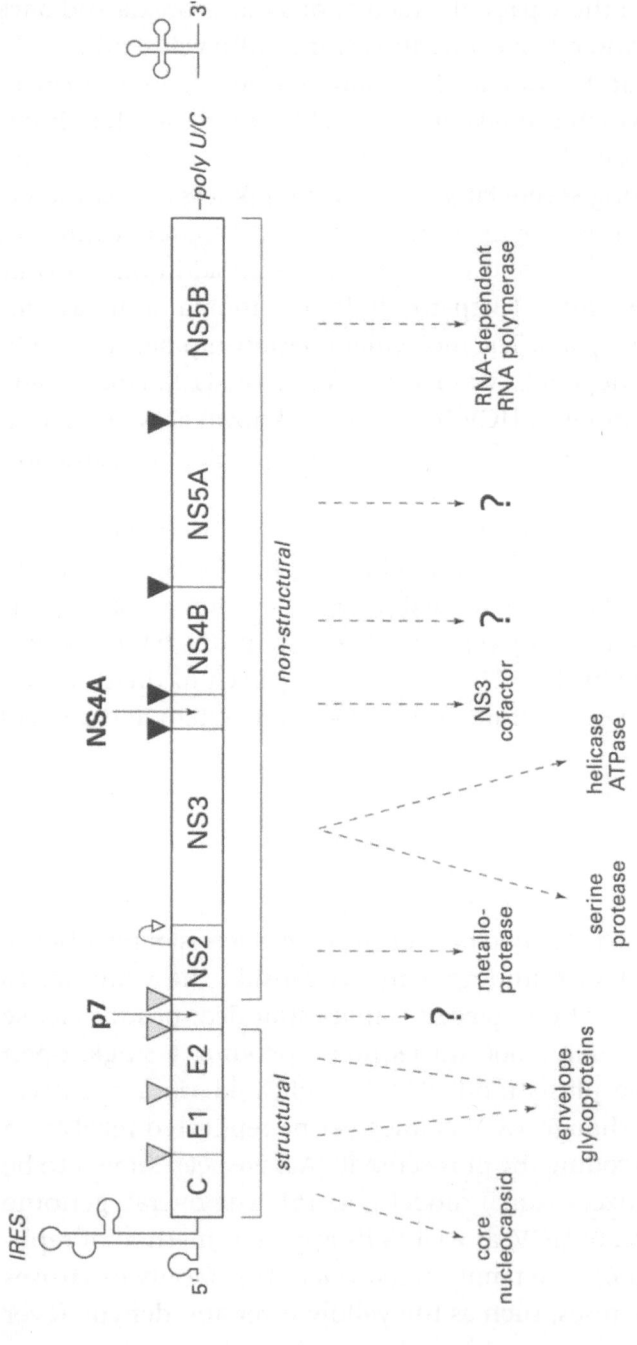

Fig. 1

Schematic of HCV genome organization and processing of viral proteins. Boxes represent the coding regions; stem-loop structures represent the 5'- and 3'-NTRs. Cleavages mediated by host signal peptidase are indicated by grey triangles. NS3 serine protease cleavage sites are designated by black triangles. Self-cleavage at the NS2/NS3 junction is shown by a curved arrow. Proteins whose function is unknown are indicated by a question mark.

viruses, and the pestiviruses, including bovine viral diarrhea and hog cholera viruses. Recently, HCV was classified as a separate genus within this family with the name "Hepacivirus" [16]. Phylogenetic analyses have classified HCV into six major genotypes, numbered 1–6. There is a strong association with geographic distribution and HCV genotype; for example, genotype 1a is most common in North America and Europe, whereas genotypes 1b and 2 predominate in Asia [17]. Additionally, genotype 1b has been associated with more severe disease recurrence following liver transplantation than non-1b genotypes [18].

The ORF of HCV is preceded by a highly conserved 5'-nontranslated region (5'-NTR), approximately 342 nucleotides in length, whose folded structure plays at least two critical roles in virus replication. First, in its anti-sense form it controls the initiation of transcription of positive-strand RNA synthesis. Second, it governs translation of the viral polyprotein *via* an embedded IRES (internal ribosome entry site) element at approximately nucleotides #42–345 of the 5'-NTR. The translation of HCV occurs *via* a cap-independent mechanism. The IRES element functions by directing internal entry of the 40S ribosome subunits to the viral RNA at the site of the initiating AUG without scanning [19]. Thus, the HCV translation is similar to that of all picornaviral (e.g., poliovirus) and certain cellular mRNAs, such as those encoding the immunoglobulin heavy chain binding protein (BiP) and the vascular epithelial growth factor [20].

The HCV ORF translates into a single polyprotein precursor that is cleaved co- and post-translationally by both host cellular and virus-encoded proteases [21], releasing three structural and at least six nonstructural (NS) viral proteins (Fig. 1). Cleavages directed by the host cell signal peptidase produce the structural proteins, including the nucleocapsid known as core protein, two envelope proteins, E1 and E2, and a small membrane-associated protein of unknown function called p7. Signal sequences within this region direct its secretion into the endoplasmic reticulum (ER) [22]. It is known that E1 and E2 are glycosylated. The remaining six nonstructural proteins are processed by viral proteases. These include: a cis-active metalloprotease comprising the NS2 and the adjacent NS3 sequences (which cleaves the NS2/3 junction) [23], a multifunctional NS3 (containing serine protease, NTPase and unwinding helicase activities (reviewed in [24] and [25])), auxiliary factor NS4A, a cofactor for NS3 protease [26], two proteins of unknown function, NS4B and NS5A, and an RNA-dependent RNA polymerase called NS5B [27].

Downstream of the ORF is a stretch of approximately 240 bases known as the 3'-NTR. The 3'-NTR consists of three elements: a 30- to 40-nucleotide region that is poorly conserved among different genotypes, a 20- to 200-nucleotide polypyrimidine (poly U/C) tract, and a highly conserved 98-nucleotide sequence termed the 3'X region. Both the poly U/C tract and the 3'X region have been found to be essential for HCV infection in the chimpanzee model [28]. The function of the poly U/C tract is not known but is likely to be important because similar tracts are found in the untranslated regions (generally 5') of other positive-strand RNA viruses, such as cardioviruses. Additionally, the HCV poly U/C tract has been found to bind two cellular proteins: the polypyrimidine tract-binding protein, PTB, and a smaller protein known as p35 [29]. The role of the 3'X region has been explored in more detail. As determined by computer modeling and enzymatic and chemical probing, the 3'X region has been shown to form stable secondary structures [30–32]. The 3'X RNA forms a three-stem-loop structure and, like the poly U/C tract and the IRES element [33], also binds to PTB [29, 34]. The 3'X region plays a role in initiation of the synthesis of minus-strand RNA as well as the regulation of IRES-dependent translation from the 5' end of HCV RNA [35].

In infected patients, HCV tends to exist as quasi-species of closely related but distinct viral populations. This genetic heterogeneity is caused by the low fidelity of the RNA-dependent RNA polymerase which permits spontaneous nucleotide substitutions at a rate of about 10^{-2} to 10^{-3} substitutions per nucleotide per year [36]. The production of HCV quasi-species has been documented in hepatocytes, peripheral blood mononuclear cells and ascitic fluid of patients with late-stage chronic HCV [37]. As a result, therapies for HCV infection will likely be hindered by the development of viral escape mutants resistant to antiviral drugs and vaccines.

1.3   Cell culture systems

Although numerous cell-based replication assays for HCV have been reported (see [38] for review), none has yet proven to be practical and readily reproducible. This shortcoming has severely limited the possible molecular studies of HCV replication and evaluation of antiviral molecules. The majority of these approaches rely on reverse transcriptase -PCR to monitor the production of minute amounts of plus- and minus-strand RNA. Nevertheless, evidence of mutational changes in the genome of HCV during culture in hepatocytes and cell lines [39, 40] strongly suggests that HCV can replicate at a low level *in vitro*. Perhaps the most encouraging cell-based assay was recently reported by Lohmann et al. [41]. This system uses neomycin selection of hepatoma cells transfected with a bicistronic transcript encoding a subgenomic replicon of HCV lacking the structural proteins. Sufficient levels of viral RNA and protein were synthesized to permit detection by Northern blots and radioisotopic labeling, respectively. Confirmation of the significance of these results awaits reproduction of the work by other groups.

In addition, there have been recent efforts to determine the cellular receptor used by HCV during infection. The E2 glycoprotein is thought to be responsible for initiating virus attachment to its receptor [42]. Both CD81 [43] and the low density lipoprotein (LDL) receptor [44] have been implicated as the HCV receptor on target cells. In a recent study of the specificity of interaction between E2 and CD81, various forms of E2 were compared for ability to bind CD81 [45]. The authors demonstrated that monomeric rather than aggregated E2 preferentially bound to CD81, and that intracellular forms of E2 had a higher affinity for CD81 than did secreted forms. A deeper understanding of how HCV interacts with the cellular receptor must await the development of a robust cell-based viral replication assay.

1.4   Animal models

To date, chimpanzees remain the only species other than humans with known susceptibility to HCV infection. Infection in chimpanzees closely resembles that seen in humans where there is an acute phase of the disease, a host immune response, and long-term sequelae such as cirrhosis and HCC. Because the chimpanzee can be infected by injecting cDNA-derived full-length transcripts directly into the liver [14, 15], the critical role played by viral proteins or RNA structures in determining infectivity can be evaluated [46]. In addition, the chimpanzee model illustrates the basic features of pathogenesis and immunology of HCV infection (reviewed in [47]). Because the use of chimpanzees is quite limited due to high cost and low availability, alternative animal models have been intensively explored. Experimental HCV infection has been reported in tupaias (tree shrews), a species closely related to primates [48], and in immunodeficient mice [reviewed in 49]. So far, the suitability of these animal models as a replacement for the chimpanzee has not been demonstrated unequivocally.

2   Prophylactic and therapeutic vaccines for HCV

Chronic HCV infections occur at high rates despite the induction of specific humoral and cellular immune responses elicited by the host. Thus, there is a pressing need to develop new vaccination strategies. Designing a prophylactic vaccine for HCV is problematic in several respects: low levels of viremia, the existence of quasi-species due to high genetic variability in the E1 and E2 glycoproteins, and the lack of a convenient animal model. Nevertheless, there has been some encouraging progress in this area.

Vaccine candidates include recombinant subunit proteins and nucleic acids. For example, chimpanzees vaccinated with recombinant envelope proteins developed high serum titers of anti-E2 antibodies and were protected against subsequent challenge with a homologous virus [50]. Even in the cases when complete protection was not provided, the resulting infection with a challenge virus produced beneficial results (lower viremia and minimal liver disease). It has been proposed that a vaccine composed of a recombinant form of several HCV proteins including the envelope glycoprotein, should provide protection against infection by different genotypes by priming cross-neutralizing anti-envelope antibodies and wide helper and inflammatory CD4+ T-cell responses [51]. However, experience with HIV suggests that a multifaceted approach of vaccination together with antivirals may be necessary to maximize the inhibitory effect. A review of the clinical and economic issues concerning prophylactic use of immunoglobulin was recently published [52]. DNA vaccines that express viral antigens intracellularly can also serve as an immune system stimulant, especially for cytotoxic T-lymphocyte (CTL) responses. The nucleic acid may be introduced by direct injection or via a gene therapy approach. For a more complete discussion of the issues involved in the different vaccination strategies for HCV, see [53].

Currently, there are many commercial approaches underway to develop an effective HCV vaccine, some using novel methods to stimulate the immune system. Only a few examples will be described here. First, work is underway to develop technologies that deliver therapeutic proteins to stimulate a CTL response to HCV [54]. In this approach, two proteins (PA and LFn) can be inserted into the cell membrane and form a pore, facilitating the entry of peptides or protein antigens into the cytoplasm. Antigens are processed and displayed on the cell surface, eliciting a CTL response and inducing the production of cellular cytokines. Second, many novel approaches are underway to improve engineered vaccines for HCV, including epitope enhancement and the presence of cytokines in the adjuvant [55]. Clinical trials with proprietary adjuvants are underway to test vaccines that may be suitable for both prophylactic and therapeutic use [56]. In a third example, a series of vaccines is being based on proprietary immunostimulatory DNA sequences [57]. These sequences, when administered with viral antigens, are thought to redirect the immune system to elicit a CTL response instead of a humoral immune response. Pre-clinical work is underway. Similarly, an immunotherapeutic vaccine that purportedly stimulates CD4+ and CD8+ T-cells to react to HCV-infected cells is under development; clinical trials are planned for the year 2000 [58]. Fourth, an effort is underway to develop recombinant vaccine candidates based on the E1 protein of HCV 1b [59]. Pre-clinical studies in chimpanzees chronically infected with HCV indicate that the vaccine does produce antibodies to E1, resulting in the elimination of HCV antigens from the liver, restoration of normal liver enzymes and improved liver histology. Alternate approaches include DNA immunization with chimeric viruses such as Hepatitis B virus [60] and adenovirus [61], and passive immunization with immunoglobulin from HCV-infected individuals, intended for post-exposure prophylaxis and the prevention of re-infection following liver transplant [62]. In summary, much effort is underway to design and test novel prophylactic and therapeutic approaches.

3   Antiviral treatment for HCV infection

As discussed above, prevention of HCV by prophylactic vaccines has been problematic due to the presence of large numbers of HCV genotypes and subtypes. Therefore, selective inhibition of HCV replication by immune modulators or by synthetic molecules could be a very effective approach to the treatment of HCV infection. Because the clinical importance of HCV has only been recognized in recent years, the development of small-molecule therapies targeting the HCV RNA genome or proteins is still at a relatively early stage. To date, the approved treatments for chronic HCV infection consist of either interferon alone or a combination of interferon and ribavirin. The following sections summarize the interferon treatments currently available and other ongoing pre-clinical antiviral approaches.

3.1 Current treatments

In the USA, interferon-α (IFNα) was the first approved treatment for chronic HCV infections. Belonging to a group of immunomodulatory proteins also termed cytokines, IFNs are involved in the human immune defense process and can be produced/secreted by host cells following viral infections. The antiviral mechanism associated with IFNs has not been clearly defined. However, it has been proposed that IFNs act *via* a cascade of events: by binding to their specific cellular receptors, they activate certain enzymes regulating protein synthesis, and eventually initiate antiviral responses [63]. In this regard, at least two cellular enzymes are known to be activated by IFN [63]: 2',5'-oligo-adenylate synthetase (OAS) and RNA-dependent protein kinase (PKR). OAS is an enzyme responsible for the synthesis of adenylate oligomer; its activation by IFN causes viral RNA degradation. PKR is a serine/threonine protein kinase that phosphorylates initiation factor eIF2A. When PKR is activated by IFN, it will phosphorylate eIF2A, resulting in the inhibition of both mRNA translation initiation and viral replication.

The first pilot study using recombinant IFNα for treatment of chronic HCV infection was carried out in 1986 by Hoofnagle and colleagues [64]. Since then, various clinical trials have been conducted to optimize IFNα treatment of HCV-infected patients [63]. It has been concluded that approximately 40% of treated patients had an initial response to IFN therapy, and about 70% of these responders relapsed after the treatment had ended (for review see [63, 65]). Overall, the long-term response to IFNα occurred in only 10–30% of patients [66]. Interestingly, patients infected with HCV genotype 1 consistently showed a poorer response to IFNα than did the other major genotypes [63, 65]. Such a low sensitivity to IFNα might be correlated to a sequence termed the IFN-sensitivity determining region (ISDR) within the HCV NS5A gene; however, these data are highly controversial [67]. In addition, response to IFN treatment might be affected by other factors such as patient's age, ethnic differences and duration of infection [63]. Since HCV exists *in vivo* as a population of heterogeneous quasi-species, the degree of quasi-species diversity might affect a patient's response to IFN treatment. Various side-effects have been observed in patients treated with IFNα. Most patients develop a severe flu-like syndrome, with symptoms such as fever, fatigue, muscle aches and headache; some also develop more severe side effects such as depression, nausea, weight loss and diarrhea [63].

Due to the low response rate and frequent relapse associated with the IFNα monotherapy, a combination therapy of IFNα and ribavirin was explored. Ribavirin is a known antiviral agent with a broad spectrum of activity against several pathogenic DNA and RNA viruses [63, 68]. This molecule, 1-β-D-ribo-furanosyl-1,2,4-triazole-3-carboxamide, is a nucleoside guanosine analogue containing a modified base. Although the inhibitory mechanism for ribavirin is not clearly understood, it has been proposed that this molecule inhibits inosine monophosphate dehydrogenase (see below), leading to a decreased intracellular pool of guanosine triphosphate [63]. This indirectly suppresses viral RNA synthesis. Other hypothesized mechanisms of action include the direct inhibition of viral RNA-dependent RNA polymerase and the prevention of efficient translation of viral transcripts [63].

Ribavirin has been successfully used for treatment of pneumonia caused by respiratory syncytial virus infection [63, 68]. When this broad spectrum antiviral agent was used in combination with IFNα, the overall response rate increased to ~40% [69, 70]. It has been shown that the combination therapy is most effective for treatment of patients who relapsed from previous IFN treatment. Unfortunately, additional side-effects have been described in the combination treatment [69, 70]. The most significant effect was reported to be hemolytic anemia due to the accumulation of ribavirin in erythrocytes.

3.2 Emerging therapies

Efforts to improve current IFN treatments are still ongoing. In this regard, a major advance is the recent development of a pegylated version of IFNα by several groups. The pegylated IFNα is generated through modification of the lysine residues of the IFNα protein by polyethylene glycol. As compared to the native IFNα form, pegylated IFNα demonstrated improved pharmacokinetic features including an increased half-life in circulation, delayed clear-

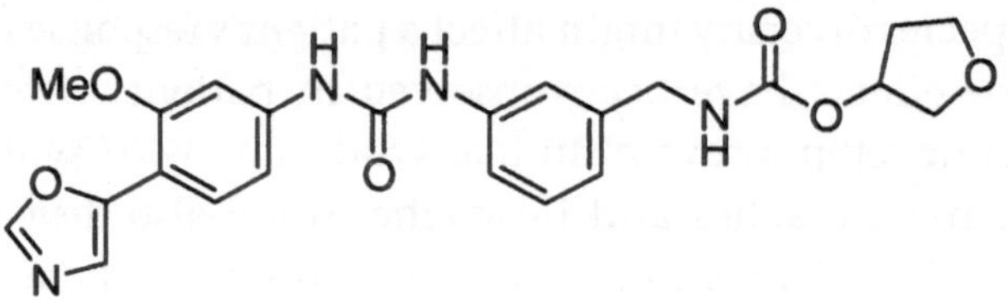

Fig. 2
VX-497

ance and reduced immunogenicity [71–73]. Therefore, the major advantage of the pegylated IFNα over the unmodified form is its properties *in vivo*, which may allow lower and less frequent doses and thus fewer side-effects. For example, the current dosage of IFNα for HCV treatment is 3 MIU administered subcutaneously or intramuscularly three times a week for 12 months, while the pegylated IFN-a could be injected once per week for the same period [73, 74]. Currently, therapeutic use of pegylated IFNα in combination with ribavirin is in phase III trials in the US and Europe.

Another emerging therapy is use of an inhibitor of cellular inosine monophosphate dehydrogenase (IMPDH) to treat HCV infections. This inhibitor, designated VX-497 (Fig. 2), was developed using structure-based drug design. VX-497 is an active site inhibitor of IMPDH and is currently in phase II clinical trials [75]. *In vitro* studies suggested that this inhibitor exerts its effects on lymphocyte migration and proliferation, and thus might prevent both virus proliferation and liver inflammation.

In a recent announcement, clinical trials have been initiated for a novel small compound that specifically inhibits a key replication activity of HCV [76]. However, no information was given regarding the compound's structure, mechanism of inhibition, or the specific target that this compound might inhibit.

3.3 Antiviral approaches in clinical and pre-clinical development

Parallel to the activities and efforts mentioned above, considerable energy has been devoted to development of specific antiviral compounds targeting the HCV genome and proteins encoded by the virus. The most recent significant advances in this regard include the identification of antisense RNAs and catalytic RNA molecules (ribozymes) that cleave the HCV genome. In addition, antiviral compounds targeting important viral enzymes such as protease, helicase, and polymerase have been discovered in recent years. Detailed information regarding progress in each of these approaches is given below.

3.3.1 Antiviral agents targeting the HCV genome

Because the sequence and structure of the HCV 5'-NTR are critical for viability and well conserved among genotypes, this region is an attractive target for the development of antivirals. The highly structured IRES in the HCV 5'-NTR controls cap-independent initiation of translation by directing ribosomes to the authentic initiation AUG upstream of the ORF. This function requires the interaction of viral RNA with proteins of cellular and, possibly, viral origin [77]. An interesting feature of the HCV IRES is that it apparently extends past the AUG into the nucleotide sequence of the core protein [78, 79]. In fact, it has been reported that the HCV core protein interacts with the 5'-NTR of the genome and modulates translation [80]. Moreover, the RNA replication signals present at the 5' terminus may also extend into the IRES element [77]. A comprehensive summary of the structure and function of the HCV IRES was recently published [81].

In the current model, the 5'-NTR folds into four structural domains, named I through IV (Fig. 3a). Domain I consists of a small stem-loop near the 5' terminus that is not critical for translation [78]. Domains II and III contain complex secondary structures. The base of Domain III forms an essential RNA pseudoknot [82]. Domain IV consists of a small stem-loop including the initiation AUG and the first 11 nucleotides of the ORF. In a recent study, chemical and enzymatic probing of the IRES in solution under various ionic conditions demonstrated that the RNA has a unique and stable three-dimensional structure at physiological salt concentrations; this folding is dependent on divalent metal ions [83]. The HCV IRES is unique in that 40S ribosomal subunits bind directly to the RNA in the absence of all initiation factors [84], including eIF4A, which is required for ribosomal attachment to capped mRNAs and the picornaviral IRES [85]. Thus, the HCV IRES first recruits the translational components, then orients the components to permit a productive interaction leading to initiation. In this way, translation initiation in HCV is similar to that of prokaryotes. The site of interaction between the IRES and p25, a component of the 40S ribosomal subunit, has been mapped using

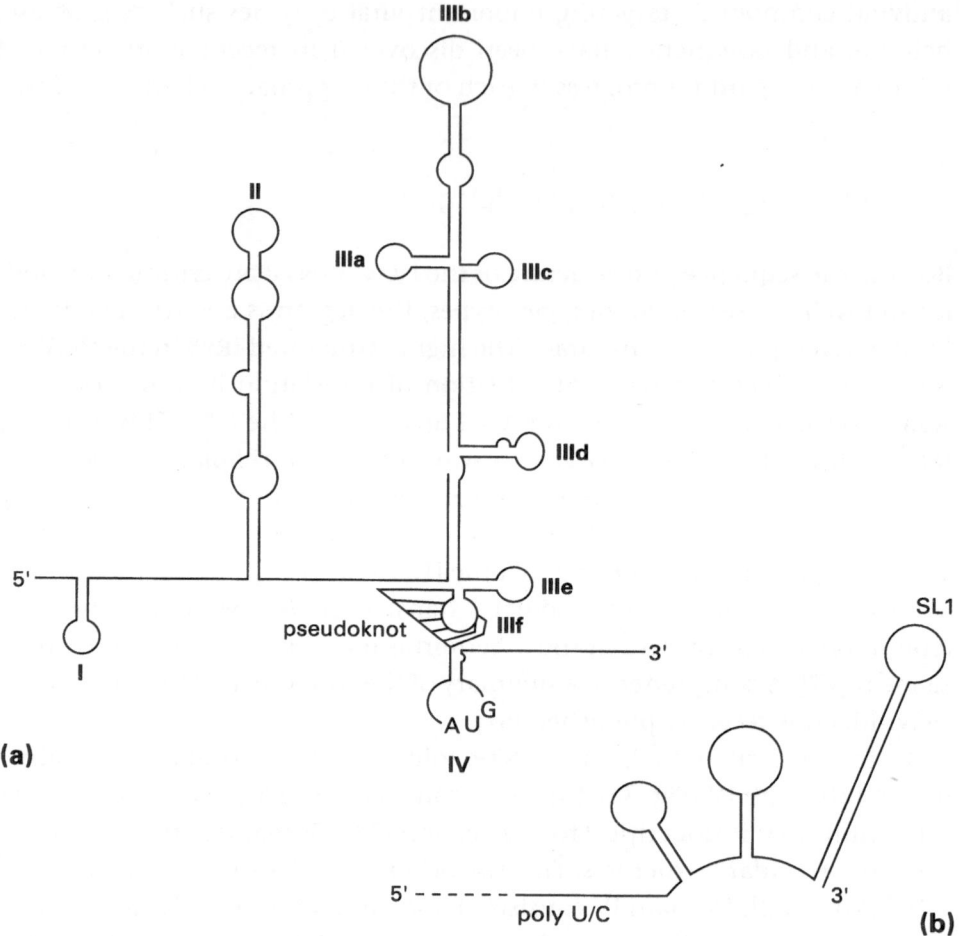

Fig. 3
Secondary and tertiary structure of the 5'- and 3'-NTRs of HCV. (a): Structure of the 3'-UTR as described in references 77, 86, and 87. Major stem-loop domains are indicated I-IV. Base-pairs involving stem-loop IIIf to form a pseudoknot structure are shown. The initiation AUG codon is indicated on stem-loop IV. (b): Secondary structure of the 98 nucleotides comprising the 3'X region of the HCV genome as identified in reference 32. The major stem-loop (SL I) is indicated.

UV cross-linking studies [86]. A detailed description of translation initiation by HCV was recently published [87].

The 98 nucleotides of the 3'X region of the 3'-NTR also fold into a conserved, stable secondary structure containing three stem-loops (Fig. 3b) [32].

This model was confirmed by chemical and enzymatic probing and temperature-dependent UV spectroscopy [32]. There is increasing evidence that the 5' and 3' termini of HCV RNA interact in ways that modulate transcription and translation [34, 88, 89].

There are many efforts underway to develop antivirals that target the 5'-NTR of HCV. Nucleic acids, in the form of antisense oligonucleotides or ribozymes, have been extensively explored in model systems. In cell culture-based assays, these molecules can be delivered in two ways: *via* liposome-mediated uptake from an extracellular source, or *via* intracellular generation using a gene therapy approach. Gene therapy using adenoviral vectors is particularly applicable to HCV infection because they can express the transgene in slowly dividing cells such as hepatocytes [90].

The use of antisense oligonucleotides against HCV has recently been investigated. The inhibitory effects of antisense molecules can be based on inhibiting translation, the induction of RNAse-H, or the inhibition of RNA splicing [91]. In recent studies, antisense oligonucleotides have been shown to inhibit HCV gene expression in *in vitro* translation assays and in transformed hepatocytes expressing the core protein [92, 93]. In addition, some of these oligonucleotides demonstrated dose-dependent inhibition of a luciferase reporter protein fused to the HCV IRES expressed in the livers of BALB/C mice [94]. The primary shortcoming of antisense molecules as therapeutic agents derives from their sensitivity to degradation by nucleases in serum. As a result, considerable effort has been devoted to identifying chemical modifications that enhance stability. Early work with phosphorothioate oligonucleotides resulted in enhanced stability but an unfavorable toxicity profile, including immune cell stimulation, complement activation and the abnormal induction of blood clotting [92]. In subsequent studies, various chemical modifications have succeeded in maximizing potency and specificity while improving half-life and toxicity profiles [91]. More recent developments suggest that a 2'-O-methoxyethyl-modified oligonucleotide may represent the next generation of antisense therapeutic agents [92]. A clinical trial to test safety and efficacy of this class of antisense oligonucleotide was recently announced [95].

A second antiviral approach based on a nucleic acid therapeutic agent is the use of hammerhead ribozymes directed against the HCV 5'-NTR [see 96 for review of antiviral ribozymes]. In surrogate cell culture systems, cleavage of this critical region results in the inhibition of IRES-driven protein translation [97]. This inhibition caused decreased infectivity in cell culture of an infectious HCV-poliovirus chimera [98]. Phase I clinical trials of a ribozyme for HCV are currently underway [99]. In other experimental approaches, the inhibition of translation results from ribozymes delivered *via* adenoviral gene therapy in cultured cells [100] and in a transgenic mouse model [101]. Similarly, the hairpin ribozymes are being developed as a potential gene therapy for HCV [102]. In this approach, a single therapeutic vector expresses several ribozymes targeting conserved regions of the viral genome.

In addition to nucleic acid-based approaches, several companies are screening the HCV IRES using libraries of small molecules. Ligand binding can be detected using a biochemical approach (that is, inhibition of translation of a reporter gene) or *via* biophysical methods. To date, no small-sized molecules have been reported as effective inhibitors targeting HCV IRES.

An additional strategy to target the HCV RNA genome is suggested by the interaction of RNA-binding proteins of cellular origin [103]. These include PTB and the La autoantigen, which have been found to bind specifically *in vitro* to either the 5'-NTR and/or 3'-NTR regions of the genome [33, 34, 104]. The relevance of these interactions was strengthened by a recent report showing that the La protein present in cytoplasmic extracts from human liver biopsies could interact specifically with the poly U/C tract of the 3'-NTR [105]. The significance of this presence is not certain, however. Unlike translation of the picornaviral IRES, PTB and La are apparently not required for the initiation of translation on the HCV IRES [84]. It is likely that a clear understanding of the role for these RNA-binding proteins will not be possible until a robust HCV replication system becomes available.

3.3.2 Antiviral agents targeting HCV proteins

As shown in Figure 1, the entire HCV genome encodes at least ten viral proteins in the following order: C-E1-E2-p7-NS2-NS3-NS4A-NS4B-NS5A-NS5B [106–109]. The six NS proteins are believed to be non-structural and involved in the viral genome replication process. In principle, each of these viral encoded proteins could serve as potential targets for antiviral therapy, assuming they are essential for viral replication and/or infection. However, the roles of some of the HCV nonstructural proteins, such as NS4B and NS5A, are not fully understood and thus no functional assays are available for these potential targets [67, 107, 110]. Consequently, development of antiviral agents that specifically interact with these viral proteins has been greatly hampered.

On the other hand, nonstructural proteins, such as NS3 and NS5B, have been studied extensively and their functions have been elucidated [106–113]. Various functional assays have been developed, which allow the measurement of their enzymatic activity in the presence of candidate antiviral compounds. As discussed below, several novel compounds demonstrating inhibitory activity against these enzymes have been identified and viewed as potential anti-HCV agents.

Development of NS3 protease inhibitors

NS3 is a multi-functional enzyme with the protease activity constrained in the N-terminal 180 amino acids and the RNA unwinding helicase and ATPase activity in the C-terminal 451 amino acids [106–109]. Sequence and structural analyses of the N-terminal domain of the NS3 protein have revealed that it represents a chymotrypsin-type serine protease with its catalytic triad identified as His-Asp-Ser [16, 26, 114]. The NS3 serine protease is responsible for generation of four mature viral proteins including NS4A, NS4B, NS5A and NS5B, which are the key components of the HCV replication complex [106–109]. It has been found that the catalytic activity of NS3 protease is stimulated by NS4A through formation of a stable complex between the two proteins [26, 115]. Recently, it has been shown that NS3 serine protease is essential for HCV replication and infection in the chimpanzee model [46]. Taken together, these observations indicate that the HCV NS3 protease, especially complexed with the NS4A cofactor, is one of the most attractive targets for chemotherapeutic intervention [24, 110, 111, 113].

Generation of active HCV NS3 protease in different recombinant systems has been reported widely (for review see [107]). Additionally, various accurate and convenient assays that employ small peptides derived from the NS3 processing sites as substrates have become available. Furthermore, the crystal structures for the full-length NS3 protein and the protease domain, alone or complexed with the NS4A fragment, have been solved [26, 114, 116, 117]. These efforts have greatly facilitated identification of viral protease inhibitors through both large-scale screening and/or rational design approaches. To date, structurally divergent molecules that inhibit the HCV NS3 protease have been described. These molecules can be classified into two major groups: nonpeptidic and peptidic.

Table 1.
Nonpeptidic inhibitors for HCV NS3 serine protease

Inhibitor	Structure	Potency	Inhibition mechanism
Phenathrenequinone (Sch68631)		$IC_{50} = 7.7\ \mu M$	ND
Thiazolidine (RD46205)		$IC_{50} = 14\ \mu M$	Noncompetitive
THNB (RD24039)		$IC_{50} = 77\ \mu M$	Mixed
Halogenated benzanilide		$IC_{50} = 6.5\ \mu M$	Noncompetitive
Hemiketal lactone (Sch351633)		$IC_{50} = 25\ \mu M$	ND

Note: for a convenient comparison, inhibition potency of the indicated compound has been converted to molar concentrations. ND, not determined; THNB, 2,4,6-trihydroxy,3-nitrobenzamide.

As seen in Table 1, several nonpeptidic molecules have been reported to inhibit HCV NS3 protease activity. These include a quinone-type compound isolated from the microorganism *Streptomyces* sp (Sch68631) [118], a thiazolidine derivative (RD46205) [119], 2,4,6-trihydroxy-3-nitrobenzamides

Table 2.
Competitive peptidic inhibitors for HCV NS3 protease

Source	Structure	Inhibition potency	Refs.
5A/5B	D-D-I-V-P-C-OH	IC_{50} = 71 µM	[123]
5A/5B	Ac-D-D-I-V-P-C-OH	IC_{50} = 28 µM	[123]
5A/5B	Ac-D-d-I-V-P-C-OH	IC_{50} = 4.0 µM	[123]
5A/5B	Ac-D-d-I-V-P-Nva-OH	IC_{50} = 17 µM	[124]
5A/5B	Ac-D-d-I-V-P-Nva-H	IC_{50} = 1.1 µM	[124]
5A/5B	Ac-D-d-I-V-P-Nva-CONHBn	IC_{50} = 0.64 µM	[124]
4A/4B	Ac-D-E-M-E-E-C-OH	IC_{50} = 1.01 µM	[125]
4A/4B	Ac-D-E-Dif-D-Cha-C-OH	IC_{50} = 0.05 µM	[126]
4A/4B	Ac-D-Gla-L-I-Cha-C-OH	IC_{50} = 0.0015 µM	[126]

Note: d is for D-Aspartic acid. The followings represent modified amino acids: Nva, norvaline; Dif, 3,3-diphenylalanine; Gla, D-γ-carboxy glutamic acid, Cha, β-cyclohexylalanine

(RD24039) [120], halogenated benzanilides [121], and a hemiketal lactone isolated from the fungus *Penicillium griseofulvum* (Sch351633) [122]. All of these molecules displayed potencies in the low micromolar range against the NS3 protease *in vitro*. These data together with their inhibitory mechanisms are summarized in Table 1.

The peptidic inhibitors thus far described for HCV NS3 are summarized in Table 2. These inhibitors were designed to mimic the peptides that represent the NS3 cleavage sites on the viral polyprotein. Some of them were identical to the NS3 cleavage products of the peptide substrates; thus they served as reversible competitive inhibitors for the viral protease. For example, a hexapeptide DDIVPC-OH, corresponding to the N-terminal cleavage product of the peptide derived from the NS5A/5B site for NS3 protease, was able to inhibit NS3 protease with an IC_{50} of 71 µM and K_i of 14 µM [123]. Potency was enhanced slightly by capping this peptide with an acetyl group at the N-terminus (Tab. 2). Further structure-activity relationship (SAR) studies revealed that replacement of P5 glutamic acid with the isomeric D-counterpart could enhance the potency several fold, while various modifications of the P1 cysteine side chain resulted in less potent compounds [124]. When norvaline was introduced into the P1 position, the resulting peptide Ac-DdIVP-Nva-OH exhibited improved inhibitory activity (Tab. 2). In a parallel investigation, NS3 inhibition by the products of peptide substrates derived from the NS4A/4B and NS4B/5A site was also observed [125]. A detailed SAR study was conducted on the hexapeptide Ac-DEMEEC-OH using a combinatorial chemistry approach [126]. After a sequential optimization at positions P2 through P5, several potent inhibitors with low-nanomolar IC_{50} were identified as summarized in Table 2 [126]. Of these, peptide Ac-D-Gla-L-I-Cha-C-OH demonstrated an IC_{50} of 1.5 nM against the purified HCV NS3 protease [126].

Similar to the approaches employed for other serine proteases, peptide analogues containing various electrophilic carbonyl groups that could serve as warheads to attack the active site serine hydroxyl group were also developed [124]. To date, aldehyde, α-ketoamide and fluorine-containing carbonyl derivatives have been explored [124]. However, these modifications to the core peptides provide only a marginal improvement in potency (Tab. 2). The most potent compound in this series is the modified peptide Ac-DdIVP-Nva-CONHBn with an IC_{50} of 0.64 μM; unfortunately, this compound lacks specificity in that it also inhibits human and porcine elastase efficiently [124]. In addition, synthesis of cyclic biphenyl ethers based on a tetrapeptide inhibitor Ac-Dif-Glu-Cha-Cys-OH has been recently reported [127]; however, no biological data are currently available for these peptidic ether analogues.

In addition to the small peptides mentioned above, a panel of macromolecular inhibitors for HCV NS3 has been disclosed. In general, these molecules are protein ligands which inhibit HCV NS3 protease through its direct binding to the viral enzyme. For example, a group of minimized antibody-like proteins, also termed minibodies, were identified through a phage-displayed synthetic repertoire. They could bind and inactivate the NS3 protease selectively with low micromolar IC_{50} and kinetic values [128–130]. Additionally, selective NS3 protease inhibitors have been designed and synthesized on the basis of eglin c protein [131]. Eglin c, a 70 amino acid protein isolated from leeches, is a well-known potent inhibitor of several serine proteases including chemotrypsin and subtilisin [132]. Several engineered eglin c mutant proteins demonstrated nanomolar potency against HCV NS3 [131]. In addition to identifying potent ligand inhbitors, these studies have provided information that will be useful for designing more potent and smaller-sized antivirals [130].

Development of HCV ATPase/helicase inhibitors
As discussed above, the C-terminal portion of the HCV NS3 protein defines an ATP-dependent helicase activity which is independent of the protease domain located at the N-terminus. Because the HCV helicase domain contains a conserved motif -DECH- box, it has been classified into the RNA heli-

Table 3.
HCV NS3 helicase inhibitors.

Piperidine derivatives	Heterocyclic carboxamide
$IC_{50} = 7~\mu M$	$IC_{50} = 0.7~\mu M$

case superfamily II (for review see [133, 134]). It is believed that HCV helicase activity is responsible for RNA unwinding during the viral replication process and its essential role has been demonstrated in the chimpanzee model [46, 107]. Due to its importance in the viral life cycle, great attention has been given to this enzyme. Generation of active recombinant HCV helicase proteins, assay development and biochemical characterization studies have been extensively described in the literature (for review see [107, 109]). In addition, the crystal structure for the HCV helicase domain, first described in 1998 [134–136], is expected to have a positive impact on the design and development of selective HCV ATPase/helicase inhibitors.

The development of specific inhibitors against the HCV helicase and/or ATPase activity has lagged behind our basic understanding of this enzyme; to date, only a few small-molecule inhibitors have been reported. Two closely related compounds, piperidine derivatives and heterocyclic substituted carboxamides, have been claimed to inhibit HCV helicase *in vitro* [137–139]. As summarized in Table 3, both compounds showed low micromolar IC_{50}s against HCV helicase activity. Macromolecular inhibitors that block HCV helicase activity have also been reported. For example, RNA aptamers rich in secondary structures were found to interact with the NS3 protein and thus inhibited both the protease and helicase activities of NS3 [140].

The ATPase activity of the HCV NS3 protein, which is required for its unwinding helicase activity, has also been viewed as a target suitable for antiviral therapy. In this regard, two compounds were recently reported to inhibit the NS3 ATPase activity. These two molecules, paclitaxel and trifluoperazine, inhibited the NS3 ATPase activity by interacting with the enzyme's ATP binding site [141]. Paclitaxel, an antimitotic agent isolated from the western yew plant, inhibited the NS3 ATPase activity competitively with an IC_{50} determined to be 17 μM, and trifluoperazine, a calmodulin antagonist, inactivated the viral ATPase by a noncompetitive mechanism with an IC_{50} of 105 μM [141]. On the other hand, paclitaxel and trifluoperazine are known for their interaction with the ATP-binding sites of other proteins, which suggested that their inhibitory activity against HCV NS3 ATPase activity was not specific.

Development of HCV polymerase inhibitors

The NS5B protein encoded by the HCV genome is associated with the RNA-dependent RNA polymerase activity [21, 142]. Recombinant NS5B expressed in both bacterial and insect cells demonstrated RNA synthesis activity using either homopolymeric RNAs or the HCV RNA genome as templates [142–144]. In the viral life cycle, the NS5B protein might assume the responsibility for viral genome replication by interacting with other viral and cellular proteins (for review see [112]). The viral polymerase has been proposed as the key component of the viral replicase complex and its essential function in HCV infection has been confirmed in the chimpanzee model [46]. Recently, several groups solved the X-ray crystallographic structure of the HCV NS5B [145–147].

HCV NS5B polymerase has also been considered an attractive target for antiviral therapy due to its critical role in viral replication and the lack of any known cellular counterparts. Notwithstanding the quantity of biochemical and structural information available for this viral polymerase, there have been no specific inhibitors that target the HCV NS5B reported so far. Nevertheless, it is noteworthy that several groups have examined the effects of known polymerase inhibitors and antiviral agents on HCV NS5B polymerase activity *in vitro*. NS5B activity was not sensitive to phosphonoacetic acid and phosphonoformic acid, inhibitors for DNA-dependent DNA polymerase and reverse transcriptases [148–150]. It has also been found that certain triphosphates of deoxynucleotide analogues which are active against other viral polymerases, such as AZT and 3TC, do not significantly inhibit the NS5B activity [148–150].

On the other hand, the presence of cerulenin and gliotoxin resulted in moderate inhibition of HCV NS5B activity [148, 151]. Interestingly, both cerulenin, a specific inhibitor of lipid and sterol biosynthesis, and gliotoxin, a fungal metabolite, have been reported to inhibit other viral RNA-dependent

RNA polymerases [148, 152]. In addition, transition state metals such as Ni^{2+} and Zn^{2+} could inhibit the NS5B RNA synthesis activity with IC_{50} in low micromolar range [150, 151]. It was proposed that these inhibitory metals compete with the required divalent cation Mg^{2+} for binding to the enzyme [150]. Certain positively charged polymers such as heparin and polylysine could also inhibit HCV NS5B polymerase activity in vitro [150]. However, their inhibition mechanism has not been clearly defined.

More recently, several groups reported that purified HCV NS5B polymerase is capable of synthesizing RNA using a primer-independent *de novo* mechanism of initiation [153–155]. It is generally accepted that a *de novo* RNA initiation pathway is likely to be the mode of viral RNA genome replication that takes place in infected cells. Therefore, NS5B polymerase assays developed based on this function might promote the discovery of novel inhibitors that specifically block the initiation step.

Inhibitor development for other HCV proteins and enzymes
In the absence of an efficient cell culture system for HCV replication, antiviral research targeting HCV proteins with no known function or with no functional assay available, such as NS4B and NS5A, has been hindered. Consequently, there have been no specific inhibitors reported for these proteins to date.

It is worth mentioning that NS4A, a cofactor for the NS3 serine protease, could be an interesting target for antiviral development [24, 107, 109]. It has been proposed that a direct interaction between NS3 and the NS4A cofactor might be important for NS3 proteolytic activity [26, 115]. From this point of view, inhibitors that block the protein-protein interaction between NS3 and NS4A would have the potential to interfere with viral polyprotein processing catalyzed by NS3 protease [26, 109, 115]. Several peptides derived from NS4A demonstrated inhibitory activity against HCV NS3 protease activity *in vitro* with low micromolar IC_{50} values [110, 156]. They apparently inhibited the NS3 enzyme by competing with the cofactor NS4A for binding to the enzyme [110].

In addition to the viral proteins discussed above, HCV NS2 protein is also of particular interest. No known cellular homologues of NS2 have been identified. Its N-terminal portion is responsible for membrane association, and its C-terminus together with NS3 is believed to catalyze the cleavage of NS2/3 site on the viral polyprotein ([107] for review). Unlike the NS3 serine protease, the catalytic mechanism of the NS2/3 protease has not been clearly defined. It functions either as a metalloprotease requiring metals such as Zn^{2+} for activity or as a cysteine protease [157, 158]. Interestingly, cleavage product-derived peptides or peptides resembling the NS2/3 cleavage site did not inhibit the NS2/3 protease activity, while peptides derived from NS4A were found to inactivate NS2/3 activity with K_i values as low as 3 µM [159].

4   Conclusions

As the major cause of chronic hepatitis in humans, HCV is closely associated with cirrhosis and hepatocellular carcinoma. At present, no effective prophylactic vaccines or antivirals are available for either prevention or treatment of HCV-related infections. The major challenges for vaccine development include the existence of divergent HCV genotypes and quasi-species and the induction of persistence despite the presence of specific immune responses. Current treatment options, which are limited to interferon alone or in combination with ribavirin, provide only limited efficacy and/or unfavorable side effects for a large proportion of patients. Unfortunately, the lack of an efficient cell culture system and a convenient animal model to study HCV replication and *in vivo* infection has greatly impeded efforts to develop HCV-specific antivirals. In spite of these obstacles, two different approaches have been intensively explored in recent years. One approach is to target well-characterized HCV enzymes and the other is to target the HCV RNA genome itself.

To date, peptidic inhibitors active in the nanomolar range for HCV NS3 protease have been described. However, the non-peptidic inhibitors identified thus far demonstrated only moderate activity. It is hoped that extensive SAR studies based on these core structures may result in more potent compounds. As compared to the NS3 protease, developments of specific inhibitors against the HCV polymerase and helicase are proceeding at a much slower rate. The expectation is that the availability of their crystal structures will facilitate identification of novel inhibitors against these enzymes. On the other hand, significant progress has been made in developing inhibitors that target the HCV genome. In this regard, two molecules targeting the HCV IRES have recently entered phase I clinical trials: an antisense oligonucleotide, ISIS 14803 [95], and a catalytic hammerhead ribozyme,

LY466700 [99]. This progress provides optimism that an effective antiviral agent will emerge within the next few years for treatment of HCV infections.

Acknowledgment

The authors would like to thank Dr. Joseph Colacino for reviewing this paper and providing helpful suggestions.

References

1   Choo Q.-L., G. Kuo, A.J. Weiner, R.L. Overby, D.W. Bradley and M. Houghton: Science *244*, 359 (1989).
2   Saito I., T. Miyamura, A. Ohbayashi, H. Harada, T. Katayama, S. Kikuchi, Y. Watanabe, S. Koi, M. Onji, Y. Ohta et al.: Proc. Natl. Acad. Sci. USA *87*, 6547 (1990).
3   Consensus Development Panel. National Institutes of Health Consensus Development Conference Panel statement: Hepatology *26*, Suppl. 1, 2S (1997).
4   Berenguer, M. and T.L. Wright: Proc. Assoc. Amer. Phys. *110*, 98 (1998).
5   World Health Organization: Weekly Epidemiological Record *72*, 65 (1997).
6   Alter, M., D. Kruszon-Moran, O.V. Nainan, G.M. McQuillan, F. Gao, L.A. Moyer, R.A. Kaslow and H.S. Margolis: New Engl. J. Med. *341*, 556 (1999).
7   Wright, T., H. Hollander, X. Pu et al.: Hepatology *20*, 1152 (1994).
8   Thomas, D.L.: Curr Top Microbiol Immunol. *242*, 25 (2000).
9   Hoofnagle, J.H.: Hepatology *26*, 15S (1997).
10   Hayashi, J., H. Aoki, Y. Arakawa and O. Hino: Intervirology *42*, 205 (1999).
11   Hadziyannis, S.J.: J. Viral Hepatitis *4*, 9 (1997).
12   Cerny, A. and F.V. Chisari: Hepatology *30*, 595 (1999).
13   Lau, J.Y.N., X. Xie, M.M.C. Lai and P.C. Wu: Seminars in Liver Disease *18*, 169 (1998).
14   Kolykhalov, A.A, A.A. Agapov, K.J. Blight, K. Mihalik, S.M. Feinstone and C.M. Rice: Science *277*, 570 (1997).
15   Yanagi, M., R.H. Purcell, S.U. Emerson and J. Bukh: Proc. Natl. Acad. Sci. USA *97*, 8738 (1997).
16   Miller, R.H. and R.H. Purcell: Proc. Natl Acad. Sci. USA *87*, 2057 (1990).
17   Mizokami M. and E. Orito: Intervirology *42*, 159 (1999).
18   Gordon, F.D., J.J. Poterucha, J. Germer, N.N. Zein, K.P. Batts, J.B. Gross Jr., R. Wiesner and D. Persing: Transplantation *63*, 1419 (1997).
19   Honda, M., E.A. Brown and S.M. Lemon: RNA *2*, 955 (1996).
20   Houdebine L.M. and J. Attal: Transgenic Res. *8*, 157 (1999).
21   Major, M.E. and S.M. Feinstone: Hepatology *25*, 1527 (1997).
22   Hijikata, M., H. Mizushima, Y. Tanji, Y. Komoda, Y. Hirowatari, T. Akagi et al.: Proc. Natl. Acad. Sci. USA *90*, 10773 (1993).
23   Grakoui A., D.W. McCourt, C. Wychowski, S.M. Feinstone and C.M. Rice: Proc. Natl. Acad. Sci. USA *90*, 10583 (1993).

24   Kwong A.D., J.L. Kim, G. Rao, D. Lipovsek and S.A. Raybuck: Antiviral Res. *41*, 67 (1999).

25   Kwong, A.D., J.L. Kim and C. Lin: Curr. Top. Microbiol. Immunol. *242*, 171 (2000).

26   Kim, J.L., K.A. Morgenstern, C. Lin, T. Fox, M.D. Dwyer, J.A. Landro et al.: Cell *87*, 343 (1996).

27   DeFrancesco, R., S.E. Behrens, L. Tomei, S. Altamura and J. Jiricny: Meth. Enzymol. *275*, 58 (1996).

28   Yanagi, M., M.St. Claire, S.U. Emerson, R.H. Purcell and J. Bukh: Proc. Natl. Acad. Sci. USA *96*, 2291 (1999).

29   Luo G.: Virology *256*, 105 (1999).

30   Kolykhalov, A.A., S.M. Feinstone and C.M. Rice: J. Virol. *70*, 3363 (1996).

31   Tanaka, T., N. Kato, M.-J. Cho, K. Sugiyama and K. Shimotohno: J. Virol. *70*, 3307 (1996).

32   Blight K.J. and C.M. Rice: J. Virol. *71*, 7345 (1997).

33   Ali, N. and A. Siddiqui: J. Virol. *69*, 6367 (1995).

34   Tsuchihara, K., T. Tanaka, M. Hijikata, S. Kuge, H. Toyoda, A. Nomoto, N. Yamamoto and K. Shimotohno: J. Virol. *71*, 6720 (1997).

35   Ito, T., S.M. Tahara and M.M.C. Lai: J. Virol. *72*, 8789 (1998).

36   Fang, J.W.S., V. Chow and J.Y.N. Lau: Clin. Liver Dis. *1*, 493 (1997).

37   Hsu, C.-W., C.-T. Yeh, P. G.-C. Chen and Y.-F. Liaw: J. Infect. Dis. *180*, 992 (1999).

38   Kato, N. and K. Shimotohno: Curr. Top. Microbiol. Immunol. *242*, 261 (2000).

39   Rumin, S., P. Berthillon, E. Tanaka, K. Kiyosawa, M.-A. Trabaud, T. Bizollon, C. Gouillat, P. Gripon, C. Guguen-Guillouzo, G. Inchauspe et al.: J. Gen. Virology *80*, 3007 (1999).

40   Kato, N., M. Ikeda, T. Mizutani, K. Sugiyama, M. Noguchi, S. Hirohashi and K. Shimotohno: Jpn. J. Cancer Res. *87*, 787 (1996).

41   Lohmann, V., F. Korner, J.-O. Koch, U. Herian, L. Theilmenn and R. Bartenschlager: Science *285*, 110 (1999).

42   Rosa, D., S. Campagnoli, C. Moretto, E. Guenzi, L. Cousens, M. Chin, C. Dong, A.J. Weiner, J.Y.N. Lau, Q.-L. Choo et al.: Proc. Natl. Acad. Sci. USA *93*, 1759 (1996) .

43   Pileri, P., Y. Uematsu, S. Campagnoli, G. Galli, F. Falugi, R. Petracca, A.J. Weiner, M. Houghton, D. Rosa, G. Grandi et al.: Science *282*, 938 (1998).

44   Agnello, V., G. Abel, M. Elfahal, G. B. Knight and Q.-X. Zhang: Proc. Natl. Acad. Sci. USA *96*, 12766 (1999).

45   Flint, M., J. Dubuisson, C. Maidens, R. Harrop, G.R. Guile, P. Borrow and J.A. McKeating: J. Virol. *74*, 702 (2000).

46   Kolykhalov A., K. Mihalik, S.M. Feinstone and C.M. Rice: 6th Intl Symposium on HCV. A40 (1999).

47   Walker, C.M.: Springer Semin. Immunopathol. *19*, 85 (1997).

48   Xie, Z-C., J.-I. Riezu-Boj, J.-J. Lasarte, J. Guillen, J.-H. Su, M.-P. Civeira and J. Prieto: Virology *244*, 513 (1998).

49   Schinazi, R.F., E. Ilan, P.L. Black, X. Yao and S. Dagan: Antiviral Chem. Chemother. *10*, 99 (1999).

50   Choo, Q.-L., G. Kuo, R. Ralston, A.J. Weiner, D.Y. Chien, G. Van Nest, J. Han, K. Berger, K. Thudium, C. Kuo et al.: Proc. Natl. Acad. Sci. USA *91*, 1294 (1994).

51   Abrignani, S. and D. Rosa: Clin. Diag. Virol. *10*, 181 (1998).

52   Piazza, M., L. Sagliocca, G. Tosone, V. Guadagnino, M.A. Stazi, R. Orlando, G. Borgia, D. Rosa, S. Abrignani, F. Palumbo et al.: BioDrugs *12*, 291 (1999).

53   Houghton, M.: Curr. Top. Microbiol. Immunol. *242*, 327 (2000).

54   AVANT Immunotherapeutics, 1999.

55   Berzofsky, J.A., J.D. Ahlers, M.A. Derby, C.D. Pendleton, T. Arichi and I.M. Belyakov: Immunological Reviews *170*, 151 (1999).
56   Chiron Press Release, February 16, 1998.
57   IMSWorld R&D Focus, 9/30/99.
58   Pharmaprojects, Record No. 028455, 1999.
59   IMSWorld R&D Focus, 9/6/99.
60   R & D Insight, p. 15–16, Accession No. 11242, September 15, 1999.
61   R & D Insight, p. 21–23, Accession No. 4742, September 15, 1999.
62   R & D Insight, p. 1–2, Accession No. 4347, November 10, 1999.
63   Damen, M. and D. Bresters, in: H.W. Reesink (ed.): Curr. Stud. Hematol. Blood Transf. Karger Publishers 1998, Basel.
64   Hoofnagle, J.H., K.D. Mullen, D.B. Jones, V. Rustgi, A. Di Bisceglie, M. Peters, J.G. Waggoner, Y. Park and E.A. Jones: N. Engl. J. Med. *315*, 1575 (1986).
65   Davis, G.L. and J.H. Hoofnagle: Hepatology *6*, 1038 (1986).
66   Houghton, M., in: B.N. Fields et al. (eds.): Fields Virology. Raven Publishers 1996, Philadelphia.
67   Pawlotsky, J.M. and G. Germanidis: J. Viral Hepatitis *6*, 343 (1999).
68   Rankin, J.T. Jr., S.B. Eppes, J.B. Antczak and W.K. Joklik: Virology *168*, 147 (1989).
69   Christie, J.M. and R.W. Chapman: Hosp Med. *60*, 357 (1999).
70   Slater, M.J. and B.E. Clarke: Exp. Opin. Ther. Patents *6*, 739 (1996).
71   Hoffmann-La Roche, EP809996, 1997.
72   Hoffmann-La Roche, WO9964016, 1997.
73   Schering-Plough Press Release, Nov. 9, 1999.
74   Pharmaceutical News Daily, Jan. 7, 2000.
75   Wright, T., M.L. Shiffman, S. Knox, E. Ette, R.S. Kauffman and J. Alam: AASLD Meeting, a990 (1999).
76   Pharmaceutical News Daily, Feb. 29, 2000.
77   Lemon, S.M. and M. Honda: Seminars in Virology *8*, 274 (1997).
78   Honda, M., L-H. Ping, R.C.A. Rijnbrand, E. Amphlett, B. Clarke, D. Rowlands and S.M. Lemon: Virology *222*, 31 (1996).
79   Honda, M., R. Rijnbrand, G. Abell, D. Kim and S.M. Lemon: J. Virol. *73*, 4941 (1999).
80   Shimoike, T., S. Mimori, H. Tani, Y. Matsuura and T. Miyamura: J. Virol. *73*, 9718 (1999).
81   Rijnbrand, R.C.A. and S.M. Lemon: Curr. Top. Microbiol. Immunol. *242*, 85 (2000).
82   Wang, C., S.Y. Le, N. Ali and A. Siddiqui: RNA *1*, 526 (1995).
83   Kieft, J.S., K. Zhou, R. Jubin, M.G. Murray, J.Y.N. Lau and J.A. Doudna: J. Mol. Biol. *292*, 513 (1999).
84   Pestova, T.V., I.N. Shatsky, S.P. Fletcher, R.J. Jackson and C.U.T. Hellen: Genes Dev. *12*, 67 (1998).
85   Pestova, T.V., C.U.T. Hellen and I.N. Shatsky: Mol. Cell Biol. *16*, 6859 (1996).
86   Fukushi, S., M. Okada, T. Kageyama, F.B. Hoshino and K. Katayama:Virus Genes *19*, 153 (1999).
87   Hellen, C.U.T. and T.V. Pestova: J. Viral Hep. *6*, 79 (1999).
88   Ito, T. and M.M.C. Lai: Virology *254*, 288 (1999).
89   Ito, T., S.M. Tahara and M.M.C. Lai: J. Virol. *72*, 8789 (1998).
90   Connelly, S.: Curr. Opinion in Molec. Therapeutics *1*, 565 (1999).
91   Caselmann, W.H., S. Eisenhardt and M. Alt: Intervirology *40*, 394 (1997).

92   Brown-Driver, V., T. Eto, E. Lesnik, K.P. Anderson and R.C. Hanecak: Antisense & Nucleic Acid Drug Dev. *9*, 145 (1999).
93   Wakita, T., D. Moradpour, K. Tokushihge and J.R. Wands: J. Med. Virology *57*, 217 (1999).
94   Zhang, H., R. Hanecak, V. Brown-Driver, R. Azad, B. Conklin, M.C. Fox and K.P. Anderson: Antimicrob. Agents Chemother. *43*, 347 (1999).
95   ISIS Press Release, March 1, 2000.
96   Menke, A. and G. Hobom: Molec. Biotechnol. *8*, 17 (1997).
97   Sakamoto, N., C.H. Wu and G.Y. Wu: J. Clin. Invest. *98*, 2720 (1996).
98   Macejak, D.G., K.L. Jensen, S.F. Jamison, K. Domenico, E.C. Roberts, N. Chaudhary, I. von Carlowitz, L. Bellon, M.J. Tong, A. Conrad et al.: Hepatology *31*, 769 (2000).
99   RPI Press Release, February 16, 2000.
100   Lieber, A., C.Y. He, S.J. Polyak, D.R. Gretch, D. Barr and M.A. Kay: J. Virol. *70*, 8782 (1996).
101   Lieber, A. and M.A. Kay: J. Virol. *70*, 3153 (1996).
102   R & D Insight, p. 3–4, Accession No. 11542, February 17, 1999.
103   Yen, J.H., S.C. Chang, C.R. Hu, S.C. Chu, S.S. Lin, Y.S. Hsieh and M.F. Chang: Virology *208*, 723 (1995).
104   Ali, N. and A. Siddiqui: Proc. Natl. Acad. Sci. USA *94*, 2249 (1997).
105   Spangberg, K. Goobar-Larsson, M. Wahren-Herlenius and S. Schwartz: J. Human Virol. *2*, 296 (1999).
106   Clarke, B.: J. Gen. Virol. *78*, 2397 (1997).
107   Reed, K.E. and C.M. Rice, in: H.W. Reesink (ed.): Curr. Stud. Hematol. Blood Transf. Karger Publishers 1998, Basel.
108   Suzuki, R., T. Suzuki, K. Ishii, Y. Matsuura and T. Miyamura: Intervirology *42*, 145 (1999).
109   Littlejohn, M., S. Locarnini and A. Bartholomeusz: Antiviral Therapy *3*, 83 (1999).
110   Walker, M.A.: Drug Discov. Today *4*, 518 (1999).
111   Shoemaker, K.R.: Curr. Opin. Anti-infect. Invest. *1*, 559 (1999).
112   Hagedorn, C.H., E.H. van Beers and C. De Staercke: Curr. Top. Microbiol. Immunol. *242*, 225 (2000).
113   Bartenschlager, R.: Viral Hepat. *6*, 165 (1999).
114   Love, R.A., H.E. Parge, J.A. Wickersham, Z. Hostomsky, N. Habuka, E.W. Moomaw, T. Adachi and Z. Hostomska: Cell *87*, 331 (1996).
115   Bartenschlager, R., V. Lohmann, T. Wilkinson, J.O. Koch: J. Virol. *69*, 7519 (1995).
116   Yan, Y., Y. Li, S. Munshi, V. Sardana, J.L. Cole, M. Sardana, C. Steinkuehler, L. Tomei, R. De Francesco, L.C. Kuo and Z. Chen: Protein Sci. *7*, 837 (1998).
117   Yao, N., P. Reichert, S.S. Taremi, W.W. Prosise and P.C. Weber: Structure Fold Des. *7*, 1353 (1999).
118   Chu, M., R. Mierzwa, I. Truumees, A. King, M. Patel, R. Berrie, A. Hart, N. Butkiewicz, B. Mahapatra, T.M. Chan and M.S. Puar: Tetrahedron Lett. *37*, 7229 (1996).
119   Sudo, K., Y. Matsumoto, M. Matsushima, M. Fujiwara, K. Konno, K. Shimotohno, S. Shigeta and T. Yokota: Biochem. Biophys. Res. Commun. *238*, 643 (1997).
120   Sudo, K., Y. Matsumoto, M. Matsushima, K. Konno, K. Shimotohno, S. Shigeta and T. Yokota: Antiviral Chem. Chemother. *8*, 541 (1997).
121   Kakiuchi, N., Y. Komoda, K. Komoda, N. Takeshita, S. Okada, T. Tani and K. Shimotohno: FEBS Lett. *421*, 217 (1998).
122   Chu, M., R. Mierzwa, L. He, A. King, M. Patel, J. Pichardo, A. Hart, N. Butkiewicz and M.S. Puar: Bioorg. Med. Chem. Lett. *9*, 1949 (1999).

123   Llinas-Brunet, M., M. Bailey, G. Fazal, S. Goulet, T. Halmos, S. Laplante, R. Maurice, M. Poirier, M. Poupart, D. Thibeault et al.: Bioorg. Med. Chem. Lett. *8*, 1713 (1998).

124   Llinas-Brunet, M., M. Bailey, R. Ddziel, G. Fazal, V. Gorys, S. Goulet, T. Halmos, R. Maurice, M. Poirier, M. Poupart et al.: Bioorg. Med. Chem. Lett. *8*, 2719 (1998).

125   Steinkuhler, C., G. Biasiol, M. Brunetti, A. Urbani, U. Koch, R. Cortese, A. Pessi and R. De Francesco: Biochemistry *37*, 8899 (1998).

126   Ingallinella, P., S. Altamura, E. Bianchi, M. Taliani, R. Ingenito, R. Cortese, R. De Francesco, C. Steinkuhler and A. Pessi: Biochemistry *37*, 8906 (1998).

127   Marchetti, A., J.M. Ontoria and V.G. Matassa: Synlett, SI, 1000 (1999).

128   Dimasi, N., F. Martin, C. Volpari, M. Brunetti, G. Biasiol, S. Altamura, R. Cortese, R. De Francesco, C. Steinkuhler and M. Sollazzo: J Virol. *71*, 7461 (1997) .

129   Martin, F., C. Volpari, C. Steinkuhler, N. Dimasi, M. Brunetti, G. Biasiol, S. Altamura, R. Cortese, R. De Francesco and M. Sollazzo: Protein Eng. *10*, 607 (1997).

130   Martin, F., C. Steinkuhler, M. Brunetti, A. Pessi, R. Cortese, R. De Francesco and M. Sollazzo: Protein Eng. *12*, 1005 (1999).

131   Martin, F., N. Dimasi, C. Volpari, C. Perrera, S. Di Marco, M. Brunetti, C. Steinkuhler, R. De Francesco and M. Sollazzo: Biochemistry *37*, 11459 (1998).

132   Qasim, M.A., P.J. Ganz, C.W. Saunders, K.S. Bateman, M.N. James and M. Laskowski Jr.: Biochemistry *36*, 1598 (1997).

133   de la Cruz, J., D. Kressler and P. Linder: TIPS *24*, 192 (1999).

134   Kadare, G. and A. Heanni: J. Virol. *71*, 2583 (1997).

135   Cho, H.S., N.C. Ha, L.W. Kang, K.M. Chung, S.H. Back, S.K. Jang and B.H. Oh: J. Biol. Chem. *273*, 15045 (1998).

136   Kim, J.L., K.A. Morgenstern, J.P. Griffith, M.D. Dwyer, J.A. Thomson, M.A. Murcko, C. Lin and P.R. Caron: Structure *6*, 89 (1998).

137   Viropharma Inc. WO9736554 (1997).

138   Viropharma Inc. WO9736866 (1997).

139   Clarke, B.E. and M.J. Slater: Exp. Opin. Ther. Patents *7*, 979 (1997).

140   Kumar, P.K., K. Machida, P.T. Urvil, N. Kakiuchi, D. Vishnuvardhan, K. Shimotohno, K. Taira and S. Nishikawa: Virology *237*, 270 (1997).

141   Borowski, P., R. Kuehl, O. Mueller, L.H. Hwang, J. Schulze Zur Wiesch and H. Schmitz: Eur. J. Biochem. *266*, 715 (1999).

142   Behrens, S.E., L. Tomei and R. De Francesco: EMBO J. *15*, 12 (1996).

143   Lohmann, V., F. Korner, U. Herian and R. Bartenschlager: J. Virol. *71*, 8416 (1997).

144   Oh, J.W., T. Ito and M.M. Lai: J. Virol. *73*, 7694 (1999).

145   Ago, H., T. Adachi, A. Yoshida, M. Yamamoto, N. Habuka, K. Yatsunami and M. Miyano: Structure Fold Des. *7*, 1417 (1999).

146   Bressanelli, S., L. Tomei, A. Roussel, I. Incitti, R.L. Vitale, M. Mathieu, R. De Francesco and F.A. Rey: Proc. Natl. Acad. Sci. USA *96*, 13034 (1999).

147   Lesburg, C.A., M.B. Cable, E. Ferrari, Z. Hong, A.F. Mannarino and P.C. Weber: Nat. Struct. Biol. *6*, 937 (1999).

148   Lohmann, V., A. Roos, F. Korner, J.O. Koch and R. Bartenschlager: Virology *249*, 108 (1998).

149   Ishii, K., Y. Tanaka, C.C. Yap, H. Aizaki, Y. Matsuura and T. Miyamura: Hepatology *29*, 1227 (1999).

150   Johnson, R.B., X.L. Sun, M.A. Hockman, E.C. Villarreal, M. Wakulchik and Q.M. Wang: Arch. Biochem. Biophys.; in press (2000).

151   Ferrari, E., J. Wright-Minogue, J.W. Fang, B.M. Baroudy, J.Y. Lau and Z. Hong: J. Virol. *73*, 1649 (1999).

152   Rodriguez, P.L. and L. Carrasco: J Virol. *66*, 1971 (1992).

153   Luo, G., R.K. Hamatake, D.M. Mathis, J. Racela, K.L. Rigat, J. Lemm and R.J. Colonno: J. Virol. *74*, 851 (2000).

154   Sun, X.L., R.B. Johnson, M.A. Hockman and Q.M. Wang: Biochem. Biophys. Res. Commun. *268*, 798 (2000).

155   Zhong, W., A.S. Uss, E. Ferrari, J.Y. Lau and Z. Hong: J. Virol. *74*, 2017 (2000).

156   Schering Corp. WO9743310 (1997).

157   Wu, Z., N. Yao, H.V. Le and P.C. Weber: TIPS *23*, 92 (1998).

158   Gorbalenya, A.E. and E.J. Snijder: Perspect Drug Discov. Des. *6*, 64 (1996).

159   Darke, P.L., A.R. Jacobs, L. Waxman and L.C. Kuo: J. Biol. Chem. *274*, 34511 (1999).

Progress in Drug Research, Vol. 55 (E. Jucker, Ed.)
©2000 Birkhäuser Verlag, Basel (Switzerland)

The effects of morphine on cell proliferation

By Jay A. Glasel

Global Scientific Consulting LLC
15 Colton St., Farmington, CT
06032, USA

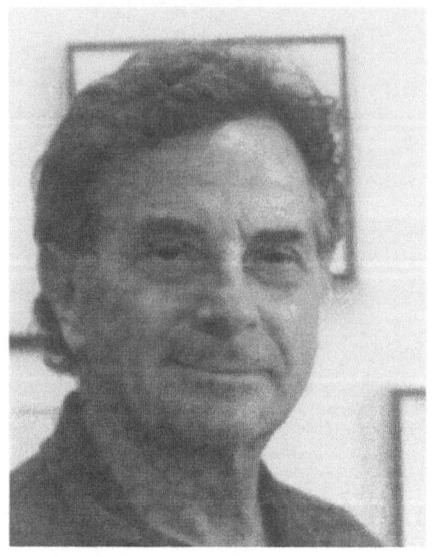

Jay A. Glasel

studied Chemistry and Physics at the California Institute of Technology and received his Ph.D. in Chemical Physics at the University of Chicago. He is the managing member of Global Scientific Consulting LLC in Farmington, Connecticut. He is senior author of an extensive list of research articles, invited chapters and reviews in scientific publications.

Summary

There is increasing evidence that endogenous opioid peptides ("enkephalins") and other neurotransmitters have widespread, receptor-mediated roles as growth regulators in non-neuronal cells and tissues. For example, it is now believed that enkephalins produced in placental trophoblast giant cells have multiple roles in supporting embryo growth, and in maternal adaptation to pregnancy. Since plant and synthetic narcotics (e.g., morphine) bind to the same receptors, the questions immediately arise: Do narcotics also have actions as growth regulators? If so, do these actions have physiological significance in addicts? Recent work on the first of these questions is covered in this review. While the greatest volume of research has been focused on the proliferative effects of narcotics for cells of the immune system, the roles of opioid peptides and narcotics on the growth of a variety of other cells has come under study recently.

Contents

Keywords

Morphine, narcotics, cell proliferation, neurotransmitters, opioids, opiates, growth regulation, enkephalins, endorphins.

Glossary of abbreviations

AchE, acetylcholinesterase; AIDS, acquired immune deficiency syndrome; BrdU, bromodeoxyuridine; cAMP, cyclic adenosine monophosphate; c-*fos* and c-*jun*, proto-oncogenes; Con-A, concanavalin A; CNS, central nervous system; CTL, cytotoxic T lymphocyte; DADLE, [D-Ala2,D-

Leu5]enkephalin; DAMGO, [D-Ala2, N-Me-Phe4-Gly-ol]enkephalin; DMPP,1,1-dimethyl-4-phenylpiperazinium; DPDPE, ([D-Pen2,D-Pen5]enkephalin); DSLET, [D-Ser2,Leu5]enkephalin-Thr6; EBV, Epstein-Barr virus; EGF, epidermal growth factor; EGL, external granular layer; ERK, extracellular-regulated kinase; GFAP, glial fibrillary acidic protein; GM-CSF, granulocyte/macrophage colony stimulating factor; GPCR, G-protein coupled receptor; HB-EGF, heparin-binding epidermal growth factor; HIV-1, human immunodeficiency virus-1; HPA, hypothalamic-pituitary-adrenal axis; HTLV-I, human T-cell leukemia virus type I; i.c.v., intracerebroventricular; IFN, interferon; IgG, immunoglobulin; IL, interleukin; JNK, c-Jun N-terminal kinase; LH-RH, luteinizing hormone releasing hormone; LPS, lipopolysaccharide; M-CSF, macrophage colony stimulating factor; Mab, monoclonal antibody; MAPK, mitogen-activated protein kinase; met-enkephalin, methionine-enkephalin; MOR-KO, μ-opioid receptor knockout (mice); NK cells, natural killer cells; NO, nitric oxide; PAG, periaqueductal gray; PBMC, human peripheral blood mononuclear cells; PHA, phytohemagglutinin; PMA, phorbol myristate acetate; RT-PCR, reverse transcription polymerase chain reaction; s.c., subcutaneous; TGFβ, transforming growth factor β; TNFα, tumor necrosis factor α; TSST-1, toxic shock syndrome toxin.

1   Introduction

Opioids initiate intracellular effects by binding to opioid receptors at cellular surfaces. Both enkephalins and narcotics non-selectively activate the two major subclasses (δ- and μ-) of opioid receptors. Recently, using knockout mice [1, 2], it was found that all of the classical physiological effects of narcotics treatment (analgesia, withdrawal, respiratory depression, immunosuppression, reward and constipation) are due solely to activation of the μ-opioid receptors. This leads to the conclusion that activation of δ-opioid receptors by narcotics, enkephalins – or both – in cells expressing this class of opioid receptor leads to non-classical physiological responses (i.e., responses to narcotics not recognized until recently).

Recent research has made it evident that the enkephalins play non-classical roles in cell proliferation. For example, enkephalin expression is highly correlated with the proliferative state of numerous types of cells [3–6] and enkephalins have been shown to down-regulate proliferation of various non-neural [6–10] and neural [11–14] cells both *in vivo* and *in vitro*. A current focus is on the proliferative roles of enkephalins in fetal growth [14–18].

This review concentrates entirely on the proliferative effects of morphine on *in vivo* and *in vitro* systems. Research on the cellular effects of narcotics is an area that has been relatively neglected by basic scientists after the discovery, now 25 years ago, of the opioid peptides. This is unfortunate because:

(1) most of the early work on the intracellular effects of morphine (and other plant and synthetic opioids) was done before the era of many molecular and cell biological discoveries and techniques; (2) drug abuse is still a major health and societal problem and, although these exogenous narcotics bind to the same cellular receptors as the endogenous opioid peptides, it is certainly not clear that narcotics and opioid peptides produce the same cellular and physiological sequelae.

Although the effects of narcotics on cell proliferation had been previously noticed [19], research in this area was stimulated by the discovery of the endogenous opiate peptides. This review concentrates on the rapidly increased quantity of research, mostly reported in the last decade, that has examined the cellular effects of acute and chronic exposure to narcotics. During this period the three major classes, μ, δ, and κ, of opiate receptors were cloned, and work on the intracellular signaling evoked by receptor-specific binding of opiate peptide and narcotic ligands has led to more understanding of their short-term effects. Work on the long-term cellular consequences of exposure to narcotics is just beginning.

1.1 Effects of neurotransmitters on gene expression in nervous tissue

In the central nervous system (CNS), it has been found that cell phenotype may influence neurotransmitter activity by selectively suppressing expression of some genes – for example, proenkephalin gene transcription in neuroepithelioma cells – during different developmental stages [20]. Conversely, neurotransmitter reception may influence the developmental state of a cell [21] and growth regulatory signals in the nervous system [22, 23] by regulating gene expression. Furthermore, it is known that certain neurotransmitters (for example, dopamine) have pleotropic effects on gene expression in the brain [24]. Thus, in the nervous system, it has become accepted that neurotransmitter-mediated processes such as learning, memory and development involve intracellular changes that must, in part, result from long-term changes in levels of expression of specific genes. The identification of these genes is just beginning. Whether or not long-term use of opiate narcotics has effects on the expression of the same or different genes will surely be an answerable question as this work progresses.

Figure 1 shows the general scheme for signaling pathways from neuro-transmitter to genome. The figure simplifies the complex pathways that result in regulation of gene expression.

2   Cells of the immune system

By far the largest literature on the proliferative effects of narcotics has resulted from work on the immune system where, from both *in vitro* and *in vivo* evidence, it is well-established that narcotics have a variety of effects. At pharmacological concentrations, narcotics suppress cell-mediated immunity, as reflected by depressed T-dependent antibody production by B lymphocytes, altered T lymphocyte functions such as proliferation, delayed-type hypersensitivity, graft-versus-host responses and decreased cytotoxic natural killer (NK) cell activity [25]. Also, early studies indicated that binding sites for opiate peptides exist on T lymphocytes and that, depending on the ligand, these peptides can act as immunodepressants (e.g., β-endorphin) or immunostimulants (met-enkephalin) [26]. We first survey work done on the cell-type dependence of narcotic-induced proliferative effects.

2.1   Dependence of effects on cell type

The immunosuppressive effects of morphine on different cell types has been studied [27]. The influence of morphine on proliferation of human tumor K562 and lymphoid cells was studied and compared with that on the mitogen-induced proliferation of human peripheral blood mononuclear cells (PBMCs). Morphine was shown to act as a suppressor of both cellular DNA synthesis and the cellular population growth of mitogen-induced PBMC, B-lymphoma Namalva cells and Epstein-Barr virus (EBV)-transformed lymphocytes. Morphine activated proliferation of myeloid K562 and T-lymphoma Yurkat cells 1.5-fold. Presumably, the opposite effects of morphine on proliferation of cell lines of immune origin reveal the difference in modulation of diverse immune cell types by morphine.

Studies on other cell types have been reported. In murine B6C3F1 splenic lymphocytes or peritoneal macrophages were cultured *in vitro* at concentrations of 0.0001–100 μM morphine sulfate, morphine-3-glucuronide, mor-

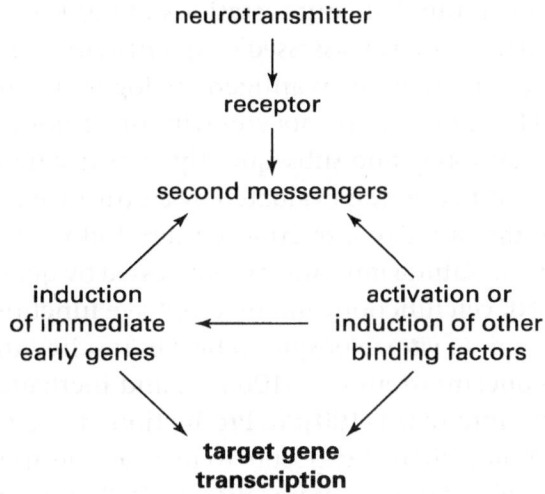

Fig. 1
Neurotransmitter signaling to nucleus. Binding of a neurotransmitter to its cell surface receptor evokes a series of intracellular events. Second messengers are small molecules (e.g., cAMP) whose actions can be exerted on two pathways: (1) They can induce expression of "intermediate-early" genes. The protein products encoded by these genes interact with regulatory regions of target genes and up- or down-regulate their expression. (2) Second messengers can also activate constitutively expressed DNA-binding proteins which then regulate the expression of intermediate-early genes or target genes. At least some of the pleotropic effects of some neurotransmitters can be attributed to activation of common regulatory factors for different genes.

phine-6-glucuronide, or normorphine. B-cell proliferation was significantly suppressed following exposure to all drugs [28]. Production of interleukin (IL)-2, IL-4 and IL-6 was affected only moderately by all drugs except morphine-6-glucuronide, which produced a marked suppression at 100 µM. Both basal and augmented NK cell function were unaffected by any drug except morphine-6-glucuronide, which enhanced NK cell activity at concentrations between 0.0001 and 1.0 µM. In contrast, both morphine-3-glucuronide and morphine-6-glucuronide significantly inhibited cytotoxic T-lymphocyte (CTL) induction at concentrations between 0.0001 and 100 µM, whereas morphine and normorphine were inactive in this assay. Thus, in the absence of direct cellular cytotoxicity, a differential immunomodulation was observed following *in vitro* exposure of these cells to morphine and its metabolites.

Similarly, the immunomodulatory effect of the drugs of heroin and methadone were studied *in vitro* [29]. Murine splenocytes or peritoneal macrophages were cultured at concentrations of 0.0001–100 μM heroin or methadone. B-cell function was assessed by quantifying cellular proliferation in response to stimulation with an antigen analogue. T-cell regulatory function was assessed by culturing splenocytes with or without drugs in the presence of anti-CD3 antibody and subsequently quantifying cytokine production. T-cell effector function was evaluated by culturing lymphocytes with or without drugs during a 5-day induction culture followed by assessment of specific CTL activity. Natural immunity was assessed by quantifying basal and IL-2-augmented NK cell function, and macrophage function was assessed by cytokine production. *In vitro* exposure to heroin resulted in decreased B-cell proliferation at concentrations of 1–100 μM, and methadone had a similar effect at concentrations of 0.1–100 μM. Production of IL-2 was suppressed by 0.1–100 μM of heroin, whereas exposure to methadone appeared to result in a generalized modulation, with suppression of IL-2 at most concentrations. In contrast, IL-4 production was only affected at the 100 μM concentration of both drugs. CTL was suppressed by exposure to 100 μM heroin, whereas NK cell activity was suppressed by high concentrations of both heroin and methadone and macrophage function was also differentially affected. In summary, these results indicate that both heroin and methadone display immunomodulatory potential.

2.2   Lymphocytes

The endogenous opioid peptides, β-endorphin and met-enkephalin, have been shown to modulate human lymphocyte proliferation, mononuclear cell locomotion, NK cell activity and neutrophil locomotion.

All of the work on the effects of narcotics on lymphocyte proliferation should be regarded in the context that work on the opioid peptides by many workers has shown consistently that mitogenic stimulation of lymphocyte proliferation is enhanced by opioid peptides *in vivo* and *in vitro* (see e.g. [30–34]).

The work reviewed in this section describes the down-regulation of proliferation of cells due to morphine exposure. However, it must be noted first that the conclusion that morphine has any proliferative effects on the mitogen-stimulated proliferation of immune-system cells has not gone uncontested. An investigation of the influence of morphine, morphine-3-glucuronide and morphine-6-glucuronide on phytohemagglutinin (PHA)-stimulated proliferation of an *in vitro* culture of peripheral mononuclear cells from healthy humans concluded there was no effect [35]. The effects of a 1-week treatment with morphine in a range of 30–240 mg/day on proliferation of lymphocytes from patients with chronic pain syndromes were further studied and, in addition, human peripheral mononuclear cell membranes were tested for specific opioid radioligand binding. The results indicated that: (1) morphine and its main metabolites do not influence mitogen-induced T-cell proliferation; (2) treatment of patients with sustained-release morphine for 1 week did not impair the lymphocyte proliferative response; and (3) no specific binding of μ-, δ- and κ-radioligands to membranes of peripheral lymphocytes obtained from healthy humans could be demonstrated. Further studies from the same laboratory did not indicate an impairment of PHA-induced T-cell proliferation during pain treatment with sustained-release morphine [36]. In considering these results, compared with others presented in this review, it should be noted that other investigators, while finding immunosuppressive effects of morphine in many *in vivo* and *in vitro* studies, have not found classical opioid receptors in peripheral lymphocytes where they have been looked for. This implies that conclusions concerning whether or not narcotics have intracellular effects based on whether or not they bind to classical receptors on the cells may not be a valid approach.

On the other hand, a detailed structure-activity study on the effects of synthetic and plant alkaloid opioids on immunosuppression has been carried out [37] and the results would presumably all be negative if the conclusions described above are correct. In this study, the potential immunosuppressive activity of morphine-derived drugs commonly used in the treatment of human pain were evaluated in the mouse. The effects of the agonists: morphine, codeine, hydromorphone, oxycodone, nalorphine, naloxone (a non-selective opioid receptor antagonist) and naltrexone (a μ-receptor selective antagonist) on antinociceptive thresholds and immune parameters (splenocyte proliferation, NK cell activity and IL-2 production) were measured (Fig. 2). It was found that:

(1) morphine displayed a potent immunosuppressive effect that was not dose-related to the antinociceptive effect;

(2) codeine possessed a weak antinociceptive effect and limited immunosuppressive activity;

(3) nalorphine (a μ-antagonist and κ-agonist) exerted a potent immunosuppressive effect, but had very weak antinociceptive activity. The pure κ-

41

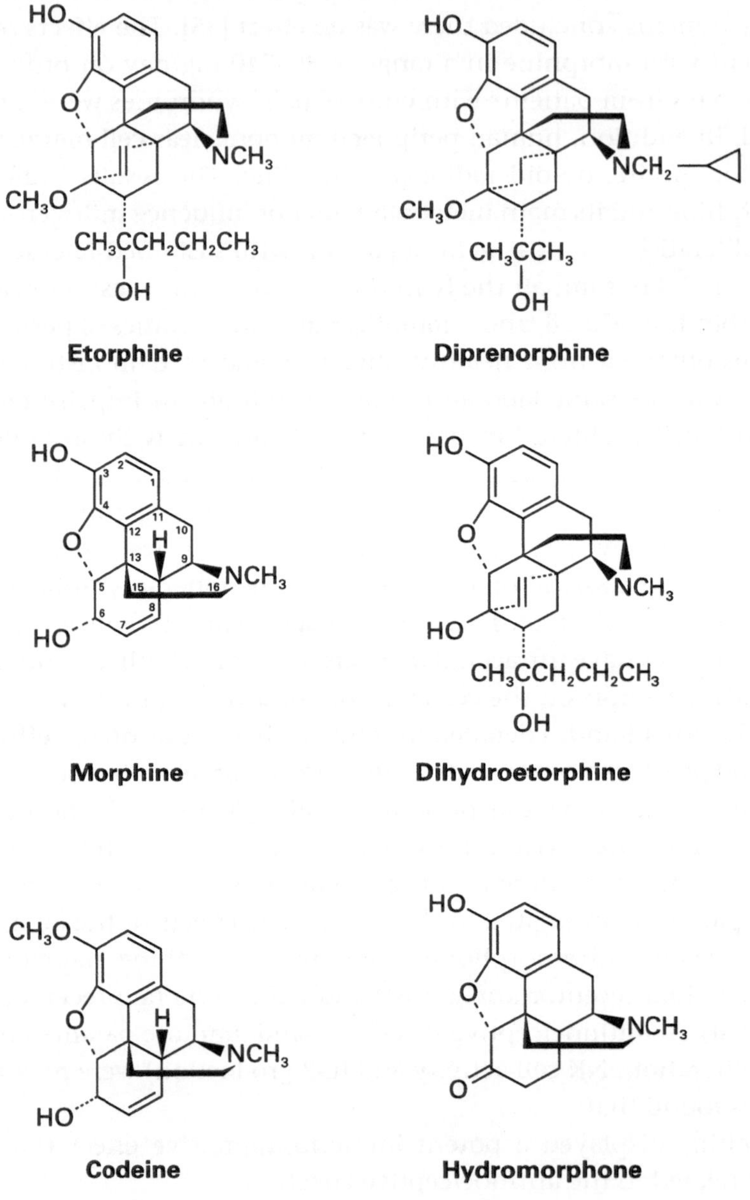

Etorphine

Diprenorphine

Morphine

Dihydroetorphine

Codeine

Hydromorphone

Fig. 2
Structures of some natural and synthetic opioids. Morphine (with ring number system), codeine, hydromorphone, oxycodone, nalorphine, naloxone, naltrexone, dihydroetorphine, etorphine, diprenorphine, and methadone.

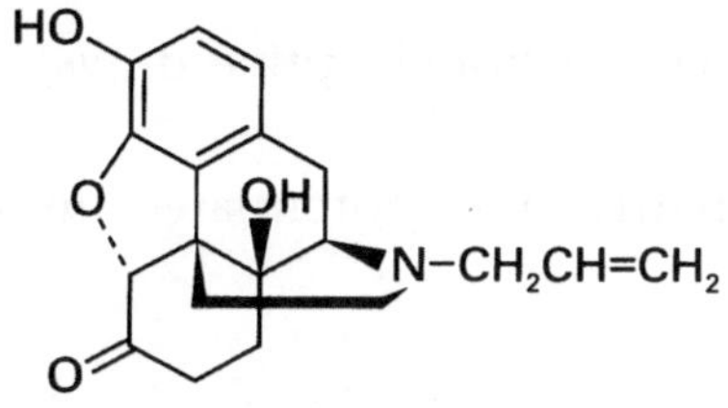

Naloxone

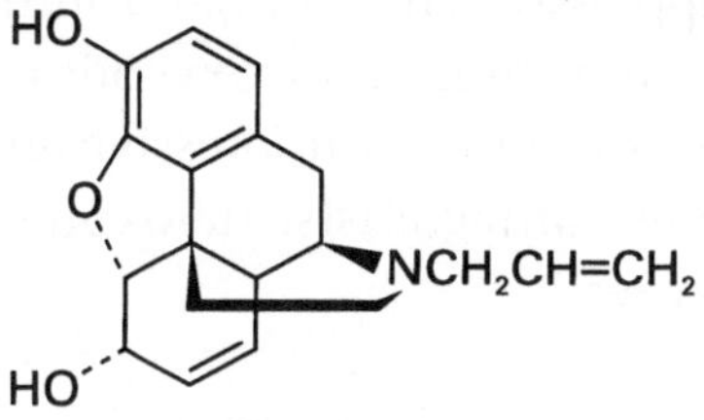

Nalorphine

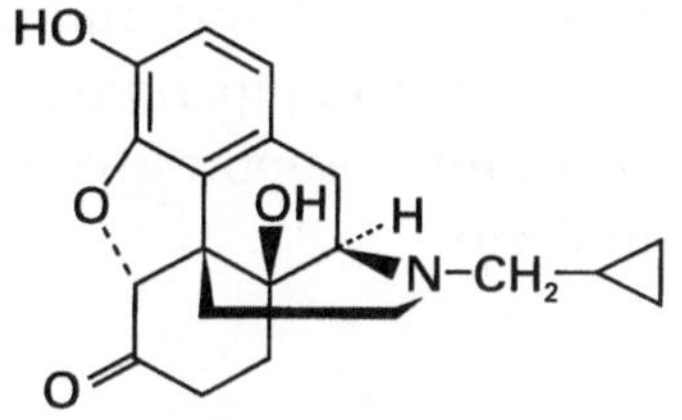

Naltrexone

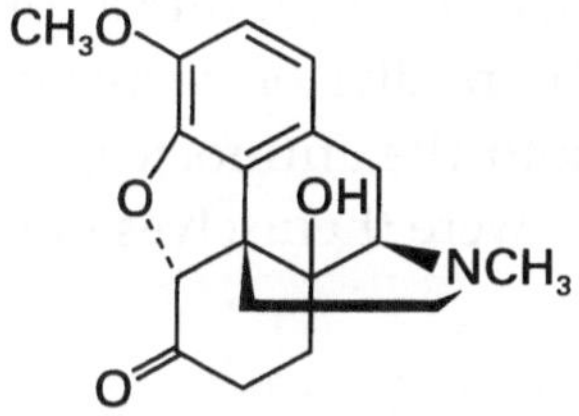

Oxycodone

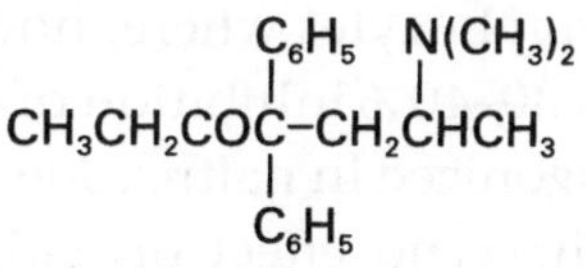

Methadone

43

antagonist nor-BNI antagonized the antinociceptive, but not the immunosuppressive effect of nalorphine;

(4) hydromorphone and oxycodone, potent antinociceptive drugs, were devoid of immunosuppressive effects;

(5) the pure antagonists, naloxone and naltrexone, potentiated immune responses.

The data are consistent with the following structural conclusions:

(1) C6 carbonyl substitution, together with the presence of a C7-8 single bond, potentiates the antinociceptive effect, but abolishes immunosuppression (hydromorphone and oxycodone);

(2) substitution of an allyl on the piperidine ring resulted in a molecule that antagonized the antinociceptive effect but maintained the immunosuppressive effect;

(3) molecules that carry modifications of C6, the C7-8 bond and C14, together with an allyl or caboxymethyl group on the piperidine ring, antagonize both the antinociceptive and the immunosuppressive effect of opiates and were themselves immunostimulants.

2.2.1 Acute treatment

Early animal model studies showed that within two hours after subcutaneous (s.c.) injection of morphine, mitogen-stimulated lymphocyte proliferation and NK cell cytolytic activity are affected [38]. Compared to saline-injected controls, blood lymphocyte proliferation was found to be 70% depressed – an effect partially antagonized in animals pretreated with naltrexone. This effect was not found in splenic lymphocytes where, however, the administration of morphine did result in a 30–40% inhibition of cytolytic activity of NK cells, an effect completely antagonized in naltrexone-pretreated animals. Naltrexone alone was found to have no effect on either proliferation of blood and splenic lymphocytes or the cytolytic activity of splenic lymphocytes. Taken together, these results demonstrated that while the effects of morphine on immune cells were dependent on the tissue source of lymphocytes, in both cases the effects were receptor-mediated. Note however that following chronic treatment with morphine, the animals become tolerant, and suppression of blood lymphocyte proliferation is no longer observed [39].

In a separate study the immunomodulatory effects of dihydroetorphine, a powerful synthetic opioid agonist, were systematically investigated in subchronically treated mice [40]. In a dose-dependent fashion, dihydroetorphine (total doses at 444.5, 889 and 1778 µg/kg) lowered the increase of body weight, decreased the weight of the spleen and thymus, weakened the delayed-type hypersensitivity, reduced the generation of antibody-forming cells, inhibited splenic lymphocyte proliferation induced by concanavalin-A (Con-A) and lipopolysaccharide (LPS) suppressed the production of IL-2 in the supernatant of splenocytes induced by Con-A, and depleted the ratio of $CD4^+$ and $CD8^+$ subpopulations. The immunosuppression due to dihydroetorphine was concomitant with addiction to the drug. Thus, subchronic treatment with dihydroetorphine dose-dependently suppresses both humoral and cell-mediated immune functions, and the immunosuppressive effects of dihydroetorphine are much more potent than those of morphine.

The work described so far raises the question of whether the immunosuppressive effect of morphine is mediated by opioid receptors located at either peripheral sites, central sites, or both. The question has been addressed [41] in work describing the effects of systemic morphine administration on analgesia, mitogen-stimulated lymphocyte proliferation and corticosterone secretion, compared to those observed after the systemic administration of N-methylmorphine, a quaternary derivative which does not readily penetrate the blood-brain barrier. It was found that, in contrast to systemically administered morphine, the i.p. injection of N-methyl-morphine (20 mg/kg) was without any effect on lymphocyte proliferation, plasma corticosterone concentrations or analgesic responses. The effects of morphine and N-methylmorphine after central administration were compared. Within 2 h after the microinjection of either morphine (10 µg/2 µl) or N-methylmorphine (15 µg/2 µl) into the third ventricle, blood lymphocyte responses were inhibited by 70%, plasma corticosterone concentrations were significantly elevated and maximal analgesic responses were present. Finally, microinjection of morphine (1 µg/0.2 µl) into the anterior hypothalamus inhibited blood lymphocyte proliferation by 50% without producing analgesia or a significant increase in plasma corticosterone. These findings suggest that central opioid pathways are involved in the immunosuppressive effects of morphine and these pathways may be distinct from those participating in opioid-induced analgesia and adrenal activation. This subject is taken up again in section 2.4 of this review.

A report describing the 24-h time course of the immunomodulatory effects of an acute s.c. injection of morphine in C57BL6 mice, and correlating these effects with the drug's analgesic properties and serum levels has appeared [42]. Acute morphine treatment had a biphasic effect on various immune parameters: there was an increase in phagocytosis and the killing of *Candida albicans* cells by peritoneal polymorphonuclear leukocytes 20 and 40 min after the injection of morphine, 20 mg/kg, when analgesia and serum morphine concentrations were at their peak. Interestingly, 24 h after morphine administration (when antinociception and morphine blood levels were no longer detectable) these parameters underwent a marked reduction. Similarly, macrophage-mediated inhibition of tumor cell proliferation was first stimulated (at 20 and 40 min) and then depressed (at 24 h). Splenic NK cell cytotoxicity, determined by standard radioassay of ^{51}Cr release from YAC-1 target cells, also was evaluated. No difference in NK activity was observed at any of the monitored time points. In addition, the immunomodulatory effects of an acute injection of methadone (a synthetic narcotic compound) were monitored at a dose inducing the same degree of analgesia as morphine. None of the tested immunoparameters were affected by the administration of methadone, which indicates the different drug-sensitivity of immunological correlates *in vivo*.

2.2.2 Chronic treatment

Implantation of s.c. morphine pellets in mice is an animal model frequently used in the study of narcotic tolerance and dependence. Mice so treated with a 75 mg morphine pellet display marked atrophy and reduced cellularity of the spleen and thymus, and an attenuated lymphocyte proliferative response to T- and B-cell mitogens (Con-A and bacterial LPS, respectively). These immunosuppressive effects were observed 72 h following implantation of the pellet, a time point by which the mice also had developed tolerance to the antinociceptive effect of the pellet. Splenic and thymic atrophy with reduced mitogen-induced lymphocyte proliferative responses and opiate tolerance were also apparent in mice subjected to a multiple pellet implantation schedule. These effects are dose-dependent because a pellet half this size did not suppress mitogen-stimulated lymphocyte proliferation. The findings concur with other observations suggesting immunosuppression with morphine tolerance [43, 44]. Later observations with the same system led to the suggestion that the mechanism of morphine-induced immunosuppression is at least partly mediated by the increase in serum corticosterone levels observed after morphine pellet implantation [45].

The question of whether or not the effects of the narcotic take place *via* an opiate receptor is left open by the studies described in the previous paragraph because they did not involve use of control animals treated with pellets of a morphine antagonist such as naloxone. This created a disagreement: a later *in vitro* study using cells taken from rhesus monkeys, and involving both morphine and naloxone, suggested that immunosuppression is not the result of direct interaction between narcotics and opiate receptors on lymphocytes [46]. On the other hand, other studies involving morphine- or naltrexone-pellet-implanted mice indicated that opioid receptors *and* β-adrenergic receptors are involved in the establishment of conditioned morphine-induced immune alterations, as well as in the expression of a subset of these conditioned alterations of immune status [47, 48].

The experimental resolution of the apparent contradiction has to face the fact that in whole animal studies, narcotics bind to, and activate, receptors in the CNS and that there may be important interactions between the CNS and putative peripheral opiate receptors on peripheral cells such as immunocytes. Therefore, it is not surprising that roles the nervous system may play in the immunosuppressive effects of morphine have begun to receive increasing attention.

In an initial study, morphine-induced suppression of lymphocyte proliferation was found to be dependent on secretions from the adrenal gland [45]. Implantation of a 75-mg morphine pellet in sham-adrenalectomized male C3H/HeN mice resulted in significant elevations of serum corticosterone levels within 6 h. Corticosterone levels remained elevated (3- to 4-fold) for 72 h and had returned to normal by 120 h post-implantation. Within 48 h of pellet implantation, morphine-pelleted mice exhibited marked reductions in spleen (35%) and thymus weight (56%) relative to values in placebo-pelleted controls. In addition, adrenal hypertrophy was observed in the morphine-pelleted shams (50% increase in adrenal weight relative to placebo). The magnitude of splenic and thymic atrophy was reduced by about 50% in adrenalectomized morphine-pelleted mice (17% and 22% reductions, respectively) compared to that in adrenalectomized mice implanted with placebo pellets. Lymphocyte proliferative responses to the T-cell mitogen Con-A and the B-cell mitogen bacterial LPS were also significantly reduced in the morphine-pelleted sham mice. Morphine-induced suppression of Con-A- or LPS-stimulated lymphocyte proliferation was absent in adrenalectomized mice. Effects similar to adrenalectomy (e.g., lessening of magnitude of morphine- induced suppression of lymphoid organ weight and lymphocyte proliferation) were found in morphine-pelleted mice given the glucocorticoid receptor antagonist RU-486 at a dose of 10 mg/kg, twice daily. These studies imply that morphine-induced immunosuppression is at least in part mediated by the increase in serum corticosterone levels after implantation of the morphine pellet.

On the other hand, a later study [49] concluded that morphine-induced immunosuppressive effects lacked either pituitary or adrenal involvement. This work examined the potential contribution of the hypothalamic-pituitary-adrenal (HPA) axis to the suppressive effects of acute morphine exposure. To assess the role of glucocorticoids, rats were pretreated with the steroid receptor antagonist RU486 (20 mg/kg) 30 min before morphine (10 mg/kg) administration. A significant inhibition of lymphocyte activity occurred with morphine in the absence or presence of RU486 pretreatment. Consistent with a mechanism independent of glucocorticoids, adrenalectomy also failed to attenuate the inhibitory actions of morphine. To examine the potential role of pituitary hormones in the suppressive effect, similar experiments were carried out in hypophysectomized animals. In sham-operated or hypophysectomized animals, morphine was found to be equally effective in suppressing lymphocyte proliferation. These results suggest that factors elaborated from intact pituitary or adrenal glands are not required for the acute inhibitory effects of morphine on peripheral blood lymphocyte activity. In view of the conflicting results between the studies just described, the involvement of pituitary and adrenal glands in immunosuppression by morphine must be regarded as undecided at present. Further work is described in section 2.4 of this review.

2.3   Thymocytes

Mouse thymocytes incubated with increasing concentrations of IL-1 in the presence of PHA exhibit a dose-dependent increase in cell proliferation, as measured by [^{3}H]-thymidine incorporation [50]. Under these conditions, there was a parallel dose-dependent increase in specific [^{3}H]-morphine binding, with a maximum increase of approximately 5-fold over basal levels. IL-2 was ineffective in promoting either cell proliferation or enhanced opioid binding, but the effects of IL-1 could be mimicked by phorbol myristate acetate (PMA), suggesting the involvement of tyrosine phosphorylation. These results indicate that morphine-binding sites on immune cells can be regulated by cytokine activation.

Although, as just stated, IL-1-induced proliferation of thymocytes is accompanied by the appearance of [^{3}H]-morphine-binding sites on the cells [50], these binding sites differ from classical opioid receptor sites in several ways: (1) lack of stereoselectivity; (2) relatively low affinity (K_d = 50 nM) and high capacity (B_{max} = 3 pmol/mg of protein); (3) binding is strongly inhibited by Ca^{2+}, Mg^{2+}, Mn^{2+} and Cl^- ions; (4) binding is inhibited by proteinase K or E and by phospholipase A2 but not trypsin treatment of thymocyte membranes; and (5) they show a preference for opioid alkaloids over opioid peptides [51].

The mechanism by which morphine inhibits PHA/IL-1-induced thymocyte proliferation [52] has been investigated. When compared to control cultures, morphine-treated thymocytes showed decreased steady-state levels of bioactive IL-2 and IL-2 mRNA. The reduced IL-2 concentration and reduced transcript levels correlated well with a decreased rate of synthesis of IL-2 mRNA as determined by nuclear runoff assays. Subsequent studies showed that morphine treatment affected transcriptional control elements of the IL-2 promoter by inhibiting the synthesis of a specific trans-activating nuclear factor, c-*fos*. c-*fos* mRNA levels measured by semiquantitative reverse transcription polymerase chain reaction (RT-PCR) were significantly decreased in thymocytes following treatment with morphine and activation with PHA and IL-1. Under identical conditions, c-Jun mRNA levels were not altered. Electrophoretic mobility shift studies with the transcription factor activator protein-1 (AP-1) consensus oligonucleotide showed significantly decreased levels of AP-1-protein complex formation in nuclear extracts prepared from morphine-treated cells. These studies demonstrated that opioid alkaloids such as morphine can impair mitogen-lymphokine-activated thymocyte proliferation by interfering with transcriptional activation of the IL-2 gene.

The effect of morphine on the release of several cytokines upon stimulation with mitogens has been studied [53]. An IL-4-dependent HT-2 cell proliferation assay was used to quantify transforming growth factor β (TGFβ). IL-6 and tumor necrosis factor α (TNFα) were measured by enzyme-linked

immunosorbent assays. Morphine (1 pM and 10 nM) alone did not significantly modulate the release of TGFβ, IL-6 or TNFα. Upon stimulation with
LPS and PHA, PBMC released more TGFβ, IL-6 and TNFα than unstimulated
PBMC. Exposure of PBMC to morphine (1 pM) for 24 h substantially amplified the release of TGFβ in the following 24-h incubation period. Morphine
did not alter the release of immunodetectable IL-6 or TNFα from stimulated
cells. The amplifying effect of morphine on the release of TGFβ was mediated
through a naloxone-sensitive mechanism. Given the fact that TGFβ has a
potent immunosuppressive effect, morphine-potentiated release of TGFβ
from PBMC may be involved in the immunomodulatory activity ascribed to
morphine.

As far as acute morphine treatment is concerned, this point has been
addressed directly [54, 55]. The results suggest that: (1) the *in vitro* immunomodulatory effects of morphine are not mediated by classical opioid receptors on immunocytes because the effects of morphine on the mitogen-stimulated proliferation of splenic and blood lymphocytes are produced only by
a very high concentration of morphine and are not naltrexone-reversible;
(2) N-methylnaltrexone (that does not gain access to the CNS, as determined
by the tail-withdrawal assay) does not antagonize the suppressive effects of
a single injection of morphine on the mitogen-stimulated proliferation of
splenic and blood lymphocytes, splenic NK cell activity and the production
of interferon-gamma by stimulated splenocytes; but (3) high doses of N-
methylnaltrexone that do gain access to the CNS (as determined by the tail-
withdrawal assay) block morphine's immunomodulatory effects. Taken
together, these results strongly suggest that it is the CNS rather than peripheral opioid receptors that plays an important role in the immune alterations
produced by acute morphine treatment in rats. On this basis, the resolution
of the seeming paradox between these later results and the ones described in
the preceding paragraph is that the antagonist used in the previous studies,
naltrexone, gains access to the CNS and exerts its actions at that level.

2.4   Involvement of the central and peripheral nervous systems

The supraspinal action of morphine in altering immune function has been
examined [56]. This study compared the effect of equianalgesic doses of s.c.
and intrathecal morphine on lymphocyte proliferative responses and phe-

notypic expression of lymphocyte cell surface markers in rats. Equianalgesic doses of s.c. (10 mg/kg) or intrathecal (30 μg, by a chronic intrathecal catheter) morphine were given twice for 5 h (time 0 and 2.5 h). Immediately after the 5-h period or 24 h after the initial injection, spleens were harvested and lymphocytes isolated. Mitogen-induced (PHA, Con-A, pokeweed, LPS) lymphocyte proliferation and monoclonal antibody labeling (Mab) of cell surface markers (T cell, B cell, CD4+, CD8+) were then performed. It was found that s.c. morphine acutely suppressed lymphocyte proliferation to the mitogens PHA, pokeweed and Con-A, but proliferative responses returned to baseline within 24 h. Morphine treatment did not alter the response to LPS. The number of splenic lymphocytes also decreased, whereas the percentage of lymphocytes expressing the CD4+ marker (T-helper/inducer cells) modestly increased. Intrathecal morphine did not alter lymphocyte proliferative responses, nor did it change phenotypic expression of cell surface markers. Thus, s.c. morphine inhibited lymphocyte proliferation, decreased splenic lymphocyte number and altered phenotypic expression of cell surface markers, whereas equianalgesic doses of intrathecal morphine did not. The results provide some support for the suggestion that spinal opioids may have theoretical benefits for the analgesic management of immunocompromised patients, but further studies are clearly indicated.

The involvement of the sympathetic nervous system (SNS) in the immunomodulatory effects of morphine has been recently reviewed [57]. In initial observations [58], sympathetic tone was elevated by s.c. administration of the ganglionic stimulant DMPP in doses of 0, 0.01, 0.1 and 1.0 mg/kg, 5 min before the s.c. administration of 15 mg/kg morphine or saline. Animals were sacrificed 1 h after the morphine injection and multiple *in vitro* immune assays were then conducted. Although DMPP did not significantly enhance morphine's suppressive effects in the spleen and blood mitogen stimulation assays or the splenic NK cell assay, DMPP alone produced effects on immune status in saline-treated animals. Therefore the immunomodulatory effects of increasing peripheral sympathetic outflow were examined in greater detail. Animals were administered a wider dose range of DMPP (0, 0.005, 0.05, 0.5 and 5.0 mg/kg, s.c.) 30 min prior to sacrifice, and an expanded repertoire of immune assays was conducted. DMPP dose-dependently suppressed the mitogenic responsiveness of splenic T lymphocytes, splenic NK cell activity and IL-2 and interferon γ (IFNγ)-production by stimulated splenocytes. DMPP did not alter the total number of splenic leukocytes or the proliferative response of splenic B lymphocytes. In the mesenteric lymph nodes, DMPP had no effect on mitogenic responsiveness, the production of IL-2 or the total number of leukocytes. In the blood, however, DMPP increased mitogenic responsiveness at intermediate doses and decreased proliferation at higher doses. DMPP also dose-dependently decreased the number of blood leukocytes/ml. Taken together, these results indicate that increasing peripheral sympathetic outflow results in profound effects on immune status that depend upon the degree to which SNS activity is altered, the compartment of the immune system and the lymphocyte subtype.

The role of the SNS in immunomodulation has been examined further by using an acetylcholinesterase (AChE) Mab-induced sympathectomy model [59]. The effects of AChE Mab treatment on the immune alterations produced by acute morphine treatment were explored. Experimental rats received tail vein injections of murine monoclonal immunoglobulin (IgG)2b antibodies against rat brain AChE, which produce a destruction of cholinergic, sympathetic preganglionic neurons and a resultant decrease in sympathetic activity. Control rats received tail vein injections of murine IgG antibodies, which do not affect sympathetic preganglionic neurons or sympathetic activity. One week after antibody treatment, rats received a s.c. injection of 15 mg/kg morphine or the saline vehicle. One hour after the morphine or saline injections, rats were sacrificed and immune assays were conducted. AChE Mab treatment increased the mitogen-stimulated proliferation of splenic T cells and IL-2 production by stimulated splenocytes, indicating that these immune measures are sensitive to the AChE Mab-induced alteration in sympathetic function. Treatment with AChE Mab did not alter the mitogen-stimulated proliferation of splenic B cells or blood T cells, splenic NK cell activity, or the production of IFNγ by stimulated splenocytes, indicating that these immune measures are relatively insensitive to the AChE Mab-induced alteration in sympathetic activity. The AChE Mab-induced alteration in sympathetic activity did not affect the suppressive effects of acute morphine treatment on the mitogen-stimulated proliferative response of splenic T and B cells and blood T cells, splenic NK cell activity, or the production of IFNγ and IL-2 by stimulated splenocytes.

Further work along the lines described in the previous paragraph showed that antagonist-reversible, morphine activation of opiate receptors in the lateral ventricle of the periaqueductal gray (PAG) was responsible for pronounced dose-dependent reductions in lymphocyte proliferation to T- and B-cell mitogens, NK cell cytotoxicity, and the production of IL-2 and IFNγ [60]. However, activation of the receptors in the caudal aspect of the PAG induced dose-dependent alterations in NK cell cytotoxicity, but had no effect on lymphocyte proliferation or cytokine production. These results indicate that opioid receptors in the PAG are involved in the regulation of NK cell activity, but are not associated with morphine's effects on proliferation or cytokine production. Thus, this study showed that activation of opioid receptors within the more caudal aspects of the PAG is required for morphine to induce alterations in splenic NK cell activity. However, the study did not identify the other brain regions responsible for morphine's effect on lymphocyte proliferation and cytokine production.

The work just described has been followed up with more extensive studies [61] on the effect of acute microinjection of morphine in the rat PAG on macrophage function. Morphine injection in the PAG was found to significantly suppress nitric oxide (NO) production by untreated, IFNγ-primed and LPS-activated splenic macrophages and did not alter macrophage viability. In contrast, IFNγ- and LPS-activated macrophages from PAG-injected saline rats generated an increased output of NO, which was associated with significant reduction in cell viability. Morphine significantly inhibited TNFα production by LPS-activated macrophages. Compared with that of macrophages from PAG-injected saline rats, morphine significantly inhibited phagocytosis of *Candida albicans* by resident macrophages. Responses of resident or activated macrophages from PAG-injected saline and untreated control groups did not differ significantly. The results of this *ex vivo* study suggest that suppressive effects of morphine on macrophage functions may contribute to increased susceptibility to infectious diseases and cancer associated with drug abuse.

Studies on the role of the autonomic nervous system in mediating the immunosuppressive effect of morphine on blood lymphocyte proliferation in rats have been reported [62]. Rats were pretreated with the ganglionic blocker chlorisondamine (5 mg/kg) prior to morphine (7 mg/kg) administration. Ganglionic blockade with chlorisondamine completely antagonized the inhibitory actions of morphine, suggesting that intact ganglionic transmission was required for the inhibition to occur. Blockade of postganglionic parasympathetic neurotransmission with atropine methylbromide (1 mg/kg) or blockade of sympathetic neurotransmission with the α-adrenoceptor antagonist phentolamine (1 mg/kg) did not attenuate the suppressive effect of morphine. Blockade of β-adrenoceptors with propranolol (2.5 mg/kg) resulted in partial antagonism, but this action was not shared by the peripherally acting β-adrenoceptor antagonist nadolol (6 mg/kg). These results suggest that the inhibitory effect of morphine on blood lymphocyte proliferation may be mediated through activation of the autonomic nervous system; however, individual blockade of either the parasympathetic or sympathetic division of the autonomic nervous system was not sufficient to antagonize this immunosuppressive effect.

Most recently, flow cytometry has been used to directly assess whether acute morphine treatment (a single s.c. dose) produces the immune alterations described in the preceding paragraph by altering the leukocyte composition of the spleen. It was found that (1) morphine suppressed the Con-A-stimulated proliferation of T cells, LPS-stimulated proliferation of B cells, and NK cell cytotoxicity in the spleen; but (2) the same morphine treatment protocol did not alter the total number of splenic leukocytes, the percentage of live splenic leukocytes, or the relative number of CD4+CD3+ T cells, CD8+CD3+ T cells, CD45RA/B+ B cells, NKR-P1A(hi)CD3- NK cells, NKR-P1A(lo)CD3+ T cells, CD11b/c+HIS48- monocytes/macrophages, or CD11b/c+HIS48+ granulocytes in the spleen. These findings indicate that the effects of a single s.c. dose of morphine on functional measures of immune status in the spleen do not result from a redistribution of splenic leukocytes; instead, morphine's effects are likely to result from direct alterations in leukocyte activities [63].

2.5 Mechanistic studies of acute and chronic effects

Work directed to roughly determining potential mechanisms by which acute morphine treatments inhibit mitogen-stimulated lymphocyte proliferation has been reported [64]. The data suggest that adrenal hormones are involved in bringing about morphine-induced lymphopenia, and coupled with the morphine-induced decrease in responsiveness to mitogenic stimulation, contribute to the overall antiproliferative effect of morphine on blood lymphocytes. In hypophysectomized animals, morphine is still effective in suppressing proliferative responses to mitogens, implying that intact pituitary glands are not required for the effects of acute morphine treatment [49]. Carrying this type of work forward, more recently evidence has been found that morphine acts primarily through central μ receptors to modulate peripheral blood lymphocyte proliferation responses. Further, the antinociception and blood lymphocyte effects show greater sensitivity to opioids than either NK cell cytolytic activity or activation of the HPA axis [30].

Morphine increases the synthesis and extracellular release of NO from macrophages in Con-A-stimulated splenocyte cultures [65]. The results suggest that the formation of the oxidant peroxynitrite through a reaction between NO and a superoxide anion does not contribute significantly to the suppression of lymphocyte proliferation; instead, the activation of soluble guanylate cyclase by NO in target cells, most likely the lymphocytes, accounts more completely for the morphine-induced suppression of lymphocyte proliferation. In the *in vivo* case using a rat model, results of intracerebroventricular (i.c.v.) administration of receptor-selective opioid agonists indicate that μ-opioid receptors within the CNS are involved in the regulation of splenic NO production [66].

Using BALB/c mice as the subjects, macrophages have been shown to be involved with inhibition of T-cell proliferation during subchronic *in vivo* treatments with morphine [67]. The mice were exposed to multiple s.c. injections of morphine in increasing doses twice a day for 4 days. T-lymphocyte proliferation in response to alloantigen was significantly affected by morphine, but the treatment failed to suppress PMA/A23187-induced macrophage-depleted lymphocyte proliferation. It was further shown that Con-A-stimulated T-cell proliferation was suppressed only when morphine-treated macrophages were combined with control or morphine-treated lymphocytes. Addition of exogenous IL-1 and IL-2 promoted the proliferative responses of lymphocytes obtained from morphine-treated mice to Con-A. Studies of the mechanism of suppression showed that macrophages are the primary target cells. The results demonstrate that morphine-triggered release of inhibitory macrophage metabolites and decrement in soluble cytokine production are involved in the immunosuppressive effects caused by subchronic *in vivo* morphine treatment.

The question of whether or not morphine's immunomodulatory effects are dose-dependent and antagonist-reversible has been addressed and answered in the positive using Lewis rats as the test animal [68]. In addition, the same study showed that (1) for splenic lymphocytes, morphine induced a dose-dependent suppression of lymphocyte function as measured by mitogen-induced proliferation, NK cell cytotoxicity, IL-2 production and IFN production; (2) for blood lymphocytes, the mitogen-induced proliferative response was suppressed in a dose-dependent manner; (3) but, in contrast, morphine did not alter the capability of lymphocytes in the mesenteric lymph nodes to proliferate or produce cytokines. Thus, the immunomodulatory effects of morphine are compartmentalized.

Using a rat model, the time course for the onset of morphine-induced proliferatory changes in NK cells, splenic T and B lymphocytes and cytokine production have been measured [69]. Morphine's immunomodulatory effects on NK cell activity begin within 30 min, continue for at least 12 h, and return to control values by 24 h. In contrast, proliferation of splenic T and B cells and IFNγ production are not altered within 30 min; maximal suppression occurs at 1 h, and recovery begins within 2 h. In all immune measures, therefore, maximal suppression is present at the 1-h time point, and recovery is complete within 24 h.

2.6   Tolerance and withdrawal

Development of tolerance in the immunosuppressive effects of morphine has been investigated [70]. In this study, a variety of *in vitro* immune measures were examined in groups of Lewis rats that chronically consumed either tap water or a 0.2, 0.4 or 0.6 mg/ml morphine drinking solution. Rats received a s.c. injection of either saline or 15 mg/kg morphine sulfate 1 h before sacrifice. In the drinking groups, the acute morphine injection significantly suppressed splenic NK cell activity, mitogen-stimulated splenic T- and B-cell proliferation and IFNγ production. A single, acute injection of morphine did not suppress NK cell activity in rats that drank the two highest concentrations of morphine, whereas it did suppress the mitogen-stimulated splenic T- and B-cell proliferation and IFNγ production. These results suggest that rats that drank morphine for 20 days developed tolerance to morphine's suppressive effect on NK cell activity but not to other measures of immune status. Morphine-drinking rats also developed tolerance to morphine's antinociceptive effects and revealed signs of physical dependence when the morphine solution was withdrawn or when naltrexone was administered.

The same group investigated opioid withdrawal-induced immunomodulation and the mechanism by which that process may be mediated [71].

They examined the immunomodulatory properties of morphine with-drawal alone and in the presence of the α2-adrenergic agonist, clonidine. The rats drank a morphine solution for 20 days and withdrawal was induced on day 21 by replacing the morphine solution with plain tap water. Measurements of withdrawal-induced weight change and immunomodulation were obtained at several time points after withdrawal induction. Immune status was assessed by determining Con-A, toxic shock syndrome toxin (TSST)-1, and LPS-stimulated splenocyte proliferation, splenic Con-A-stimulated IFNγ production and splenic NK cell activity. In a separate series of experiments, systemic injections of clonidine (0.001–0.01 mg/kg) were administered during a 12-h withdrawal episode and all measures of immune status were reassessed. This study concluded that weight change was time-dependent, with peak decreases in weight occurring 24 h following withdrawal induction. Rats also exhibited a time-dependent suppression of immune status in all assays except LPS-stimulated proliferation; immunomodulation was most evident 12 h following withdrawal induction. Clonidine dose-dependently prevented withdrawal-induced suppression of Con-A and TSST-1-stimulated splenocyte proliferation, Con-A-stimulated splenocyte IFNγ production and splenic NK cell activity. Taken together, the findings show that opioid withdrawal significantly suppresses a subset of immune parameters and that these effects can be prevented by clonidine.

2.7   Gene knockout animal studies

The role of the μ-opioid receptor (MOR) in immune function has been investigated using MOR-knockout (KO) mice. Morphine modulation of several immune functions, including macrophage phagocytosis and macrophage secretion of TNFα, was not observed in the MOR-KO animals, suggesting that these functions are mediated by the classical μ-opioid receptor. In contrast, morphine reduction of splenic and thymic cell number and mitogen-induced proliferation are unaffected in MOR-KO mice, as is morphine inhibition of IL-1 and IL-6 secretion by macrophages. These latter results are consistent with morphine action on a naloxone-insensitive morphine receptor, a conclusion supported by the previous studies characterizing a nonopioid morphine binding site on immune cells [51]. Alternatively, morphine may act either directly or indirectly on these cells, by a mechanism mediated by either δ- or κ-opioid receptors.

Work with a mouse model in which the μ-receptor gene was disrupted by targeted homologous recombination [72] is related to the studies described above. Mice homozygous for the disrupted gene developed normally, but their motor function was altered. Drug-naïve homozygotes displayed reduced locomotor activity, and morphine did not induce changes in locomotor activity observed in wild-type mice. Pertinent to this review is the finding that the lack of a functional receptor resulted in changes in both the host defense system and the reproductive system. Increased proliferation of granulocyte-macrophage, erythroid and multipotential progenitor cells in both bone marrow and spleen was observed.

2.8   Acquired immune-deficiency syndrome (AIDS)

The clinical consequences of the suppressive effects of narcotics on the immune system are seen in the striking increase in the incidence of infections suffered by intravenous narcotics abusers, including AIDS and complications of AIDS (for example, human T-cell leukemia virus (HTLV)-I infection).

In one approach, a mouse model has been developed to study the effects of long-term morphine administration on mice with murine retrovirus infection [73, 74]. For these mice, retrovirus infection-induced splenocyte proliferation was down-regulated by chronic (11 week) morphine treatment.

Human immunodeficiency virus (HIV)-1 and the HTLV-I oncoretrovirus share a common host in $CD4^+$ T lymphocytes. The result of HIV-1 infection is a dramatic decrease of these lymphocytes, whereas HTLV-I infection results in an increased proliferation of infected cells. Using an *in vitro* coinfection system (HIV-1 + HTLV-I), morphine treatment was found to enhance the levels of HTLV-I p19 while indicators of *in vitro* infection by cell-free HIV-1 were reduced by morphine treatment in both single and dual *in vitro* infection experiments [75]. IL-2 levels in the affected cultures were found to increase with combined HTLV-I infection and morphine treatment. Thus, these *in vitro* results indicate the need to further explore the activity of HTLV-I within narcotics-treated cells, as this oncoretrovirus appears to be especially sensitive to morphine-induced alterations to its host cell environment.

2.9 Conclusions

The conclusion is that narcotics at pharmacological concentrations suppress cell-mediated immunity, as reflected by depressed T-dependent antibody production by B lymphocytes, altered T lymphocyte functions such as proliferation, delayed-type hypersensitivity, graft-versus-host responses and decreased cytotoxic NK cell activity. While macrophages appear to have binding sites for morphine, the preponderance of available evidence suggests these are non-classical opiate receptors in terms of dissociation constants, stereoselectivity, etc.

The mechanisms for the suppressive effects are not well-understood. Possible mechanisms include narcotic actions on the neurons of the central and sympathetic nervous systems. In the CNS, narcotics can activate the neuroendocrine system with a subsequent increase in serum glucocorticoid levels. In the SNS, narcotic-induced activation could result in noradrenergic inhibition of the immune system.

A summary of possible roles played by morphine and other drugs having effects on the immune system and their possible significance to critical care medicine has appeared [76]. Evidence is presented that the immunosuppressive effects of hypoprolactinemia, chronic morphine treatment and chronic glucocorticoid administration are reversed by prolactin or by drugs that stimulate endogenous prolactin release and that prolactin, synthesized by lymphocytes, plays an autocrine role in their proliferation [76].

In further work, the possible clinical significance of the time course of onset of morphine-induced effects on the immune system has been studied [69]. It was found that acute morphine treatment in rats produces immune alterations and antinociception and, although there are slight differences in morphine's maximal immunological and antinociceptive effects, morphine suppresses immune status at time points concordant with its antinociceptive effects. On the basis of these observations it was suggested that these effects should be considered when administering morphine to patients whose systems are immunocompromised.

3 Cells of the nervous system

While there is an enormous literature on the mechanisms for receptor-mediated intraneuronal signaling elicited by narcotics, there have been relatively few reports on the effects of the long-term molecular biological effects of morphine on nervous tissue. As mentioned at the beginning of this review, part of the problem has been that such studies were exceedingly difficult before the era of modern molecular biological techniques. However, the lack of attempts is still somewhat surprising, given the possible clinical importance of such work. For example, it would be supposed a priori that the potential long-lasting effects of the drug on fetal brains in embryos carried by addicted pregnant women, and on the differentiated CNS of addicted adults, would have potentially important clinical impact.

3.1 Tissue studies

Early work concentrated on ultrastructural examination of the brain after morphine treatment. For example, in male rats, it was found [77] that one cross-sectional level (middle 1/3) of the arcuate nucleus of the hypothalamus after two weeks of morphine treatment exhibited a marked increase in lamellar whorls of endoplasmic reticulum in the neurons of this nucleus in each group. Castrated rats exhibited the same phenomenon. A comparable incidence of whorls was not detected in rats treated with lactose, those treated for only 1–3 days with morphine, or in those given testosterone plus morphine for 2 weeks. It was suggested that the testosterone deficiency following either castration or chronic morphine treatment stimulated the observed increase in whorls. A close correspondence was noted between the distribution within the arcuate nucleus of the hypothalamus of neurons containing whorls and those previously reported to contain luteinizing hormone-releasing hormone (LH-RH).

The study just described was followed by one in which the arcuate nucleus of the hypothalamus of male rats that had been treated either with estradiol benzoate (which acts both peripherally and centrally to limit testosterone production), or cyproterone acetate (an anti-androgen), was examined ultrastructurally for the presence of whorls of endoplasmic reticulum [78]. It was found that the incidence of whorl containing neurons in this nucleus was 2–4 times higher in animals treated for 2–3 weeks with estradiol benzoate or for 2 weeks with cyproterone acetate than in the nuclei of oil-treated controls. These findings, together with previous evidence that whorls proliferate in male rats deprived of androgen by morphine treatment or castration [79,

80], suggest that steroid feedback (androgen alone or both androgen and estrogen) plays an important role in whorl proliferation.

Qualitative observations on the effects of morphine on brain cell development have also been reported [81]. Perinatal morphine administration affects neuronal growth in the developing animal. Neuronal packing density was reduced by morphine treatment in both the primary somatosensory cortex and the preoptic area of the hypothalamus. However, glial packing density was increased, but only in the hypothalamus, which could reflect greater severity of opiate-induced neurotoxicity in the hypothalamus. Cortical pyramidal neurons show morphine-induced reduction of basilar dendritic growth limited to late-developing terminal branches. This effect is completely reversed by concurrent naltrexone administration. This selective effect could be caused by morphine acting at opiate receptors to inhibit extrinsic determinants of dendritic growth (e.g., afferent supply). The ontogeny of opiate receptors is also affected by perinatal morphine administration in a regionally dependent manner. μ-receptors are down-regulated by morphine in the hypothalamus, but not in the cortex. Differential maturity of receptors in these regions could be a factor in such differential drug effects. Therefore, different critical periods for opiate action in different regions of the developing brain could exist.

Quantitative morphological characteristics of cells in the primary somatosensory cortex of 6-day-old rats have been examined following continuous maternal administration of morphine (10 mg/kg/day), naltrexone (10 mg/kg/day), or saline vehicle from gestation day 12 [82]. Naltrexone reduced neuronal packing density and significantly increased cortical thickness but had no effect on neuronal number, while morphine reduced neuronal packing density and the number of neurons without affecting cortical thickness. The results suggest that blockade of endogenous opioid function during development enhances neuronal maturation in this brain region, while perinatal morphine administration might act to restrict cortical cell proliferation and maturation. Thus, the effect of ontogenetic activation of opioid receptors by endogenous opioid compounds could be similar to but less severe than the effect of exogenous opiate exposure on cortical cell development.

The possible effects of morphine on nerve fiber regeneration had been examined earlier [83]. Rat facial nerve trunks from saline, acute morphine and continuous morphine-treated animals were examined by light and electron microscopy at 3, 7 and 14 days after crush injury. The number of axonal sprouts/unit area and the diameters of regenerating axons were quantified at each survival interval. Both saline-treated and acute morphine-treated facial nerves demonstrated myelin degradation and Schwann cell hypertrophy (at 3 days post-axotomy), sprout outgrowth (at 7 days) and axon maturation and myelination (at 14 days). In the chronic morphine-treated animals, a retardation of the regenerative process was evident. Axon sprout outgrowth and axonal diameters were reduced at 3 and 7 days post-axotomy. In treated 14-day animals, axon diameters were normal; however, significantly fewer axon profiles/unit area were observed. After chronic morphine exposure, Schwann cell hypertrophy and proliferation, as well as myelin debris removal, were inhibited at all survival periods.

Endogenous opioid peptides and morphine have been found to inhibit the proliferation of cerebellar external granular layer (EGL) neuroblasts by mechanisms that are incompletely understood [84]. Multiple extracellular factors regulate granule cell neurogenesis and these undoubtedly act in concert with opioids to shape developmental outcome. Heparin-binding epidermal growth factor (HB-EGF), a recently described member of the EGF family, was examined to see if it might compete with an inhibitory opioid signal. The results confirmed that morphine inhibited neuroblast proliferation, while HB-EGF enhanced cell replication. HB-EGF not only counteracted the antiproliferative morphine signal, but invariably enhanced DNA synthesis irrespective of morphine treatment. The findings suggest that regional and temporal differences in the availability of endogenous HB-EGF may serve to limit the response of EGL neuroblasts to opioids, and HB-EGF may be neuroprotective in opiate drug abuse. If similar responses occur *in vivo*, then the EGF family and the opioid system may represent distinct and contrasting components of an extracellular signaling system serving to coordinate EGL neurogenesis.

The effect of morphine on DNA synthesis by EGL neuroblasts has been examined in whole-mount organotypic cultures isolated from 10-day-old rat cerebella using incorporation of bromodeoxyuridine (BrdU) to measure DNA synthesis [85]. After 24 h, explants were treated for 24 h with 10 nM, 1 or 100 μM morphine, morphine plus 30 nM, 3 or 300 μM of naloxone, respectively, or those concentrations of naloxone alone. BrdU was added during the last 4 h of drug treatment. EGL neuroblasts were unambiguously identified by size and morphology, location and by protein kinase C II immunocytochemistry. The proportion of EGL neuroblasts incorporating BrdU was significantly reduced in the presence of 1 μM morphine, while 100 μM morphine had little additional effect. The concentration of morphine predicted to cause a half-maximal reduction in the BrdU labeling index was 22.5 nM. Morphine's ability to reduce BrdU incorporation by EGL neuroblasts was concentration-dependent and was prevented by concomitant treatment with naloxone, implicating the involvement of opioid receptors. The results suggest that morphine can directly regulate the growth of the developing cerebellum by inhibiting neuroblast proliferation within the EGL.

3.2 Glial and glioma cells

Work on the proliferative effects of morphine on rat brain began with a study of tritiated thymidine uptake [86]. It was found that acute morphine administration (10 mg/kg; 30 min prior to [^{3}H]-thymidine) increased incorporation of [^{3}H]-thymidine into DNA of rat striatum. This effect was antagonized by naloxone (1 mg/kg). The observed change in incorporation of [^{3}H]-thymidine into DNA in striatum could not be accounted for by differences in the local availability of the label in morphinized rats. An autoradiographic study revealed that the [^{3}H]-thymidine was localized in nuclei in cells of the subependymal layer lining the lateral ventricles, an area of glial cell proliferation in adult rats. No change in [^{3}H]-thymidine incorporation into DNA was observed in any area of the brain in morphine-addicted rats or in rats undergoing naloxone-precipitated withdrawal. The results suggest that narcotics may induce permanent anatomical changes in the brain, including alterations of neuroglial interactions.

More recently, the effects of morphine on astrocyte proliferation and differentiation in primary cultures of murine glial cells have been studied [87]. Morphine decreases glial cell production in a dose-dependent, naloxone-reversible way and gliogenesis virtually ceased in the presence of micromolar morphine during the first week in culture. In addition, morphine treatment inhibited [^{3}H]-thymidine incorporation by glial fibrillary acidic protein (GFAP) immunoreactive, flat (type 1) astrocytes, and caused significant increases in both cytoplasmic area and process elaboration. These observations suggest that opiate drugs can directly modify neural growth by influencing two critical developmental events in astrocytes, i.e., inhibiting proliferation and inducing morphologic differentiation. A later investigation examined whether or not morphine at micromolar concentrations is toxic to glia [88] and found that morphine-induced reductions in glial numbers did not result from an increased rate of cell death, suggesting that morphine inhibits the production of flat, polyhedral astrocytes solely by decreasing their rate of proliferation.

It has been found that morphine can affect the proliferative rate of astrocytes from diverse brain regions [89]. Astrocyte-enriched cultures from striatum, hippocampus and cerebral cortex derived from newborn mouse brains were studied. Cultures from each region were continuously incubated in media alone (controls), or in media treated with 1 µM morphine, 1 µM morphine plus 3 µM naloxone, or 3 µM naloxone alone. Before harvesting at 6 days, cultures were exposed to [^{3}H]-thymidine. The thymidine-labeling index was determined autoradiographically in flat, polyhedral (type 1) GFAP-immunoreactive astrocytes. Morphine significantly inhibited [^{3}H]-thymidine incorporation in astrocytes from all three brain regions, although regional differences in labeling indices were noted.

The idea that astrocytes simply provide structural and trophic support to neurons has been challenged by recent evidence demonstrating that astrocytes exhibit a form of excitability and communication based on intracellular Ca^{2+} variations and intercellular Ca^{2+} waves, which can be initiated by neuronal activity. These astrocyte Ca^{2+} variations have now been shown to induce glutamate-dependent Ca^{2+} elevations and slow inward currents in neurons [90].

In view of the importance of Ca^{2+} in astrocyte function, the possible role of morphine in altering Ca^{2+} levels in astrocytes has been investigated [91]. Astrocyte-enriched cultures were derived from newborn ICR mouse cerebra. Quantitative fluorescent measurements of intracellular free Ca^{2+} ($[Ca^{2+}]_i$) using Fura-2 as well as fluo-3 and computer-aided image analysis showed that 1 µM morphine significantly increased $[Ca^{2+}]_i$ in flat, polyhedral, GFAP-immunoreactive astrocytes at 2 and 6 min, and at 72 h. Co-administration of 3 µM naloxone blocked morphine-dependent increases in $[Ca^{2+}]_i$. Treatment with 1 µM concentrations of the κ-opioid receptor agonist, U69,593, but not equimolar amounts of µ- (DAMGO) or δ- (DPDPE) opioid receptor agonists, significantly increased $[Ca^{2+}]_i$ in astrocytes. The role of Ca^{2+} in morphine-induced astrocyte differentiation was also investigated: Untreated and

1 μM morphine-treated astrocyte cultures were incubated for 5 days in 0.01, 0.3, 1.0 or 3.0 mM extracellular Ca^{2+} ($[Ca^{2+}]_o$), or incubated with 1.0 mM $[Ca^{2+}]_o$ in the presence of 1 μM of the Ca^{2+} ionophore, A23187. The areas of single astrocytes were measured and there was a positive correlation between astrocyte area and $[Ca^{2+}]_o$. Morphine had an additive effect on area and form factor measures when $[Ca^{2+}]_o$ was 1.0 mM. High $[Ca^{2+}]_o$ (3.0 mM) alone mimicked the action of morphine. Morphine alone had no effect on astrocyte area in the presence of low (< 0.01 mM) or high (3.0 mM) Ca^{2+}. However, 1 mM A23187 without any additions did mimic the effects of morphine. The authors suggested that the actions of morphine in increasing $[Ca^{2+}]_i$ may be mediated by κ-opioid receptors in astrocytes despite the high K_d exhibited by this class of receptor for morphine.

More recently, the work discussed in the previous paragraph has been amplified to concentrate on the question of which opioid receptor type mediates the effects of morphine on Ca^{2+} levels. The same astrocyte preparation was used. Morphine (1 μM) and non-morphine-exposed cultures enriched in murine astrocytes were incubated in Ca^{2+}-free media supplemented with < 0.005, 0.3, 1.0 or 3.0 mM Ca^{2+} ($[Ca^{2+}]_o$), or in unmodified media containing Ca^{2+} ionophore (A23187), nifedipine (1 μM), dantrolene (10 μM), thapsigargin (100 nM), or L-glutamate (100 μM) for 0–72 h. μ-Opioid receptor expression was examined immunocytochemically using receptor-specific antibodies. Intracellular Ca^{2+} ($[Ca^{2+}]_i$) was measured by microfluorometric analysis using fura-2. Astrocyte morphology and BrdU incorporation were assessed in GFAP immunoreactive astrocytes. In direct contrast to previous work [91], the results showed that morphine inhibited astroglial growth by activating μ-opioid receptors. Astrocytes expressed MOR1 immunoreactivity and morphine's actions were mimicked by the selective m agonist PL017. In addition, morphine inhibited DNA synthesis by mobilizing $[Ca^{2+}]_i$ in developing astroglia. At normal $[Ca^{2+}]_o$, morphine attenuated DNA synthesis by increasing $[Ca^{2+}]_i$; low $[Ca^{2+}]_o$ (0.3 mM) blocked this effect, while treatment with Ca^{2+} ionophore or glutamate mimicked morphine's actions. At extremely low $[Ca^{2+}]_o$ (< 0.005 mM), morphine paradoxically increased BrdU incorporation. Although opioids can increase $[Ca^{2+}]_i$ in astrocytes through several pathways, not all affect DNA synthesis or cellular morphology. Nifedipine (which blocks L-type Ca^{2+} channels) did not prevent morphine-induced reductions in BrdU incorporation or cellular differentiation, while thapsigargin (which depletes IP3-sensitive Ca^{2+} stores) severely inhibited DNA synthesis and cellular differentiation – irrespective of morphine treatment. However, dantrolene (an inhibitor of Ca^{2+}-dependent Ca^{2+} release) selectively blocked the effects of morphine. Although the findings of both studies indicate that morphine suppresses astroglial DNA synthesis and promotes cellular hypertrophy by inhibiting Ca^{2+}-dependent Ca^{2+} release from dantrolene-sensitive intracellular stores [91, 92], it is puzzling why the identification of the activated opioid receptor involved is so uncertain.

Two earlier, and somewhat tantalizing, initial studies on generalized proliferative effects of morphine and naltrexone in the developing brain have evidently never been followed up. One study reported that repeated administration of morphine in increasing doses delayed normal cell death in the ciliary ganglion of the chick embryo, an effect completely blocked by naloxone. Survival of spinal motor neurons was not affected [93]. Using histological and autoradiographic methods, the effect of naltrexone on the proliferation of the 4–12-week-old rat forebrain subependymal layer was examined [94]. When administered daily throughout the weaning period, this antagonist evoked a long-lasting increase of the mitotic rate and the [^{3}H]-thymidine labeling index, an effect most significant about 8–10 weeks after ending the naltrexone treatment. A direct influence of naltrexone on long-term subependymal cell proliferation could not be ruled out, although the authors discuss evidence of an indirect effect *via* suppression of noradrenergic activity in the forebrain.

4   Organs and tissues

4.1   Angiogenesis

The effect of morphine sulfate (MS), in the presence and absence of naloxone, on chicken chorioallantoic membrane as a function of blood vessel proliferation has been reported [95]. A 50% reduction in blood vessel proliferation occurred by 10 µg of β-endorphin (β-EP) or by 5 µg of MS per egg compared to controls. However, the effect is not naloxone-reversible, suggesting that although morphine may be involved in the proliferation of vascular endothelial cells, the effect may be mediated by immunity factors such as interferons, interleukins and prostaglandin E2.

4.2 Kidney

Morphine and nalaxone have been reported to modulate water excretion (see [96] and references therein) and focal glomerulosclerosis is the predominant glomerular lesion in heroin nephropathy. Also, renal interstitial scarring is an important feature of HIV-associated nephropathy and intravenous drug abuse has been demonstrated to be a risk factor for the development of HIV-associated nephropathy in patients with HIV infection. Since mesangial expansion is considered to be a precursor of glomerulosclerosis, the effects of morphine on mesangial cell proliferation have been studied [97–102].

In primary cultures, mesangial cells incubated with micromolar morphine show enhanced incorporation of [^{3}H]-thymidine compared with controls when intermittently exposed to the drug. This growth-stimulating effect of morphine was also observed at time points of one- and one and a half-week-old cultures and thereafter. Higher concentrations of morphine (by factors of 10 and 100) showed a suppressive effect on proliferation that changed to a proliferation enhancement after one and a half weeks. Naloxone attenuated the effect of morphine in one and a half week-old cultures [97].

The effect of morphine-activated macrophages on mesangial cell proliferation and matrix synthesis has also been reported [99] using conditioned media containing either macrophage secretory products or secretory products of morphine-treated macrophages. Treatment with the latter media increased proliferation of the mesangial cells compared with the control and also significantly increased synthesis of laminin and collagen type IV by the cells compared to controls. The proliferative effect was decreased by anti-TGFβ antibodies. Since media containing morphine-activated macrophage secretory products also increased mRNA expression for TGFβ by mesangial cells, the effect of the medium on proliferation may be mediated through the generation of TGFβ.

The HIV aspect has been studied by observing the effect of tubular cell-morphine and/or HIV-1 gp120 envelope protein interaction products on kidney fibroblast (KF) proliferation and apoptosis [100]. Tubular cell-morphine and/or gp120 interaction products were prepared by incubating confluent human proximal tubular cells with buffered, millimolar morphine (I), gp120 at 0.01 μg/ml (II), or a mixture of the two (III). The effect of tubular cell interaction products on fibroblast proliferation was studied with growth-arrested kidney fibroblasts treated with variable concentrations (5%, 10%, 20%, 30%

and 50%) of (I), (II) or (III) for 48 h. The role of cytokines in induced fibroblast proliferation, cells were studied by adding cytokine-neutralizing antibodies (anti-TGFβ, anti-TNFα, anti-fibroblast growth factor (anti-FGF), or anti-IL-6) to the (I), (II) and (III) mixtures for 48 h. Cell counting assays were then performed. To assay for apoptosis, cells were treated with the morphine/gp120 interaction products for 24 h and then appropriately stained and counted. The role of early growth genes in induced fibroblast proliferation were assayed by probing with cDNA for c-*fos* and c-*jun*.

At a lower concentration (20%) (II) enhanced proliferation of KF when compared with control (buffer alone), but (I) did not. Beginning at the same concentration, (III) promoted proliferation in a dose-dependent way when compared with control, (I), or (II) and it also enhanced mRNA expression of c-*fos* and c-*jun*. All tubular cell interaction products at a higher concentration (50%) promoted apoptosis of KF. From these results it was concluded that tubular cell-gp120 interaction products stimulated KF proliferation and that morphine amplified the effect of tubular cell-gp120 interaction on the proliferation. The (III)-induced proliferation may be mediated through the expression of early growth genes, whereas the lack of growth stimulation in (II)-treated cells may be mediated through the induction of apoptosis.

The effect of morphine on cultured rat renal medullary interstitial cell proliferation and matrix accumulation was studied by exposing growth-arrested cells to submicromolar concentrations of the drug [101]. Treatment with 10^{-12} M drug resulted in a maximum proliferation enhancement of 30% relative to control, which decreased to 0% at 1 micromolar as monitored 48 h after starting incubation. On the other hand, nalbuphine, a non-addicting alkaloid, did not modulate the proliferation of the same cells. [^{3}H]-thymidine and BrdU incorporation studies confirmed the mitogenic effect of morphine. Morphine also enhanced mRNA expression for c-*jun* and c-*myc* on these cells. Neutralizing antibody to IL-6 inhibited the effect of morphine on the proliferation of the cells as did a protein kinase C inhibitor. These studies provide some preliminary basis for a hypothesis that morphine may be playing a role in the development of renal interstitial pathology in patients with heroin addiction.

The effect of morphine on the proliferation of KF has also been studied [102]. At a concentration of 10^{-12} M, morphine enhanced the proliferation of KF by approximately 100% vs control. The result was further confirmed by [^{3}H]-thymidine incorporation studies. At concentrations of 10^{-12} M to

10^{-10} M, morphine also modulated mRNA expression of c-*fos*, c-*jun* and c-*myc* early growth-related genes. At concentrations of 10^{-8} to 10^{-4} M, morphine promoted apoptosis of KF and also enhanced the synthesis of p53 by KF. The results suggest that it is possible that morphine-induced KF proliferation may be mediated through the activation of early growth-related genes, whereas morphine-induced KF apoptosis may be mediated through the generation of p53. Taken as a whole, the results in this section provide some evidence that morphine may play a role in the development of renal interstitial scarring in patients with heroin-associated nephropathy.

4.3 Bone marrow

Although opioids have been shown to have diverse effects on the immune system, both *in vivo* and *in vitro*, their interactions on immature progenitor cells have been little studied. Three reports on the effects of morphine treatment of mice on colony formation by bone marrow cells *in vitro* have appeared [103–105].

Bone marrow cells from mice implanted with morphine pellets for 72 h showed a 65% decrease in their response to macrophage colony-stimulating factor (M-CSF), but chronic morphine treatment had no effect on the response of bone marrow cells to granulocyte/macrophage (GM)-CSF [103]. Removal of the morphine pellets from the mice resulted in a time-dependent reversal of the inhibition of macrophage colony formation, and the inhibition was completely blocked by simultaneous administration of naloxone and morphine pellets to the mice. No inhibition of colony formation was observed in bone marrow cells from mice treated with a single acute dose of morphine. Incubation of bone marrow cells from untreated mice for 7 days with *in vitro* morphine concentrations as low as 25 µM also reduced macrophage colony formation, and the opioid peptide β-endorphin was even more potent, significantly reducing macrophage colony formation at concentrations as low as 0.25 µM. In agreement with the *in vivo* effects, neither opioid *in vitro* had a significant effect on GM-CSF. The results suggest that opioids may significantly alter the maturation of immune cells, which could result in potent effects on overall immune competence.

In the second report [104] it was shown that either dynorphin A-(1-13) or dynorphin A-(1-10) amide, though having no effect on proliferation by

Jay A. Glasel

themselves at concentrations less than 0.1 mM, can block the inhibitory effect of morphine both *in vivo* and *in vitro*, in a dose-dependent manner. Naloxone can also block morphine's inhibitory effect on bone marrow cell proliferation *in vivo*, but has no effect *in vitro*. Dynorphin A-(1-13) was also able to block the dramatic reduction of spleen weight observed in animals chronically treated with morphine. Thus dynorphin, which has previously been shown to antagonize morphine analgesia, is also able to antagonize some of the immunosuppressive effects of morphine.

To understand the molecular mechanisms involved in morphine-mediated suppression of myeloid cell differentiation, a macrophage cell line, Bac 1.2 F5, was investigated [105]. *In vitro* proliferation of this cell line is dependent on the exogenous supply of M-CSF. Treatment of Bac 1.2F5 cells with morphine showed a dose-dependent inhibition of proliferation which was associated with morphological changes. Characterization of the binding site revealed that the binding site for morphine on these cells is different from the classical opioid receptors described in the brain. In addition to the putative novel class of morphine receptors, Bac 1.2F5 cells also express the delta opioid receptors as determined by RT-PCR analyses. These studies suggest that Bac 1.2F5 cells are suitable for the molecular characterization of opioid effects on the proliferation and differentiation of myeloid progenitor cells.

4.4 Adrenal gland

Implantation of a 75-mg morphine pellet in sham-adrenalectomized male C3H/HeN mice have been reported to result in significant elevations of serum corticosterone levels within 6 h [43]. Corticosterone levels remain elevated (3- to 4-fold) for 72 h and then return to normal by 120 h post-implantation. Within 48 h of pellet implantation, morphine-pelleted mice exhibited marked reductions in spleen (35%) and thymus weight (56%) relative to values in placebo-pelleted controls. In addition, adrenal hypertrophy was observed in the morphine-pelleted shams (50% increase in adrenal weight relative to placebo). The magnitude of splenic and thymic atrophy was reduced by about 50% in adrenalectomized morphine-pelleted mice (17% and 22% reductions, respectively) compared to that in adrenalectomized mice implanted with placebo pellets. Lymphocyte-proliferative responses to the T-cell mitogen Con-A and the B-cell mitogen bacterial LPS were also significantly reduced in the morphine-pelleted sham mice. Morphine-induced suppression of Con-A- or LPS-stimulated lymphocyte proliferation was absent in adrenalectomized mice. Effects similar to adrenalectomy (e.g., lessening of magnitude of morphine-induced suppression of lymphoid organ weight and lymphocyte proliferation) were found in morphine-pelleted mice given the glucocorticoid receptor antagonist RU-486 at a dose of 10 mg/kg, twice daily. These studies imply that morphine-induced immunosuppression is at least in part mediated by the increase in serum corticosterone levels after implantation of the morphine pellet.

4.5 Lung

It has been reported that morphine and codeine are synthesized in the rat at detectable levels [106, 107]. Following this work, data were presented purporting to show that mammalian lung tissue contain the opiate alkaloids morphine and codeine and that these alkaloids are also to be found in normal lung cell lines. However, analysis of both small-cell and non-small-cell lung cancer cells indicated that they did not contain these opiate alkaloids endogenously [108]. Unfortunately, the primary method for assaying the opioid alkaloids in these three reports was radioimmunoassay using a polyclonal anti-morphine antibody. Since the results report levels of "endogenous" morphine that may be calculated to yield a concentration in a cell of over 1 molar, the specificity of the antibodies must be called into question.

Nonetheless, in work not dependent on the antibodies described above [109], lung cancer cell lines of diverse histologic types have been reported to express multiple, high-affinity (K_d = 10^{-9}–10^{-10} M) membrane receptors for μ-, δ- and κ-opioid agonists and for nicotine and α-bungarotoxin. These receptors were considered biologically active on the basis of decreases in cAMP levels in the lung cancer cells after opioid and nicotine application. Nicotine at concentrations (approximately 100 nM) found in the blood of smokers had no effect on *in vitro* lung cancer cell growth, whereas μ-, δ- and κ-opioid agonists at low concentrations (1–100 nM) inhibited growth. It was also found that lung cancer cells expressed various combinations of immunoreactive opioid peptides (β-endorphin, enkephalin, or dynorphin), suggesting the participation of opioids in a negative autocrine loop or tumor-suppressing system. It was found that nicotine at concentrations of

100–200 nM partially or totally reversed opioid-induced growth inhibition in 9/14 lung cancer cell lines. Since nicotine is often found in patients suffering from lung cancer, the authors suggest that their *in vitro* results imply that opioids could function as part of a "tumor suppressor" system and that nicotine can function to circumvent this system in the pathogenesis of lung cancer.

The possible relationship between opioid and nicotinic receptor activation on the immune system has been investigated further [110] by comparing the effects of morphine with both nicotine and the highly selective nicotinic agonist, epibatidine. Male Sprague-Dawley rats were treated with either morphine (10 mg/kg, s.c.), nicotine (2.85 mg/kg, s.c. = 1 mg/kg freebase), or epibatidine (5 µg/kg, s.c.) and sacrificed 2 h later. Each drug increased plasma corticosterone levels and decreased the magnitude of the peripheral blood lymphocyte proliferation response to Con-A. None of the treatments had a significant effect on splenic or thymic lymphocyte responses. The effects of nicotine treatment were dose-dependent. Pretreatment with the quaternary ganglionic antagonist chlorisondamine (0.5 mg/kg, i.p.), completely blocked the effect of epibatidine on blood lymphocytes without altering the elevation of corticosterone levels. Although naltrexone (10 mg/kg, s.c.) blocked all effects of morphine, the effects of epibatidine were not blocked by the opioid receptor antagonist. Furthermore, in contrast to morphine, central injection of neither nicotine (30 or 240 nmol) nor epibatidine (5, 50, or 500 ng) altered blood lymphocyte responses. These results suggest that, like morphine, nicotinic agonists decrease blood lymphocyte proliferation responses, apparently independent of elevated corticosterone. However, unlike morphine, nicotinic agonists appear to act predominantly at peripheral receptors, suggesting that nicotinic receptors are downstream of opioid receptors in a centrally mediated opioid-induced immunomodulatory pathway [110].

Despite the work described above, the presence of classical opioid receptors on lung cells must be regarded as controversial. The small-cell lung carcinoma cell line U-1690 was found to bind β-endorphin *via* nonopioid binding sites also recognized by the C-terminal part of this opioid peptide (Lys-Lys-Gly-Glu), but not by naloxone and morphine or other opioid peptides [111]. However, this does not mean that observations on the suppression of proliferation of lung cancer by morphine cannot be true: while the β-endorphin binding to the U-1690 cells did not affect the production of cAMP, it was enhanced by dexamethasone pretreatment and the observed β-endorphin-stimulated proliferation of the cells was inhibited by Lys-Lys-Gly-Glu and increased by dexamethasone pretreatment. The cells were also found to produce β-endorphin, suggesting an autocrine mechanism [111].

5   Transformed cells

5.1   Prostatic cancer

Opioid agonists (ethylketocyclazocine, etorphine, DADLE, DAMGO, DSLET and morphine) have been found to inhibit the proliferation of human prostate cancer cell lines (LNCaP, DU145 and PC3), in a dose-dependent manner [112]. The 50% inhibitory concentrations (IC_{50}) were in the picomolar range. In many cases, this effect was antagonized by the general opioid antagonist, diprenorphine, indicating the existence of specific opioid binding sites. Saturation binding experiments with selective ligands and effectors showed no opioid sites on the LNCaP cell line, κ1 and μ sites on the PC3 cell line, and κ1, κ3 and μ sites on the DU145 cell line. In other cases, the opioid effect was not antagonized by diprenorphine, indicating that the action of opioids might be mediated through other membrane receptors. Furthermore, casomorphin peptides, issued from bovine α- (α-casein-90-95 and α-casein-90-96) and β-caseins (β-casomorphin and β-casomorphin-1-5), and human αS1-casein (α-casomorphin and αS1-casomorphin amide) inhibited cell proliferation of human prostate cell lines, also by a mechanism partly involving opioid receptors. These findings suggest a role for opioids in prostate cancer cell growth because opioid neurons can be found in the prostate gland, and casomorphin peptides could reach the gland through the general circulation.

5.2   Breast cancer

The action of opioid receptor agonists on the proliferation of cells of the T47D human breast cancer cell line, grown in the absence of exogenously added steroids and growth factors, has been reported [113]. The opioid receptor agonists ethylketocyclazocine, morphine, DADLE, DSLET and etorphine inhibit in a dose-dependent way. The opioid receptor antagonist diprenorphine had no significant effect *per se*, but it was able to reverse the action of all opioid receptor agonists except morphine. In order to investigate the mechanism of action of opioids on T47D cells, the opioid receptors present on this cell line were characterized by saturation binding using radiolabeled receptor-selective agonists. Opioid binding sites belonging mainly to the κ-type (κ1, κ2 and κ3), a few δ-opioid receptor sites, but no μ-opioid receptors, were found. These results indicate that the inhibitory effect of opioids on T47D cell growth is mediated through κ- and δ-opioid receptors and that the effect of morphine may not be mediated through the classical opioid receptors.

6   Special cultured cell lines

6.1   OK cells

As discussed in section 4.2, opioids (and somatostatin and analogues) have been implicated in the modulation of renal water handling, but whether their action is accomplished through central and/or peripheral mechanisms remains controversial. In different cell systems, on the other hand, opioids and somatostatin inhibit cell proliferation. The OK cell line has been used to characterize opioid and somatostatin receptors and to investigate the action of opioids and somatostatin on tubular epithelial tissue. The results show the presence of one class of opioid binding sites with k- selectivity (K_D 4.6 ± 0.9 nM, 57,250 sites/cell), whereas δ, μ or other subtypes of the κ-site were absent. Somatostatin also presents a high affinity site on these cells (K_D 24.5 nM, 330,000 sites/cell). No effect of either opioids or somatostatin on the activity of the Na^+/P_i cotransporter was observed, indicating that these agents do not affect ion transport mechanisms. However, opioid agonists and somatostatin analogues decrease OK cell proliferation in a dose-dependent manner; in the same nanomolar concentration range, they displayed reversible specific binding for these agents. The addition of diprenorphine, a general opioid antagonist, reversed the effects of opioids, with the exception of morphine. Furthermore, morphine interacts with the somatostatin receptor in this cell line too, as was the case in the breast cancer T47D cell line. The results indicate that in the proximal tubule, opioids and somatostatin do not affect transport, but they might have a role in the modulation of renal cell proliferation either during ontogenesis or in kidney repair.

6.2 Fibroblasts

The G0/G1 to S-phase transition in quiescent EL2 rat fibroblast cells stimulated by mitogens such as EGF can be blocked by the addition of morphine to the system [114]. The drug must be actively present when quiescent EL2 cells are induced to enter the proliferative state. Even when morphine is added after mitogenic stimulus, an exposure only within 6 h is required to inhibit DNA synthesis. These results suggest that morphine can directly influence the proliferation of the nonlymphoid cell system, particularly during the establishment of a competence state (i.e., G0/S phase transition).

In other work, a novel clonal NIH3T3 fibroblast-derived cell line transfected with the δ-opioid receptor encoding gene, has been used to study morphine-activated regulation of cell proliferation [115–117]. These new cell lines, designated with the suffix 3T3DA, can be cultured stably in serum-free, hormone-defined medium: insulin is the only exogenous growth factor added to the culture medium of proliferating 3T3DA cell lines, and their proliferation can be stopped and started by the respective removal or addition of insulin. Micromolar concentrations of morphine were used to activate the δ-opioid receptor over periods extending to 6 days. Distinct patterns of G-protein coupled receptor (GPCR)-specific, agonist-activated growth regulation in serum-free cultures, but not in serum-supplemented cultures were observed [116]. At concentrations > 10 μM, morphine inhibits growth of cells by 40% with respect to control cells not expressing the opioid receptor. Opioid agonist-induced inhibition of cAMP production as well as growth down-regulation are pertussis toxin-sensitive, indicating that the exogenously expressed delta-opioid receptors demonstrate classical opioid receptor signaling. Neither the untreated nor the agonist-treated cells form colonies in soft agar, indicating that they retain anchorage-dependent growth control. These cell lines provide a simple system that could be used as a tool for probing the complex molecular mechanisms associated with opioid agonist-activated growth control.

Computer simulation of cell cycle kinetics was used to analyze the observed rates of proliferation of these cells in the presence and absence of morphine, and after withdrawal of morphine treatment [117]. The question under study was whether the difference in cell kinetics observed for the cell populations under the different treatments could be due to changes in the length of the cell cycle, withdrawal of cells from the cycle into a quiescent state, or differences in cell renewal. This was investigated by comparing observed cell numbers as a function of time with the results of different computer simulations using different values for these parameters. It was found that a satisfactory explanation of the experimental observations could be made on the basis of changes in a small set of parameters: (1) untreated cells experience a slowdown of cell proliferation at about the culture density where multiple cell-cell contacts are made; (2) beginning then, a large fraction is shunted from G1 into a quiescent state. Chronic morphine treatment inhibits proliferation by slowing passage through G1, but the cells remain as sensitive to cell-cell contacts as the untreated cells. After drug withdrawal following a 6-day treatment with morphine, the cells exhibit a large temporary increase in their rate of proliferation compared with control or chronically treated cells but about 48 h after withdrawal, when cell-cell contacts just begin to be made, the cells return to almost their pre-treatment total cell cycle time and, as before, a large fraction is shunted into a quiescent state. Taken in conjunction with previously discussed results, these indicate a possible interaction between morphine-induced and insulin-induced nuclear signaling pathways to the nucleus.

In this cell line, endogenous β2-adrenergic receptors (AR) are coexpressed with the exogenous δ-opioid receptors [115]. While chronic morphine treatment inhibits cell proliferation, chronic procaterol activation of the β2-AR stimulates it. Chronic morphine treatment with the individual agonists is accompanied by differential activation of the MAPK isozymes, ERK and JNK. The findings suggest that chronic β2-AR activation stimulates proliferation by interacting with the ERK signalling cascade independent of a cAMP-mediated pathway. In contrast to treatment with individual agonists, chronic dual agonist treatment suppresses procaterol-induced stimulation of ERK activity and stimulation of proliferation indicating that a cross-regulatory interaction occurs between the opioid and adrenergic signaling systems in the cells under these conditions.

References

1   H.W. Matthes, R. Maldonado, F. Simonin, O. Valverde, S. Slowe, I. Kitchen, K. Befort, A. Dierich, M. Le Meur, P. Dolle et al.: Nature 383, 819 (1996).
2   B.L. Kieffer: Trends Pharmacol. Sci. 20, 19 (1999).
3   H. Rosen and Z. Bar-Shavit: J. Cell Biochem. 55, 334 (1994).

4   P.M. Villiger and M. Lotz: Embo J. *11*, 135 (1992).
5   A. Bottger and B. A. Spruce: J. Cell Biol. *130*, 1251 (1995).
6   K.M. Linner, H.E. Quist and B.M. Sharp: J. Immunol. *154*, 5049 (1995).
7   Z. Vertes, J.L. Kornyei, S. Kovacs and M. Vertes: J. Steroid Biochem. Mol. Biol. *59*, 173 (1996).
8   G. Weisinger, O. Zinder and R. Simantov: Biochem. Biophys. Res. Commun. *214*, 530 (1995).
9   I.S. Zagon, J.W. Sassani and P.J. McLaughlin: Am. J. Physiol. *268*, R942 (1995).
10   P.J. McLaughlin: Am. J. Physiol. *271*, R122 (1996).
11   P.J. McLaughlin and I.S. Zagon: Life Sci. *41*, 1465 (1987).
12   T. Isayama, P.J. McLaughlin and I.S. Zagon: Vis. Neurosci. *13*, 695 (1996).
13   I. S. Zagon and P. J. McLaughlin: Brain Res. *542*, 318 (1991).
14   F.M. Leslie, Y. Chen and U.H. Winzer-Serhan: Can. J. Physiol. Pharmacol. *76*, 284 (1998).
15   Y. Zhu and J.E. Pintar: Biol. Reprod. *59*, 925 (1998).
16   I.S. Zagon, Y. Wu and P.J. McLaughlin: Brain Res. *839*, 313 (1999).
17   W. Bryant, J. Janik, M. Baumann and P. Callahan: Brain Res. *807*, 228 (1998).
18   Y. Zhu, M.S. Hsu and J.E. Pintar: J. Neurosci. *18*, 2538 (1998).
19   R. Pabst: Dtsch. Med. Wochenschr. *101*, 293 (1976).
20   M.A. Verbeeck, M. Draaijer and J.P. Burbach: J. Biol. Chem. 265, 18087 (1990).
21   T.M. Esterle and E. Sanders-Bush: Trends Pharmacol. Sci. *12*, 375 (1991).
22   J.M. Lauder: Psychoneuroendocrinology 8, 121 (1983).
23   J.M. Lauder: Trends Neurosci. *16*, 233 (1993).
24   A.M. Graybiel, R. Moratalla and H.A. Robertson: Proc. Natl. Acad. Sci. USA *87*, 6912 (1990).
25   B. Rouveix: Therapie *47*, 503 (1992).
26   H.N. Bhargava: NIDA Res. Monogr. *96*, 220 (1990).
27   M.G. Sergeeva, Z.V. Grishina and S.D. Varfolomeyev: Immunol. Lett. *36*, 215 (1993).
28   P.T. Thomas, H.N. Bhargava and R.V. House: Pharmacology *50*, 51 (1995).
29   P.T. Thomas, R.V. House and H.N. Bhargava: Gen. Pharmacol. *26*, 123 (1995).
30   R.D. Mellon and B.M. Bayer: Brain Res. *789*, 56 (1998).
31   S.C. Gilman, J.M. Schwartz, R.J. Milner, F.E. Bloom and J.D. Feldman: Proc. Natl. Acad. Sci. USA *79*, 4226 (1982).
32   W. Gilmore and L.P. Weiner: Immunopharmaco.l *17*, 19 (1989).
33   F.H. Hucklebridge, B.N. Hudspith, P.M. Lydyard and J. Brostoff: Immunopharmacol. 19, 87 (1990).
34   A.W. Kusnecov, A.J. Husband, M.G. King, G. Pang and R. Smith: Brain Behav. Immun. *1*, 88 (1987).
35   S. Palm, C. Mignat, K. Kuhn, H. Umbreit, J. Barth, F. Stüber and C. Maier: Methods Find. Exp. Clin. Pharmacol. *18*, 159 (1996).
36   S. Palm, S. Lehzen, C. Mignat, J. Steinmann, G. Leimenstoll and C. Maier: Anesth. Analg. *86*, 166 (1998).
37   P. Sacerdote, B. Manfredi, P. Mantegazza and A.E. Panerai: Br. J. Pharmacol. *121*, 834 (1997).
38   B.M. Bayer, S. Daussin, M. Hernandez and L. Irvin: Neuropharmacology *29*, 369 (1990).
39   B.M. Bayer, M.C. Hernandez and X.Z. Ding: Pharmacol. Biochem. Behav. *53*, 227 (1996).
40   W.R. Wu, J.W. Zheng, N. Li, H.Q. Bai, K.R. Zhang and Y. Li: Eur. J. Pharmacol. 366, 261 (1999).

41   M.C. Hernandez, L.R. Flores and B.M. Bayer: J. Pharmacol. Exp. Ther. *267*, 1336 (1993).

42   R. Pacifici, G. Patrini, I. Venier, D. Parolaro, P. Zuccaro and E. Gori: J. Pharmacol. Exp. Ther. *269*, 1112 (1994).

43   H.U. Bryant, E.W. Bernton and J.W. Holaday: Life Sci. *41*, 1731 (1987).

44   H.U. Bryant, B.C. Yoburn, C.E. Inturrisi, E.W. Bernton and J.W. Holaday: Eur. J. Pharmacol. *149*, 165 (1988).

45   H.U. Bryant, E.W. Bernton, J.R. Kenner and J.W. Holaday: Endocrinology *128*, 3253 (1991).

46   L.F. Chuang, K.F.J. Killam and R.Y. Chuang: In Vivo *7*, 159 (1993).

47   M.E. Coussons-Read, L.A. Dykstra and D.T. Lysle: J. Neuroimmunol. *55*, 135 (1994).

48   M.E. Coussons-Read, L.A. Dykstra and D.T. Lysle: Brain Behav. Immun. *8*, 204 (1994).

49   L.R. Flores, M.C. Hernandez and B.M. Bayer: J. Pharmacol. Exp. Ther. *268*, 1129 (1994).

50   S. Roy, B.L. Ge, S. Ramakrishnan, N.M. Lee and H.H. Loh: FEBS Lett. *287*, 93 (1991).

51   S. Roy, B.L. Ge, H.H. Loh and N.M. Lee: J. Pharmacol. Exp. Ther. *263*, 451 (1992).

52   S. Roy, R.B. Chapin, K.J. Cain, R.G. Charboneau, S. Ramakrishnan and R.A. Barke: Cell Immunol. *179*, 1 (1997).

53   C.C. Chao, S. Hu, T.W. Molitor, Y. Zhou, M.P. Murtaugh, M. Tsang and P.K. Peterson: J. Pharmacol. Exp. Ther. *262*, 19 (1992).

54   K. Fecho, K.A. Maslonek, L.A. Dykstra and D.T. Lysle: J. Pharmacol. Exp. Ther. *276*, 626 (1996).

55   K. Fecho, K.A. Maslonek, L.A. Dykstra and D.T. Lysle: J. Pharmacol. Exp. Ther. *277*, 633 (1996).

56   J.G. Hamra and T.L. Yaksh: Anesthesiology *85*, 355 (1996).

57   D.M. Hall, J.L. Suo and R.J. Weber: J. Neuroimmunol. *83*, 29 (1998).

58   K. Fecho, K.A. Maslonek, L.A. Dykstra and D.T. Lysle: Brain Behav. Immun. *7*, 253 (1993).

59   K. Fecho, K.A. Maslonek, L.A. Dykstra and D.T. Lysle: Brain Behav. Immun. *11*, 167 (1997).

60   D.T. Lysle, K.E. Hoffman and L.A. Dykstra: J. Pharmacol. Exp. Ther. *277*, 1533 (1996).

61   R. Gomez-Flores, J.L. Suo and R.J. Weber: Brain Behav. Immun. *13*, 212 (1999).

62   L.R. Flores, K.L. Dretchen and B.M. Bayer: Eur. J. Pharmacol. *318*, 437 (1996).

63   K. Fecho and D.T. Lysle: Cell Immunol. *195*, 137 (1999).

64   L.R. Flores, S.M. Wahl and B.M. Bayer: J. Pharmacol. Exp. Ther. *272*, 1246 (1995).

65   K. Fecho, K.A. Maslonek, L.A. Dykstra and D.T. Lysle: J. Pharmacol. Exp. Ther. *272*, 477 (1995).

66   G.M. Schneider and D.T. Lysle: J. Neuroimmunol. *89*, 150 (1998).

67   Z.W. Lu, W.J. Dai, G.L. Wang and Z.B. Lin: Brain Behav. Immun. *10*, 351 (1996).

68   D.T. Lysle, M.E. Coussons, V.J. Watts, E.H. Bennett and L.A. Dykstra: J. Pharmacol. Exp. Ther. *265*, 1071 (1993).

69   C.J. Nelson, L.A. Dykstra and D.T. Lysle: Anesth. Analg. *85*, 620 (1997).

70   J.P. West, D.T. Lysle and L.A. Dykstra: Drug Alcohol Depend. *46*, 147 (1997).

71   J.P. West, L.A. Dykstra and D.T. Lysle: Psychopharmacology (Berl) *146*, 320 (1999).

72   M. Tian, H.E. Broxmeyer, Y. Fan, Z. Lai, S. Zhang, S. Aronica, S. Cooper, R.M. Bigsby, R. Steinmetz, S. J. Engle et al.: J. Exp. Med. *185*, 1517 (1997).

73   M.C. Lopez, L.L. Colombo, G.J. Chen, B. Watzl, H.R. Darban, D.S. Huang and R.R. Watson: Int. J. Immunopharmacol. *15*, 899 (1993).

74   M.C. Lopez, G.J. Chen, L.L. Colombo, D.S. Huang, H.R. Darban, B. Watzl and R.R. Watson: Int. J. Immunopharmacol. *15*, 909 (1993).

75   S.B. Nyland, S. Specter and K.E. Ugen: DNA Cell Biol. *18*, 285 (1999).

76   J.W. Holaday: Klin. Wochenschr. *69*, 13 (1991).

77   M.T. Price, J.W. Olney and T.J. Cicero: Cell Tissue Res. *171*, 277 (1976).

78   M.T. Price, J.W. Olney and T.J. Cicero: Cell Tissue Res. *182*, 537 (1977).

79   M.T. Price, J.W. Olney and T.J. Cicero: Cell Tissue Res. *171*, 277 (1976).

80   R. Kato: Xenobiotica *7*, 25 (1977).

81   R.P.J. Hammer, A.A. Ricalde and J.V. Seatriz: Neurotoxicology *10*, 475 (1989).

82   J.V. Seatriz and R.P.J. Hammer: Brain Res. Bull. *30*, 523 (1993).

83   R.S. Sinatra and D.H. Ford: Brain Res. *175*, 315 (1979).

84   L.A. Opanashuk and K.F. Hauser: Brain Res. *804*, 87 (1998).

85   K.F. Hauser: Brain Res. Dev. Brain Res. *70*, 291 (1992).

86   R.B. Messing, C. Dodge, J.C. Waymire, G.S. Lynch and S.A. Deadwyler: Brain Res. Bull. *4*, 615 (1979).

87   A. Stiene-Martin, J.A. Gurwell and K.F. Hauser: Brain Res. Dev. Brain Res. *60*, 1 (1991).

88   J.A. Gurwell and K.F. Hauser: Brain Res. Dev. Brain Res. *76*, 293 (1993).

89   A. Stiene-Martin and K.F. Hauser: Neurosci. Lett. *157*, 1 (1993).

90   A. Araque, R.P. Sanzgiri, V. Parpura and P.G. Haydon: Can. J. Physiol. Pharmacol. *77*, 699 (1999).

91   A. Stiene-Martin, M.P. Mattson and K.F. Hauser: Brain Res. Dev. Brain Res. *76*, 189 (1993).

92   K.F. Hauser, A. Stiene-Martin, M.P. Mattson, R.P. Elde, S.E. Ryan and C.C. Godleske: Brain Res. *720*, 191 (1996).

93   S.D. Meriney, D.B. Gray and G. Pilar: Science *228*, 1451 (1985).

94   W. Schmahl, R. Funk, U. Miaskowski and J. Plendl: Brain Res. *486*, 297 (1989).

95   A. Pasi, B.X. Qu, R. Steiner, H.J. Senn, W. Bär and F.S. Messiha: Gen. Pharmacol. *22*, 1077 (1991).

96   A. Hatzoglou, E. Bakogeorgou, E. Papakonstanti, C. Stournaras, D.S. Emmanouel and E. Castanas: J. Cell Biochem. *63*, 410 (1996).

97   P.C. Singhal, N. Gibbons and M. Abramovici: Kidney Int. *41*, 1560 (1992).

98   P.C. Singhal and J. Mattana: Exp. Nephrol. *2*, 138 (1994).

99   P.C. Singhal, J. Mattana, P. Garg, M. Arya, Z. Shan, N. Gibbons and N. Franki: Kidney Int. *49*, 94 (1996).

100   P.C. Singhal, S. Sagar, K. Reddy, P. Sharma, R. Ranjan and N. Franki: J. Investig. Med. *46*, 243 (1998).

101   P.C. Singhal, P. Sharma, N. Gibbons, N. Franki, A. Kapasi and J.D. Wagner: Nephron *77*, 225 (1997).

102   P.C. Singhal, P. Sharma, V. Sanwal, A. Prasad, A. Kapasi, R. Ranjan, N. Franki, K. Reddy and N. Gibbons: Kidney Int. *53*, 350 (1998).

103   S. Roy, S. Ramakrishnan, H.H. Loh and N.M. Lee: Eur. J. Pharmacol. *195*, 359 (1991).

104   S. Roy, H.H. Loh and N.M. Lee: Eur. J. Pharmacol. *202*, 355 (1991).

105   S. Roy, M. Sedqi, S. Ramakrishnan, R.A. Barke and H.H. Loh: Cell Immunol. *169*, 271 (1996).

106   J. Donnerer, G. Cardinale, J. Coffey, C.A. Lisek, I. Jardine and S. Spector: J. Pharmacol. Exp. Ther. *242*, 583 (1987).

107   J. Donnerer, K. Oka, A. Brossi, K.C. Rice and S. Spector: Proc. Natl. Acad. Sci. USA *83*, 4566 (1986).

108   I.D. Munjal, J.D. Minna, R. Manneckjee, P. Bieck and S. Spector: Life Sci. *57*, 517 (1995).

109   R. Maneckjee and J.D. Minna: Proc. Natl. Acad. Sci. USA *87*, 3294 (1990).

110   R.D. Mellon and B.M. Bayer: J. Pharmacol. Exp. Ther. *288*, 635 (1999).

111   M.F. Melzig, I. Nylander, M. Vlaskovska and L. Terenius: Exp. Cell Res. *219*, 471 (1995).

112   M. Kampa, E. Bakogeorgou, A. Hatzoglou, A. Damianaki, P.M. Martin and E. Castanas: Eur. J. Pharmacol. *335*, 255 (1997).

113   A. Hatzoglou, E. Bakogeorgou and E. Castanas: Eur. J. Pharmacol. *296*, 199 (1996).

114   P. Di Francesco, R. Gaziano, I.A. Casalinuovo, A.T. Palamara and C. Favalli: Int. J. Tissue React. *16*, 205 (1994).

115   D. Agarwal and J.A. Glasel: Cell Prolif. *32*, 215 (1999).

116   D. Agarwal and J.A. Glasel: J. Cell Physiol. *171*, 61 (1997).

117   J.A. Glasel and D. Agarwal: Life Sci. *61*, 305 (1997).

Progress in Drug Research, Vol. 55 (E. Jucker, Ed.)
©2000 Birkhäuser Verlag, Basel (Switzerland)

Glucosamine and chondroitin sulfates in the treatment of osteoarthritis: a survey

By Gerlie C. de los Reyes, Robert T. Koda and Eric J. Lien

Department of Pharmaceutical Sciences, School of Pharmacy, University of Southern California, Los Angeles, CA 90089, USA

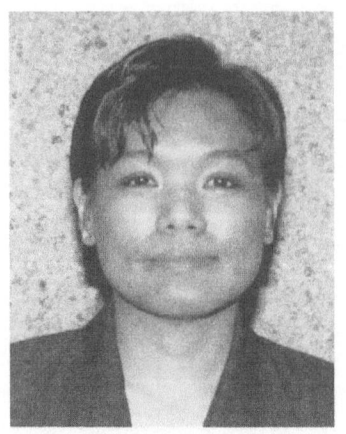

Gerlie C. de los Reyes

received her B.S. and M.S. Pharmacy degrees from the University of the Philippines Manila (UPM). Currently, she is a Ph.D. student at the School of Pharmacy, University of Southern California, where she was admitted as a teaching assistant in 1997. Her research interests include dosage form development, assay development and validation for the quantification of drugs from pharmaceutical dosage forms and biological matrices, in vivo ocular absorption, and in vitro oral absorption of phytopharmaceuticals using the Caco-2 cell system.

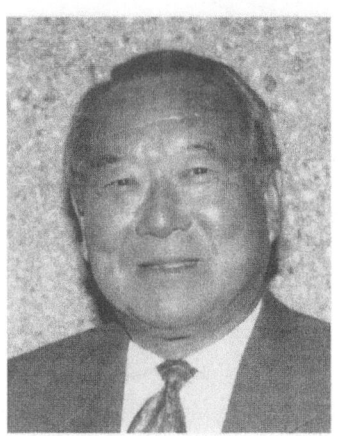

Robert T. Koda

received both the Pharm.D. and Ph.D. degrees from the University of Southern California. His primary research effort is the investigation of the pharmacokinetics of investigational drugs and novel therapies used in the treatment of cancer, HIV and its related conditions, and dosage form development. He was appointed as "Expert Analyste" by the Ministère des Affaires Sociales et de la Solidarité Nationale, France, and to the Medi-Cal Therapeutic Drug Utilization Review Committee and served as its Vice Chairman. He is a member of the Bioequivalence Advisory Panel to the Medi-Cal Therapeutics and Drug Advisory Committee of the State of California.

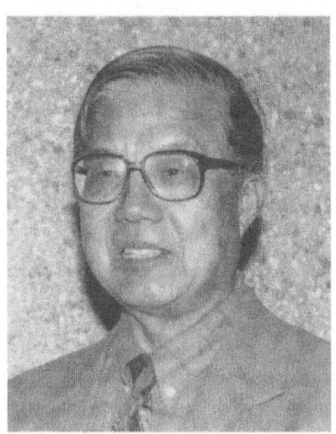

Eric J. Lien

received his Ph.D. from the University of California at San Francisco Medical Center in 1966. After his postdoctoral training at Pomona College, he joined the University of Southern California in 1968 as a faculty member. His research interests include structure-activity relationship and drug design, physical organic chemistry and natural products. Ongoing research projects include design, synthesis and testing of antiviral and anticancer agents, gastrointestinal and percutaneous absorption of drugs, correlation of side effects and toxicities with molecular structures, extrapyramidal syndrome and skin sensitization and isolation of bioactive natural products like immunostimulating polysaccharides from Chinese herbs.

Summary

For more than 30 years, non-steroidal anti-inflammatory drugs (NSAIDs) have been used as standards in the treatment of osteoarthritis (OA). Serious and often life-threatening adverse effects due to these agents are common. Clinical findings have revealed that glucosamine sulfate and chondroitin sulfate are effective and safer alternatives to alleviate symptoms of OA. Experimental evidence indicates that these compounds and their low molecular weight derivatives have a particular tropism for cartilage where they serve as substrates in the biosynthesis of component building blocks. This paper is a literature review of the chemistry, mechanism of action, pharmacokinetics, clinical efficacy and safety of these two nutraceuticals.

Contents

Keywords

Glucosamine sulfate, chondroitin sulfate, osteoarthritis, chondroprotective agents, cartilage, glycosaminoglycans, proteoglycans, pharmacokinetics, mechanism of action, chemistry, clinical trials, dosage, adverse drug reactions, toxicity.

Glossary of abbreviations
OA, osteoarthritis; GAG, glycosaminoglycans; PG, proteoglycan; NSAID, non-steroidal anti-inflammatory drug; GS, glucosamine sulfate; CS, chondroitin sulfate.

1   Introduction

Osteoarthritis (OA, osteoarthrosis) is the most prevalent musculoskeletal problem found in the elderly and is estimated to affect more than 16 million Americans, especially those over 40 years old [1]. Aging, obesity and physical injuries are contributing factors in this disorder. OA involves the erosion of the cartilage (Fig. 1) which is considered to be the protective "cushion" in the articulating surfaces between the joints of bones [2]. The degenerative process is caused by a defect in the elaboration of the component macro-molecules including glycosaminoglycans (GAGs) and proteoglycans (PGs).

For many years, non-steroidal anti-inflammatory drugs (NSAIDs) have been used to manage the articular pain and inflammation associated with the disease. However, NSAIDs are strictly palliative and are limited due to their adverse drug reactions (ADRs). It is even suspected that these drugs may exacerbate the progression of OA [4]. On the other hand, nutraceuticals, like glu-

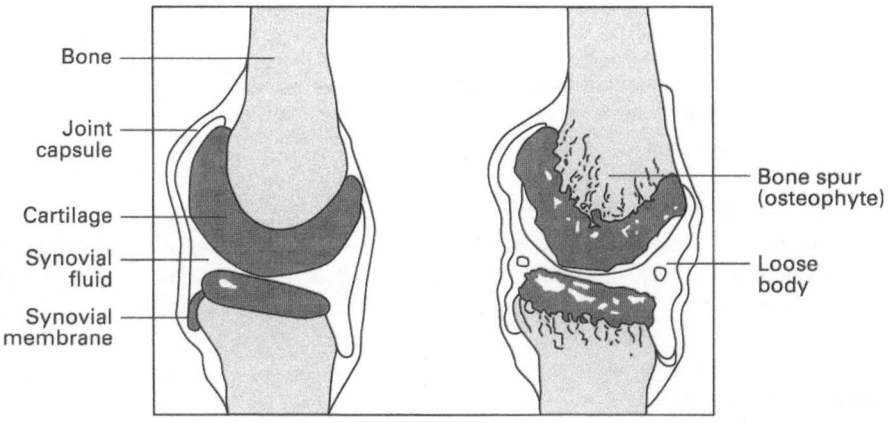

Fig. 1
Normal *versus* osteoarthritic joint. Adapted from [3].

cosamine and chondroitin sulfates, are gaining increasing favor as chon-droprotective agents because these two agents address the underlying degen-erative disorder. Both these substances are naturally occurring components of the body and as such are generally considered safer than the NSAIDs.

2   Glucosamine sulfate

2.1   Chemistry

Glucosamine sulfate (GS) is the artificially synthesized sulfate salt of 2-amino-2-deoxy-D glucopyranose (Fig. 2), a small molecule of molecular weight 179.17, and a pKa of 6.91 [5]. Glucosamine is found naturally in chitin, in mucoproteins, and in mucopolysaccharides of many animals.

2.2   Physiological role of glucosamine

Glucosamine is an aminomonosaccharide synthesized from glucose and is used by the body in the biosynthesis of GAGs and PGs (Fig. 3) [6]. In OA, there is an abnormal reduction in the formation of GAGs, PGs and other articular

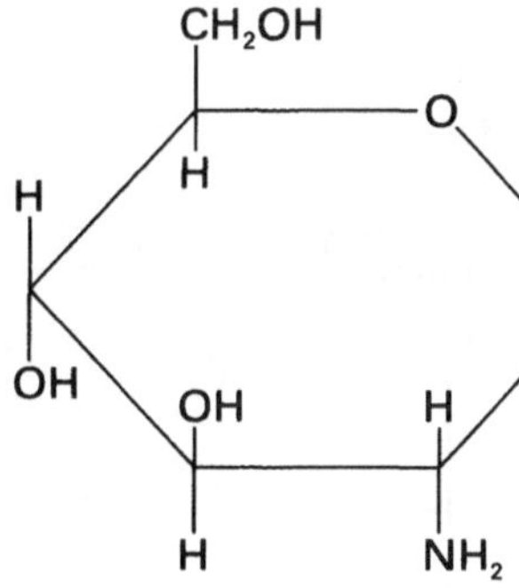

Fig. 2
Chemical structure of glucosamine.

Gerlie C. de los Reyes et al.

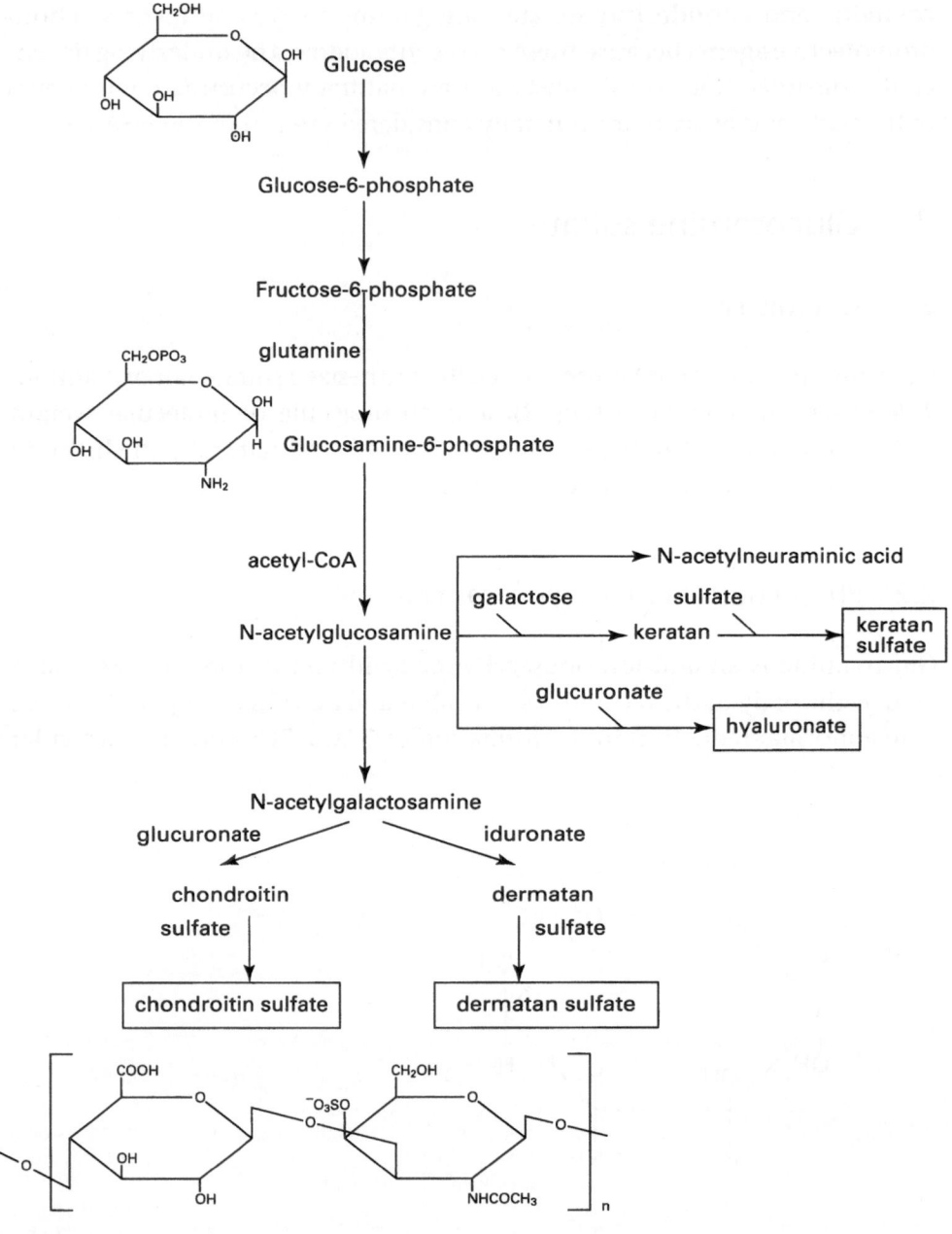

Fig. 3
Biosynthesis of glycosaminoglycans (GAGs), chondroitin sulfate, dermatan sulfate, hyaluronic acid and keratan sulfate. Adapted from [6].

cartilage components and/or an overstimulation of enzymatic processes that destroy cartilage. Exogenous glucosamine, if available, becomes a preferred source of the hexosamine precursor and the sulfate anion needed for the biosynthesis of GAGs in the articular cartilage [7].

2.3   Mechanism of action

In vitro experimental evidence suggests that GS may have a beneficial effect on cartilage metabolism. Glucosamine stimulates chondrocytes to synthesize the cartilage building blocks (GAGs, PGs, collagen) and inhibits lysosomal enzymes which degrade cartilage [8]. Its mild anti-inflammatory property is thought to be due to several processes, including stabilization of cell membranes by the addition of the newly synthesized PGs [9], inhibition of lysosomal enzymes (e.g., interleukin-induced aggrecanase) which degrade cartilage and blockage of the generation of superoxide free radicals by macrophages [10]. Unlike the NSAIDs, glucosamine is an ineffective inhibitor of cyclooxygenase and inflammatory mediators, including bradykinin, serotonin and histamine [11].

2.4   Pharmacokinetics

The pharmacokinetics of single-dose, oral and parenteral GS were investigated in healthy volunteers [7, 12]. Some of the calculated pharmacokinetic parameters are summarized in Table 1.

Following oral absorption in man, GS dissociates into glucosamine and sulfate ion. The free hexosamine is rapidly incorporated into plasma globulins and tissue proteins. Its elimination from plasma follows two-compartment kinetics similar to i.v. and i.m. administration, but the area under the curve (AUC) is about five-fold lower than by the parenteral routes. The bioavailability of glucosamine after oral administration is only 26% of that after i.v. injection. The low plasma bioavailability is presumably due to first-pass hepatic metabolism and tissue retention.

Biodistribution studies in dogs and rats indicate that after oral administration, the greatest quantity of the drug is distributed to the major elimination organs, the liver and kidneys. Glucosamine rapidly appears in the artic-

Table 1.
Pharmacokinetics of glucosamine sulfate in human subjects[*]

Parameter	Administration route	
	i.v.	oral
Relative bioavailability (%)	100	26
C_{max}, plasma proteins (μmol/l)	128	31
t_{max} (h), plasma proteins	10	8
AUC (mmol/l $\times$ h)	12.9	3.2
Terminal $t_{1/2}$, Plasma proteins (h)	70	68
Elimination in 120 h (% of dose)		
urinary	28	10
fecal	0.5	11.3

[*]obtained after administration of 50 μCi uniformly labelled ^{14}C-glucosamine sulfate: 400 mg in 2 ml water for injection (i.v.); 250 mg in 5 ml water for injection (oral). Adapted from [12].

ular cartilage and is retained in this tissue for long periods of time (Figs. 4a and 4b). The data indicate that exogenous glucosamine has an affinity for bone and cartilage where it may serve as the preferred substrate for PG biosynthesis [7, 13].

2.5 Clinical trials

A recent meta-analysis of GS in the therapy of OA suggested that this nutraceutical has the potential to improve the quality of life of OA sufferers. Towheed and coworkers reviewed nine randomized clinical trials which had a mean duration and number of subjects of 5.4 weeks and 97, respectively [14]. Seven of the studies compared GS to placebo, and two trials compared GS to ibuprofen. GS was consistently superior to placebo, extremely safe and at least equal in potency to the NSAID in reducing articular pain. In addition, McAlindon et al. evaluated 13 double-blind, placebo-controlled trials of greater than 4 weeks duration using oral or parenteral GS or chondroitin sulfate (CS) for hip or knee OA. Substantial benefits from both supplements were demonstrated: 39.5% and 40.2% reductions in global pain scores or Lequesne index relative to placebo for GS and CS respectively [15]. The details of some of these clinical trials are summarized in Table 2. The results of short-term studies indicate that a daily dose of 1.5 g GS for at least 7 days is usually sufficient to achieve noticeable improvements in OA symptoms that are signif-

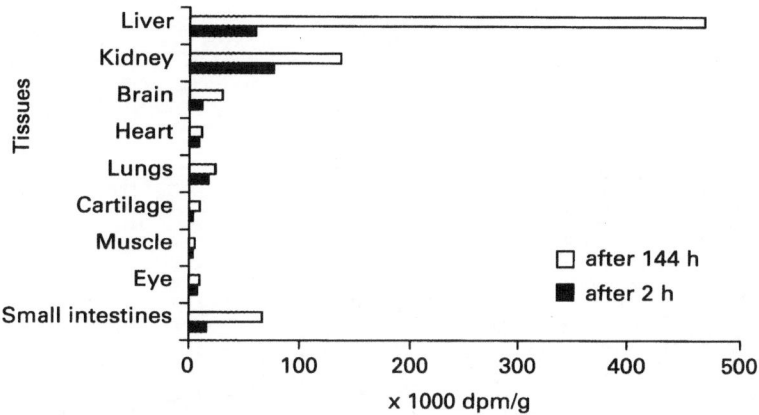

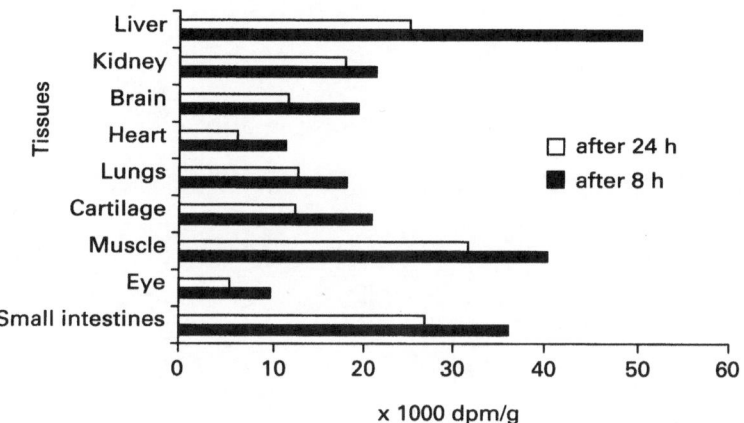

Fig. 4
(a) Radioactivity found in organs of dog after oral administration of 25 µCi/kg BW of [^{14}C]-glucosamine. Adapted from [7].
(b) Radioactivity found in organs of rat after oral administration of 20 µCi/kg BW of [^{14}C]-glucosamine. Adapted from [13].

icantly greater than placebo, or are at least as effective as 400 mg/day ibuprofen, with only mild and infrequent side-effects, if any. Additionally, although the improvements occurred more rapidly with ibuprofen, persistent reductions in symptoms were greater in patients who received GS.

Table 2. Glucosamine sulfate trials (*via* the oral route)

Study design	Dosage/duration	Number of patients Glucosamine/ placebo or NSAID	Joints evaluated	Results	Ref.
Double-blind, placebo-controlled	1.5 g daily (1 month)	40/40	General	-GS vs placebo: 72% vs 36% reduction in symptom score; improvement in articular pain (7 days), tenderness, swelling and active range of motion (14 days), passive range of motion (21 days) -Biopsies from GS-treated patients showed smooth cartilage without major discontinuities compared with the placebo group (irregular surface with cavities)	[17]
Placebo-controlled	Loading dose (LD): 400 mg injection daily (1 week) Maintenance dose (MD): 1.5 g orally (2 weeks)	15/15	General	-More rapid and marked improvement in the GS group (72% improvement in walking speed) -No drug-related complaints nor signs of interference with other illnesses or drug interactions reported	[18]
Double-blind, placebo-controlled	1.5 g /day (6–8 weeks)	10/10	Knee	GS vs placebo: 80% vs 20% improvement in pain, joint tenderness, swelling and range of motion; physician rating "excellent" in all 10 GS-treated patients -No ADRs reported	[19]

Table 2. continued

Study design	Dosage/duration	Number of patients Glucosamine/ placebo or NSAID	Joints evaluated	Results	Ref.
placebo-controlled 21 days	LD: 400 mg i.v. or i.m. (1 week) MD: 1.5 g/day (2 weeks)	15/15	General	-Joint pain at rest and in motion showed significantly greater improvement at 1 week than with placebo; continued improvement with oral GS at 3 weeks -GS well tolerated; No ADRs reported during the treatment period	[20]
Double-blind, randomized	GS: 1.5 g/day Ibuprofen: 400 mg 3/day (8 weeks)	18/20 (ibuprofen)	Knee	-Pain relief more dramatic for Ibu group; more gradual and sustained throughout 8 week trial period with GS -Minor tolerance complaints: 2 from GS group and 5 from Ibu group	[21]
Open label	1.5 g/day (7 weeks)	1208	General	-Pain (resting and in motion) relief sustained for up to 12 weeks after cessation of GS administration; physician rated GS "good" in 59% and "sufficient" in 35% of patients -No ADRs in 86% of patients; most reported ADRs disappeared upon discontinuation of GS	[22]

Table 2. continued

Study design	Dosage/duration	Number of patients Glucosamine/ placebo or NSAID	Joints evaluated	Results	Ref.
Randomized, placebo-controlled	GS: 1.5 g/day Piroxicam: 20 mg/day (3 months)	329 (piroxicam)	Knee	-Decrease in Lequesne index after 3 months: GS: 4.8 (significant); GS/Piroxicam: 4.6; Piroxicam: 2.9; Placebo: 0.8 -GS response maintained for up to 2 months after discontinuation	[23]
Randomized, double-blind	GS: 1.5 g/day Ibuprofen: 1.2 g/day (4 weeks)	100/99 (ibuprofen)	Knee	-GS equivalent to Ibu in magnitude of pain relief and improvement of range of motion (Lequesne index) -Ibu vs GS response rates: 48% vs 28% (1 week), 52% vs 48% (4 weeks) -ADRs: Ibu vs GS (35% vs 6%)	[24]
Double blind, placebo-controlled	1.5 g/day (4 weeks)	126/126	Knee	-Improvement in Lequesne index: 55% vs 38% responders (GS vs placebo)	[25]
Double-blind, placebo-controlled	GS: 1.5 g/day Ibuprofen: 1.2 g/day (4 weeks)	89/89	Knee	-GS more effective in reducing pain and swelling during treatment period; exhibited more pronounced remnant effect -Tolerance better for GS better than Ibuprofen: 6% vs 16%; 0% vs 10% drop-outs	[26]

Recently, Philippi et al. conducted a 16-week randomized, double-blind, placebo-controlled crossover trial of 1.5 mg daily GS, 1.2 mg daily CS and 228 mg daily manganese ascorbate to assess the benefit of the combination therapy in knee or low back OA patients [16]. The study demonstrated that together, the three dietary supplements relieved symptoms of knee OA, without adverse events. The value of the same combination was not unequivocally established for spinal degenerative joint disease.

2.6   Adverse drug reactions and toxicity

For over 30 years, glucosamine has been used in Germany to help alleviate symptoms of arthritis. Short-term studies conducted mostly in Europe have reported either no ADRs or mild, sporadic side-effects that include gastric problems, drowsiness, skin rash and headache [18]. These ADRs were always lower in magnitude compared to the standard NSAIDs and sometimes even less than placebo. Table 3 and Figure 5 compare the incidence of ADRs associated with the use of GS or NSAIDs [26].

Since even very high doses (5 g/kg oral, 3 g/kg i.m., 1.5 g/kg i.v.) of GS did not produce lethality in test mice and rats, there is no LD_{50} defined for GS [27]. In all reporting clinical studies GS was generally well tolerated. There is a paucity of data regarding the contraindications and drug interactions of GS. In one study, injectable and oral forms of the agent were well tolerated by inpatients suffering from other concurrent illnesses including cardiovascular disease, liver and lung disorders, depression, infections and diabetes [18]. Based on the findings, it appears that GS does not interfere with either the course of these diseases or the medications used concomitantly.

On the other hand, GS should be used cautiously by individuals with active peptic ulcers and those using diuretics because they may exhibit a lower response and tolerance to GS [22]. Likewise, Type II diabetes patients should be monitored closely while on GS, because GS has been shown to induce insulin resistance and pancreatic dysfunction in rats following parenteral administration [28]. Its hyperglycemic effect has not been corroborated in human studies following oral administration [18]. This is not surprising because the bioavailability from the oral form is much lower than from the parenteral preparations [7, 12].

Gerlie C. de los Reyes et al.

Table 3.
Reported adverse drug events: glucosamine sulfate *versus* ibuprofen

Glucosamine sulfate 500 mg 3× daily (4 weeks)	%	Ibuprofen 400 mg 3× daily (4 weeks)	%
mild stomach discomfort	3.4	mild abdominal pain	1.1
mild nausea	1.1	mild swelling of legs	1.1
mild sleepiness	1.1	mild sleepiness	1.1
		moderate vomiting	1.1
		severe stomach discomfort[*]	1.1
		severe hypertension[*]	1.1
		severe hematuria[*]	1.1
		severe vomiting[*]	1.1
		severe abdominal discomfort[*]	1.1
		severe edema (eyelids/lips)[*]	1.1
		severe edema (face/legs)	1.1
		severe skin rash[*]	1.1

[*]required discontinuation of treatment. Adapted from [26].

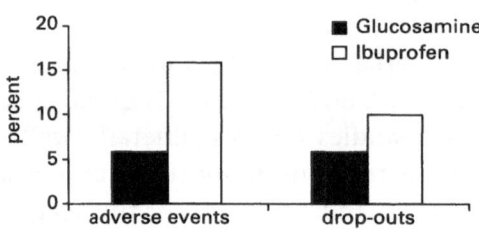

Fig. 5
Drug-related adverse events and drop-outs: glucosamine sulfate *versus* ibuprofen. Adapted from [26].

2.7 Dosage

Most clinical trials for which GS has shown marked efficacy and tolerability followed a dosage regimen consisting of 500 mg oral GS three times daily. Since the observed improvement occurred gradually and was somewhat persistent, it is recommended that the duration of the treatment be continued for at least 4 weeks. Based on results of short-term studies, the beneficial effects of GS may last up to 12 weeks after cessation of treatment depending on the duration of the preceding treatment period.

94

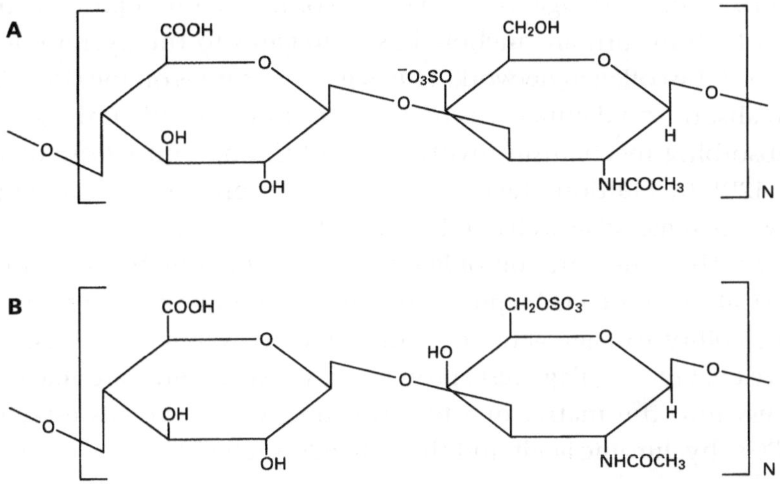

Fig. 6
Chemical structures of chondroitin-4-sulfate (A) and chondroitin-6-sulfate (B).

3 Chondroitin sulfate

3.1 Chemistry

Preparations of chondroitin sulfate are a mixture of chondroitin 4- and 6-sulfates (CS-A and CS-C, respectively) derived from bovine and calf tracheal cartilage.

Chondroitin sulfates (Fig. 6) are monosulfated GAGs consisting of disaccharide (N-acetylgalactosamine + glucuronic acid) repeating units. These compounds are very large molecules, with molecular weights of 25 to 40 kDa. The sulfates and carboxylic acid residues confer on these mucopolysaccharides their negative charges which partly account for their pharmacological roles [29].

3.2 Physiological role of chondroitin sulfate (CS)

Administered chondroitin 4- and 6-sulfates contribute to the endogenous pool of GAGs (mainly CS, and to a lesser extent keratan sulfate and hyaluronic acid). In the cartilage, the GAGs are complexed to a protein core to form PGs which in turn are anchored as aggregates to the hyaluronic acid backbone and the collagen network. The negative charges on the GAGs allow the PGs to absorb and dampen mechanical stress and strain on the joints by a shock-absorbing mechanism involving the binding and release of water molecules [29]. In addition, the fluid flux provides proper nourishment and means of waste removal as well as lubrication to the essentially avascular cartilage. In OA, the concentration of PGs is reduced mainly due to premature depolymerization of their GAG precursors, and to the synthesis of altered PGs with lesser ability to aggregate and interact with water molecules. Other degradative enzymes (collagenase, protease, glycosidase etc.) are able to gain easier access into the matrix due to fewer and weaker bonds established between PGs, hyaluronic acids and the collagen material.

3.3   Mechanism of action

In vitro and *in vivo* studies have shown that CS regulates the formation of new cartilage by stimulating chondrocyte synthesis of collagen, PG and hyaluronic acid. In addition, CS inhibits proteolytic and lysosomal enzymes (elastase, hyaluronidase) which can damage joint cartilage. For example, in a study involving OA patients, a significant increase of hyaluronan, PGs and Type 2 collagen, and a decrease of N-acetylglucosaminidase (a lysosomal enzyme) were observed in the joints after oral treatment with CS compared to the placebo group [14, 15]. In addition to metabolic regulatory activity, CS possesses anti-inflammatory properties by mechanisms involving the inhibition of complement C'1 recognition [30]. In a controlled clinical study, the oral CS treatment group showed greater anatomical improvement of the inflamed knee tissues compared with a group given salicylates [31].

3.4   Pharmacokinetics

The pharmacokinetics of CS was investigated in humans [32]. Some of the parameters calculated from the plasma levels are reported in Table 4. Following oral administration, 13.2 % of the intact CS was absorbed together with high molecular weight (HMW) and low molecular weight (LMW) poly-

Table 4.
Some plasma pharmacokinetic parameters after intravenous and oral administration of chondroitin sulfate in man

	i.v.	oral
$t_{1/2}$ elimination (h)	4.7 ± 0.53	6.1 ± 0.02
t_{max} (h)	–	3.2 ± 0.35
C_{max} (µg/ml)	–	11.4 ± 3.7
AUC $_{0-24\,h}$ experimental* (µg/ml/h)	163.3 ± 56.6	128.5 ± 37.32

*Obtained with a bolus of 0.5 g or 3 g of chondroitin sulfate administered i.v. or orally, respectively. Adapted from [32].

saccharides resulting from the depolymerization and desulfation of CS. Approximately 10% and 20% of the dose were absorbed as HMW and LMW derivatives, respectively.

Due to conflicting evidence in the literature, the impact of the metabolic fate of CS on OA remains controversial. Baici et al. reported that oral exogenous CS did not change the GAG serum levels in 18 subjects (6 healthy volunteers, 6 rheumatoid arthritis and 6 osteoarthritis patients) [33]. On the other hand, Gross showed an increase in the plasma level of CS and the subsequent increase in the concentration of CS in the synovial fluid [34]. Similarly, Conte and coworkers reported that the oral administration of commercial CS to healthy volunteers increased plasma levels of CS and its depolymerized and desulfated derivatives, although the overall concentration of the sulfated GAGs remained unchanged [32]. An increase in the concentration of hyaluronic acid and LMW derivatives of sulfated GAGs in the synovial fluid of patients was also noted. Furthermore, in separate studies using radiolabelled preparations, 70% of the radioactivity was absorbed after oral administration in rats and dogs but only 8.5% was attributed to the intact CS molecules. Radioactivity associated with molecules with molecular weight less than or equal to that of N-acetylgalactosamine persisted and increased with time. There is experimental evidence to indicate that the CS molecule is absorbed by pinocytosis, as is the case with heparin and other HMW compounds [35]. In this mode of transport, the molecule may be routed to lysosomes where it can be degraded to HMW polysaccharides and LMW derivatives such as N-acetylgalactosamine and glucuronic acid which can serve as building blocks for GAG biosynthesis. It has been shown that exogenous labelled CS (parenteral or oral) is mainly distributed into various tissues including the intestine, liver, kidneys (organs involved in the absorption,

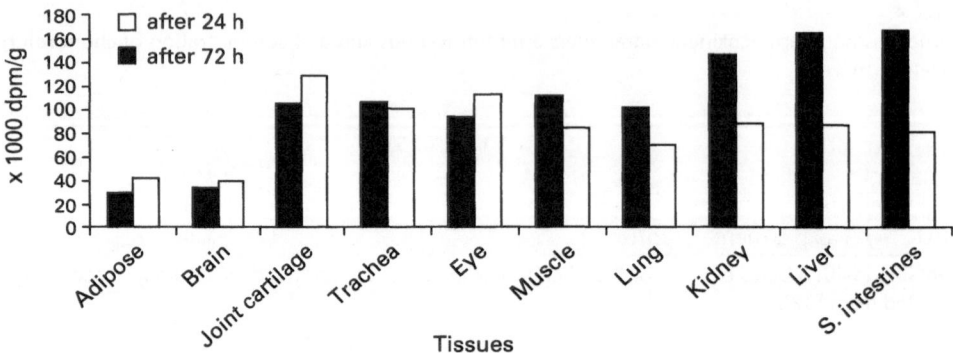

Fig. 7
Distribution of radioactivity in some tissues after oral administration of reducing end-labelled ^{3}H-chondroitin sulfate to the rat. Adapted from [36].

breakdown and excretion of oligo- and polysaccharides) with a tendency to accumulate in the synovial fluid and GAG-rich tissues such as joint cartilage (Fig. 7) [36]. In man, the kidney is the main organ of elimination for CS and its fragments after oral administration [37].

3.5 Clinical trials

In a recent meta-analysis of oral CS in OA therapy, Leeb and colleagues evaluated 4 randomized, double-blind, placebo- or NSAID-controlled trials including 227 patients on CS. All these investigations revealed that CS was at least 50% superior to placebo with respect to the Lequesne index, Visual Analog Scale (VAS) pain score and co-medication consumption [38]. Table 5 summarizes these and other controlled trials which used orally administered CS.

3.6 Adverse drug reactions and toxicity

Like GS, CS is well tolerated following an oral dose [39, 47]. In one study, only 3% of the patients had complaints of slight gastric symptoms or nausea [39]. Because of the heparinoid effect of other sulfated GAGs, there were initial

Table 5.
Chondroitin sulfate trials (*via* oral administration)

Study design	Dosage/duration	Number of patients Chondroitin/ placebo or NSAID	Joints evaluated	Results	Ref.
Open-label	1.2 g/day orally (6 months)	100	General	-Pain reduction and mobility improvement evident after 2nd week of treatment -No reported side-effects	[39]
Double-blind, placebo-controlled	200 mg 4×/day (3 months)	58/56	Knee, hips	-Improved joint pain in the CS-treated group -CS group used significantly lesser NSAIDs than the placebo group at end of 3-month trial period and at end of 2-month follow-up	[40]
Randomized, double-blind	CS: 1.2 g/day (3 months) diclofenac:150 mg/day (1 month)	74/172 (diclofenac)	Knee	-Diclofenac group showed prompt reduction in joint pain (10 days) which disappeared after cessation of treatment; CS group showed improvements (30 days) which remained up to 3 months after treatment cessation	[41]
Double-blind, placebo-controlled	800 mg/day (1 year)	25/22	Knee	-Joint pain, swelling, range of motion improved -Acetaminophen use significantly less in the CS group than in the placebo group	[42]

Table 5. continued

Study design	Dosage/duration	Number of patients Chondroitin/ placebo or NSAID	Joints evaluated	Results	Ref.
Double-blind, placebo-controlled	800 mg/day (6 months)	40/40	Knee	-Significant improvement in the Lequesne index, VAS pain scale, 20-m walk time, patient/physician efficacy ratings -Acetaminophen use significantly less in CS than placebo group	[43]
Double-blind, placebo-controlled	1.2 g/day (6 months)	40/44	Knee	-CS group had significant reduction in Lequesne index score, spontaneous joint pain (not observed in placebo group)	[44]
Double-blind, placebo-controlled; radiological progression	800 mg/day (1 year)	42	Knee (Tibio-femoral joint)	-CS significantly reduced pain and increased overall mobility; normalized biochemistry in joint and bone -Joint space in placebo group decreased significantly but did not change from baseline values in the CS-treated group	[45]
Radiological pro-gression of disease	1.2 g/day (3 years)	34/85	Hand (interphalangeal joint)	Significant decrease in erosion of of cartilage in CS-treated group (8.8%) compared to placebo (29.4%)	[9]
Placebo-controlled	800 mg/day (1 year)	104	Knee	50% decrease in Lequesne index of CS group	[46]

concerns regarding a possible anticoagulant activity, but results of clinical studies conducted in Italy, France and Switzerland disproved such speculations [48]. Unlike heparin and hypersulfated GAGs, CS does not interact with antithrombin II [49]. As expected from the absence of properties common to haptenic molecules, allergic reactions associated with CS and its metabolites are generally mild and infrequent [22]. The ability of CS to interfere with medications concurrently administered to OA patients has not been evaluated.

Technically, a LD_{50} or minimum lethal dose (MLD) cannot be defined for CS because no fatal outcomes or toxic consequences appeared following administration of very high doses, i.e., 1–2 g/kg (orally or i.v. in mice), 150 mg/kg (i.m., in mice) and 1.5 g/kg (in rats) [50]. In sub-acute and chronic toxicity studies using guinea pigs, the oral administration of 100 mg/kg CS for 5 days per week for 8 weeks did not cause death [50]. There were no observed malformations (teratogenicity) in the fetuses or the young of pregnant rats and rabbits fed with 0.1 to 1 g/ kg CS daily [50]. CS did not demonstrate mutagenicity in the *Salmonella* (Ames) and yeast test systems [51].

3.7 Dosage

Based on findings of clinical studies conducted to evaluate the efficacy and safety of CS, 800 to 1200 mg daily in 2 to 4 divided doses is sufficient to reduce pain and improve the range of motion in OA patients. Although the benefits derived from this dosage schedule will not be evident until after at least 4 weeks of treatment, the effect of CS is long-lasting.

4   Conclusion

Chondroprotective agents, particularly glucosamine and chondroitin sulfates, have efficacies similar to NSAIDs, possess more desirable safety profiles, have slower onset but longer duration of action, and work via mechanisms not involving the inhibition of the eicosanoid pathway. It seems rational to include these supplements in OA therapy based on the demonstration of absorbability and accumulation in cartilagenous fluid and tissues. However, although these agents have been used for the treatment of OA in European countries for over 30 years, it should be noted that no long-term controlled clinical efficacy and safety trials on either of these two agents have been conducted. To date, there is limited information in the literature regarding the synergistic effect, contraindications and drug interactions of a chondroitin-glucosamine sulfate combination in OA therapy. Accumulated data suggest that long-term randomized clinical trials with either of the agents, alone or in combination, are warranted.

References

1   C. Da Camara and G. Dowless: Rheumatol. *32*, 580 (1998).
2   J. Theodosakis, B. Adderly and B. Fox: The Arthritis Cure. St. Martin's Press, New York (1997).
3   C. Koop: Self-care Advisor. The Health Publishing Group, U.S.A. (1996).
4   M. Palmoski and K.Brandt: Arthrit. Rheum. *23*, 1010 (1980).
5   Martindale's the Extra Pharmacopeia, Royal Pharmaceutical Society, London (1996).
6   G. Kelley: Alt. Med. Rev. *3*, 27 (1998).
7   I. Setnikar, C. Giacchetti and G. Zanolo: Arzneim. Forsch. *36*, 729 (1986).
8   K. Wlock: Can. Phar J. Oct, 34 (1997).
9   G. Verbruggen, S. Goemaere and E.Veys: Osteoarthritis Cartilage 6, 37-38 (1998).
10   The Medical Letter *39*, 91 (1997).
11   R. Vidal y Plana, D. Bizarri and A. Rovati: Pharmacol. Res. Comm. *10*, 557 (1978).
12   I. Setnikar, R. Palumbo, S. Canali and G. Zanolo: Arzneim. Forsch. *43*, 1109 (1993).
13   I. Setnikar, C. Giacchetti and G. Zanolo: Pharmatherapeutica *8*, 538 (1984).
14   T. Towheed: Arthrit. Rheum. *41*, S198 (1998).
15   T. McAlindon, J. Guli and D. Felson: Arthrit. Rheum. *41*, S198 (1998).
16   A. Philippi, C. Leffler, S. Leffler, J. Mosure and P. Kim: Military Med. *164*, 85 (1999).
17   A. Drovanti, A. Bignamini and A. Rovati: Clin. Ther. *3*, 260 (1980).
18   G. Crolle and E. D'Este: Curr. Med. Res. Opin. *7*, 104 (1980).
19   J. Pujalte, E. Llavore and F. Ylescupidex: Curr. Med. Res. Opin. *7*, 110 (1980).
20   E. D'Ambrosio, B. Casa, R. Bompani, G. Scali and G. Scali: Pharmatherapeutica *2*, 504 (1981).
21   A. Vaz: Curr. Med. Res. Opin. *8*, 145 (1982).
22   M. Tapadinhas, I. Rivera and A. Bignamini: Pharmatherapeutica *3*, 157 (1982).
23   L. Rovati: Int. J. Tiss. React. *14*, 243 (1992).
24   A. Mueller-Fäßbendeer, G. Bach, W. Hase, L. Rovati and I. Setnikar: Osteoarthritis Cartilage *2*, 61 (1994).
25   W. Noack, M. Fischer, K. Forster, L. Rovati and I. Setnikar: Osteoarthritis Cartilage *2*, 51 (1994).
26   G. Qui, S. Gao, G. Giacovelli, L. Rovati and I. Setnikar: Arzneim. Forsch. *48*, 469 (1998).
27   P. Senin, F. Makovec and L. Rovati: Stable compounds of glucosamine sulphate. United States Patent 4,642,340 (1987).

28   A.Virkamaki, M. Daniels, S. Hamalainen T. Utriainen, D. McClain and H. Yki-Jarvinen: Endocrinology *138*, 2501 (1997).

29   E. Paroli, L. Antonilli and M. Biffoni: Drugs Exptl. Clin. Res. *17*, 9 (1991).

30   M.V. Biffoni and E. Paroli: Drugs Exptl. Clin. Res. *17*, 35 (1991).

31   P. Jenoure: Der informierte Artz/Gazette Medicinale *7*, 187 (1986).

32   A. Conte, N. Volpi, L. Palmieri, I. Bahons and G. Ronca: Arzneim. Forsch. *45*, 918 (1995).

33   A. Baici, D. Horler, B. Moser, A. Hofer, K. Fehr and F. Wagenhauser: Rheumat. Int. *12*, 81 (1992).

34   D. Gross: Therapiewoche *33*, 4238 (1983).

35   T. Sue: In: N.M. Mc Duffie (ed.): Heparin: Structure, cellular functions and clinical applications, Academic Press, New York 1979.

36   L. Palmieri, A. Conte, L. Giovanni, P. Lualdi and G. Ronca: Arzneim. Forsch. *40*, 319 (1990).

37   A. Conte, M. De Bernardi, L. Palmieri, P. Lualdi, G. Mautone and G. Ronca: Arzneim. Forsch. *41*, 768 (1991).

38   B. Leeb, H. Schweitzer, K. Montag and J. Smolen: Arthrit. Rheum. *41*, S198 (1998).

39   U. Oliviero, G. Sorrentino, P. De Paola, E. Tranfaglia, A. D'Alessandro, S. Carifi, F. Porfido, R.Cerio, A. Grasso and D. Policicchio: Drugs Expl. Clin. Res. *17*, 45 (1991).

40   B. Mazieres, G. Loyau, C. Menkes, J. Valat, R. Dreisier, J. Charlot, A. Masounable-Puyanne: Rev. Rheum. Mal. Osteoartic. *59*, 466 (1992).

41   P. Morreale, R. Manopulo, M. Galati, L. Boccanera, G. Saponati and L. Bocchi.: J. Rheumatol. *23*, 1385 (1996).

42   A. Fleish, C. Merlin and A. Imhoff: Osteoarthritis Cartilage *5*, 70 (1997).

43   L. Bucsi and G. Poor: Ostoearthritis Cartilage *6*, 39 (1998).

44   P. Bourgeois, G. Chales, J. Dehais, B. Delcarnbre, P. Dreyfus, J. Kuntz, S. Rosenberg: Osteoarthritis Cartilage *69*, 25 (1998).

45   D. Uebelhart, E. Thonar, P. Delmas, A. Chantraine and E. Vignon: Osteoarthritis Cartilage *6*, S39-46 (1998).

46   T. Conrozier: Presse Med. *27*, 1862 (1998).

47   G. Rovetta: Drugs Exptl. Clin. Res. *17*, 53 (1991).

48   A. Chistolini and F. Mandelli: Farm. Ter. *6*, 71 (1989).

49   G. Soldani and J. Romagnoli: Drugs Exptl. Clin. Res. *17*, 81 (1991).

50   J. Camus: Verificacion de l'action de l'acid chondroitine sulfurique chez des malades arthrosiques. Laboratoires Gremy-Longuet, Paris 1972.

51   La Placa M: Studio dell'azione mutagena nei confronti di popolazioni batteriche e dell' induzione di sintesi riparativa di DNA in popolazione di linfociti umani periferici ad opera dei composti 7601/7602 della ditta IRBI. Instituto di Microbiologia, Università di Bologna 1978.

Progress in Drug Research, Vol. 55 (E. Jucker, Ed.)
© 2000 Birkhäuser Verlag, Basel (Switzerland)

Multi-dimensional QSAR in drug research

Predicting binding affinities, toxicity and pharmaco-kinetic parameters

By Angelo Vedani[1] and Max Dobler[2]

[1]Biographics Laboratory 3R, Missionsstrasse 60, 4055 Basel, Switzerland
[2]Laboratory for Organic Chemistry, ETH Zürich, 8092 Zürich, Switzerland

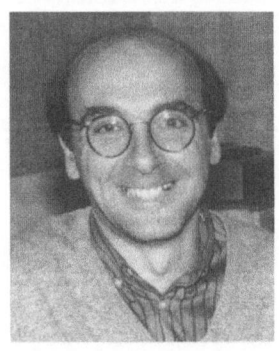

Angelo Vedani

received his Ph.D. in Chemistry in 1981 at the University of Zürich. Thereafter, he spent post-doctoral years at Texas A & M University and the Federal Institute of Technology (FIT) in Zürich. From 1986–1990 he served as assistant professor at the departments of Chemistry and Biochemistry at the University of Kansas. Since 1991 he has been director of the Biographics Laboratory in Basel – a non-profit organization aimed at replacing animal experiments by computer simulations. Since 1998 he is responsible for molecular modeling at the departments of Chemistry and Pharmacy of the University of Basel. Professional activities include all aspects of molecular modeling, in particular QSAR, pseudoreceptor modeling, and force-field development.

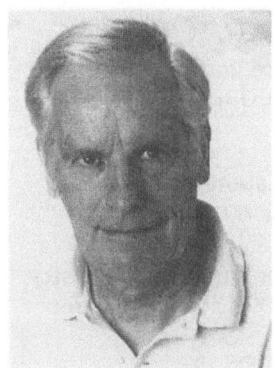

Max Dobler

received his Ph.D. in Chemical Crystallography at the Federal Institute of Technology (FIT) in Zürich. He joined the Laboratory for Molecular Biophysics at Oxford University, U.K., as a research fellow in 1969 and became lecturer at the Laboratory for Organic Chemistry of the FIT in Zürich in 1975. In 1984 he received the Werner Prize of the Swiss Chemical Society. Since 1985, he worked as a professor at the FIT until his retirement in 1999. Thereafter, he joined the Biographics Laboratory as a scientific advisor and software engineer. Professional activities include X-ray crystallography of biological molecules, especially ionophores, crystallography teaching, molecular modeling and computation chemistry.

Summary

Quantitative structure-activity relationships (QSAR) are an area of computational research which builds atomistic or virtual models to predict the biological activity or the toxicity of known or hypothetical substances. Of particular interest for the biomedical sciences are three-dimensional receptor surrogates (3D-QSAR) because they allow for the simulation of directional forces such as hydrogen bonds or metal-ligand contacts – key interactions for both molecular recognition and stereospecific ligand binding.

While more powerful approaches make use of a genetic algorithm or a neural network to evolve a receptor surrogate, its predictive power still critically depends on the spatial alignment of the ligand molecules – mirroring the pharmacophore hypothesis – used to construct it. To avoid this bias, a recent development at our laboratory includes the possibility to represent each ligand molecule by an ensemble of conformations, orientations and protonation states as the fourth dimension (4D-QSAR). In addition, it allows for a potentially flexible receptor site (mimicking local induced fit) and solvent-accessible or shallow binding pockets.

In this account, we seek to document the superiority of 4D-QSAR compared to 3D-concepts with simulations on the steroid, the aryl hydrocarbon and the neurokinin-1 receptor system. More complex, future applications of 4D-QSAR – the establishment of a virtual laboratory for the assessment of receptor-mediated toxicity and the prediction of oral bioavailability – are outlined.

Contents

Keywords
4D-QSAR, genetic algorithms, receptor-surface models, induced-fit simulation, drug design, toxicity modeling, bioavailability modeling.

Glossary of abbreviations
AMBER, assisted model building with energy refinement (software name); AMPA, α-amino-3-hydroxy-5-methyl-4-isoxazol propionic acid; CoMFA, comparative molecular field analysis; MNDO, modified neglect of differential overlap; NMDA, N-methyl D-asparate; NMR, nuclear magnetic resonance; *Quasar*, quasi-atomistic receptor modeling (software name); QSAR, quantitative structure-activity relationship; RMS, root-mean-square.

1   Introduction

A prerequisite for stimulating a side-effect-free response to a drug is believed to be the stereospecific and selective binding of a small molecule to a bioregulatory macromolecule. Soluble enzymes, antibodies, receptor proteins embedded in cell-protective lipid membranes, glycosylated marker proteins projecting similarly from enveloped viruses, ion channels and various forms of RNA and DNA represent some of the regulatory targets. The contribution of computational methodologies to the identification of small molecules binding to such bioregulators takes many forms. Quantum-mechanical and semi-empirical calculations, receptor fitting/mapping, homology modeling as well as QSAR are most frequently used.

Quantitative structure-activity relationships (QSAR) are an area of computational research which builds atomistic or virtual models to predict quantities such as the binding affinity, the toxicity, or pharmacokinetic parameters of a given molecule. The idea behind QSAR is that structural features can be correlated with biological activity. Of particular interest for biomedical research (lead finding and optimization in drug-design applications, toxicity predictions and pharmacokinetical studies) are QSAR based on three-dimensional models, because they allow for the simulation of directional forces – hydrogen bonds, metal-ligand contacts, polarization effects and the interaction between electric dipoles. Such forces are known to play a key role in both molecular recognition and ligand binding.

The need for a receptor model (or "surrogate") may arise from a situation where no experimental structure (X-Ray or NMR) is available for a target bioregulator. Atomistic binding-site surrogates can achieve an appreciable realism if they are based on the three-dimensional structure of a closely related homologue [1]. If no such data are available, a small number of amino-acid building blocks composed into a pseudoreceptor may serve to represent an extended active-site region [2]. Unfortunately, the predictive power of such a construct is limited due to the large number of structurally feasible combinations, all of which cannot be discounted based on a small training set of typically 10–30 ligand molecules. Nonetheless, the validity of pseudoreceptors has been demonstrated on several occasions [3–6].

A receptor-surface model represents a yet higher level of abstraction. Here, the essential information about the hypothetical receptor site is provided by means of a three-dimensional envelope, which surrounds the ligand molecules of the training set at the van-der-Waals distance and is populated with properties mapped onto its surface. The shape of the surface represents information about the steric nature of the receptor site; the associated properties represent other information of interest, such as hydrophobicity, partial charge, electrostatic potential and hydrogen-bonding propensity [7]. Various algorithms to generate and validate receptor-surface models have been described ([8–12]; see also [13–14]). Other notable approaches include the construction of 3-D models using a 4-D formalism [15], the use of a genetic neural network [16] as well as the utilisation of self-organizing molecular-field analysis [17].

2 Receptor models

2.1 Beginnings

In the 1990s, a number of efforts began to explore the bridge between structure-based receptor fitting and property-based receptor mapping. Receptor models of various types have been constructed around single or multiple ligands with predefined geometries [2–5, 18–21]. The corresponding complexes are termed pseudoreceptors and permit the receptor-mapping results to be exploited in a receptor-fitting context, for example, the examination of key ligand-receptor interactions, the simulation of molecular dynamics and the estimation of relative free binding energies. A pseudoreceptor concept developed at our laboratory [5–6] allows the generation of a three-dimensional peptidic receptor model – an atomistic binding-site surrogate – about any molecular framework of interest, e.g., a series of superimposed ligand molecules. As the forces controlling ligand–receptor interactions – ion-pair formation, metal-ligand contacts, hydrogen bonding and hydrophobic clustering – are more or less directional in nature [22–28], a directional force field, previously developed for modeling small-molecule protein complexes [25, 28], was incorporated in this concept [5, 6].

In contrast to the true biological receptor – where only one ligand molecule can bind at a given time – a virtual experiment (e.g., a pseudoreceptor study) is typically based on a series of ligand molecules "binding simultaneously" to an averaged receptor model. This leads to the problem of mutual functional-group obscuring within the ligand alignment. For example, the

Angelo Vedani and Max Dobler

–OCH$_3$ group of a ligand might exactly lie on top of the –OH group of another ligand within the training set. Such a three-dimensional constellation will hardly permit any H-bond donor or acceptor group to approach the –OH functionality and to establish a hydrogen bond. To remove this problem, we have devised a procedure referred to as receptor-mediated ligand alignment. It permits identification of an alternate position, orientation and conformation for each ligand molecule by means of a conformational search within a primordial receptor model, constructed around the most potent ligands of a series. To derive an energetically relaxed model with a high correlation between calculated and experimental free energies of ligand binding, we have further developed a ligand equilibration protocol. During this iterative procedure, the receptor surrogate and the ligand molecules are allowed to relax individually, with and without correlation-coupled energy minimization, until an appreciable correlation is achieved in a relaxed state [6]. The concept was tested by generating and evaluating a pseudoreceptor for the cannabinoid receptor. The binding-site surrogate was constructed around a series of 18 cannabinoid antagonists. It consists of 26 amino-acid residues and is capable of predicting the binding affinities of related compounds within a factor of 4 in K from the experiment, maximal individual deviations not exceeding a factor of 12 in K [6].

Still, two shortcomings remain associated with atomistic and receptor-surface models based on averaged receptor entities: (i) receptor-ligand adaptation (the influence of induced fit on the shape of the binding site) and (ii) H-bond flip-flop. If the ligand-receptor interaction energy is determined towards an averaged receptor model (i.e., equal for all ligand molecules), subtle effects associated with the adaptation of the receptor to the individual ligand molecules remain unaddressed. Moreover, amino-acid residues at the true biological receptor, bearing a conformationally flexible H-bond donor or acceptor (Ser, Thr, Tyr, Cys, His, Asn, and Gln residues), can engage in differently directed H-bonds with unequal ligand molecules – an effect that can also not be simulated with an averaged receptor, simultaneously binding a series of ligand molecules in a virtual experiment. Inhibitor-dependent H-bond flip-flop has been observed, for example, in the enzyme purine nucleoside phosphorylase [29].

A more fundamental problem in 3D-QSAR is associated with the mutual alignment of the ligand molecules – i.e., the identification of the bioactive conformation. Typically, this entity is found by conformational-search pro-

110

tocols combined with cluster-analysis algorithms (see for example [31]) – without any direct means to control the result. If the construction of a pseudoreceptor or a receptor-surface model is based on one or more incorrect ligand conformations, the resulting receptor surrogate is hardly of any use for predictive purposes. Of course, a variety of tools has been developed to detect such erroneous prerequisites (cf. below). While the alignment problem has long been recognized [30–32], only the most recently developed 4D-QSAR technologies provide an acceptable solution. Therefore, this account shall be mainly devoted to 4D-QSAR based on Quasi-atomistic receptor-surface models – a technology developed at our laboratory.

2.2 Quasi-atomistic receptor models

A "quasi-atomistic receptor model" refers to a three-dimensional receptor surface, populated with atomistic properties (hydrogen bonds, salt bridges, hydrophobic particles, virtual solvent) mapped onto it. The software *Quasar* and the underlying concept represent a 4D-QSAR tool – the fourth dimension being the possibility to represent each molecule by an ensemble of conformations, orientations, and protonation states, thereby reducing the bias associated with ligand alignment. In contrast to other approaches in the field, *Quasar* also allows for the simulation of local induced fit (isotropic or anisotropic), H-bond flip-flop as well as dynamic cavity shaping [11, 12]. *Quasar* is available for Macintosh, Unix and PC computer platforms and is presently used by an increasing number of pharmaceutical companies and academic research sites. Current information can be downloaded from http://www.biograf.ch.

2.2.1 Construction of quasi-atomistic receptor models

The quasi-atomistic modeling concept (software *Quasar*) developed at our laboratory allows the construction of a receptor-surface model – a three-dimensional surface (envelope), populated with atomistic properties at uniformly distributed discrete positions – about any molecular framework of interest, e.g., a pharmacophore [11, 12]. The construction of a family of receptor models includes the following steps:

(1) Construction of individually adapted receptor envelopes

First, the training set of ligand molecules is surrounded by virtual particles (e.g., radius r = 0.8 Å) defining a van-der-Waals surface. We refer to this entity as the "averaged receptor envelope". Next, an induced fit may be simulated by adapting this envelope to the topology of each ligand molecule in both training and test sets. This is achieved by first defining vectors (force- or shape-based) [33] from each point on the mean envelope to the closest point of a transiently generated "inner envelope", which snugly accommodates the individual ligand molecule, and then moving each point on the mean envelope along this vector. The magnitude of induced fit along this direction can be isotropic (linear) or anisotropic (force scaled). Finally, a regularization algorithm restores equal separations between all points on the adapted envelope. The root-mean-square (RMS) deviation from the mean envelope is used as a criterion to estimate the energy associated with the envelope adaptation. For model evaluation during the simulated evolution, this energy contributes to the total energy balance (cf. equation (1), below). As the mode and magnitude of a local induced fit cannot be estimated in the absence of the true biological receptor, it is typically necessary to perform several simulations differing in mode and magnitude, of the induced fit. For the systems so far simulated at our laboratory (β2-adrenergic receptor, dopamine β-hydroxylase, aryl hydrocarbon receptor, cannabinoid receptor, steroid receptor and neurokinin-1 receptor), the amount of induced fit is substantial (RMS shifts of 0.5–1.8 Å) and varies significantly among the individual ligand molecules.

(2) Generation of an initial family of parent structures

Points on the receptor surface are then randomly populated with atomistic properties (Tab. 1), optionally observing standard distances (2.4–3.2 Å) between H-bonding particles.

Potential H-bond sites are restricted to positions on the receptor surface which are located within a reasonable distance and at a favorable orientation with respect to any H-bond donor or acceptor moiety of the ligand molecules defining the training set. Likewise, positions suited to host a hydrogen-bond flip-flop particle are defined at spatial regions where H-extension vectors and lone-pair vectors cluster appropriately. The underlying vector concept is based on the directionality of hydrogen bonds and is discussed in [5, 6]. If there is experimental or other evidence for a solvent-accessible receptor cavity, parts of the receptor envelope may be assigned as representing solvent.

Table 1.
Properties of receptor-surface particles used in *Quasar*.

Particle (Property)	Non-bonded potential type[1]	Electric charge	Well-depth of non-bonded function
Hydrophobic, neutral	6/12	–	–0.024 kcal/mol [2]
Hydrophobic, positive	6/12 + electrostatics	+0.10	–0.09 kcal/mol [2]
Hydrophobic, negative	6/12 + electrostatics	–0.10	–0.09 kcal/mol [2]
H–bond donor	10/12	–	–5.0/–4.1/–2.3 kcal/mol [3]
H–bond acceptor	10/12	–	–5.0/–4.1/–2.3 kcal/mol [3]
Salt bridge, positive	10/12 + electrostatics	+0.25	–5.0/–4.1/–2.3 kcal/mol [3]
Salt bridge, negative	10/12 + electrostatics	–0.25	–5.0/–4.1/–2.3 kcal/mol [3]
H–bond flip–flop[4]	10/12	–	–5.0/–4.1/–2.3 kcal/mol [3]
Surface solvent	symmetric 10/12[5]	–	–0.97/–0.80/–0.46 kcal/mol [3,6]
Void (shallow pockets)	–	–	–

[1]The values i,j refer to the attractive and repulsive coefficients of the non-bonded potential function used for the ligand-receptor interaction. The general form of this potential is: $E(r) = A/r^i - C/r^j$.

[2]This function adapts the form $E(r) = A/r^{12} - C/r^6$. The coefficients A and C are calculated according to $A = -\varepsilon \cdot (r_i + r_j)^{12}$ and $C = -2 \cdot \varepsilon \cdot (r_i + r_j)^6$, respectively, and with $\varepsilon = (\varepsilon_i \cdot \varepsilon_j)^{1/2}$. The given figure represents ε_j; r_i and r_j correspond to the van-der-Waals radii of the two involved atoms.

[3]Values for $-O-H\cdots Y$, $>N-H\cdots Y$, and $-S-H\cdots Y$ H-bond interactions, respectively, where "Y" denotes a virtual H-bond acceptor. Identical values are used for the $X\cdots O$, $X\cdots N$ and $X\cdots S$ arrangement where "X" denotes a virtual H-bond donor.

[4]H-bond flip-flop particles can adapt their property (H-bond donor or acceptor) to each ligand molecule within the pharmacophore, depending on its interacting functional group.

[5]To avoid repulsive forces between surface solvent and any ligand molecule, a symmetric 10/12 potential (mirrored at $r = r°$) is used. This represents a possible approximation to a mobile solvent.

[6]As the virtual particles are different in radius from a water molecule, the associated energy must be corrected for different volumes: $E = (2 \cdot r_{vp}/2.75)^3 \cdot E°$; e.g. for $r_{vp} = 0.8$ Å $\rightarrow E = 0.197 \cdot E°$. The 2.75 Å correspond to a mean $O-H\cdots O$ H-bond distance.

Alternatively, regions may be defined as being purely hydrophobic in nature or nonexistent (void). Such assignments can be static in nature or dynamically evolved. Best results are typically obtained with an initial population of 200–500 randomly generated models.

(3) Evolution of a model family

Using a genetic algorithm (for a detailed description, see, for example, [9] or [34]), the initial family of receptor models is evolved using both cross-over and mutation events. When selecting two parents, those already fitter are more likely to be selected for a cross-over event than weaker individuals. At each cross-over step, there is a small probability (typically 0.01–0.05) of a transcription error, which is expressed by a random mutation. Only those children are retained which differ by a minimal amount of properties (typically 10% of all populated points) from any parent. Thereafter, those two individuals of the population with the highest lack-of-fit (RMS of ΔG^0_{pred}–ΔG^0_{exp} obtained from a cross-validation, combined with the sum of populated points on the receptor surface; see for example [34]) are discarded. This process is repeated until a target cross-validated r^2 (typically 0.9) or the limiting number of cross-over steps (typically 5,000–10,000) is reached.

(4) Estimation of relative free energies of ligand binding
In our concept [5–6, 11–12], we have combined the approach of Blaney et al. [35] with a method of Still et al. [36] for estimating ligand solvation energies and a term to correct for the loss of entropy upon receptor binding, following Searle and Williams [37]:

$$E_{bdg} \approx E_{lig\text{-}rec} - T\Delta S_{bdg} - \Delta G_{solv.,lig} - \Delta E_{int.,lig} - \Delta E_{env.adapt.,lig} \tag{1}$$

The term $E_{lig\text{-}rec}$ corresponds to the enthalpic contribution to the ligand–receptor interaction and is determined using a directional force field [27; 5, 11–12; 38]. $T\Delta S_{bdg}$ is estimated by assigning an amount of 0.7 kcal/mol to every freely rotatable bond, excluding terminal –CH_3 groups. The term $\Delta G_{solv.,lig}$ corresponds to the energy required to strip the solvent molecules off the ligands when binding from an aqueous environment to a hydrophobic receptor cavity. The amount is calculated using an algorithm developed and validated by Still et al. [36]. Blaney's approximation is based on the assumption that all ligands are equally buried within the receptor and, hence, that differences in the solvation energy of the ligand–receptor complexes are negligible. For systems where the ligands expose a different fraction of their surface to a solvent-accessible part of the binding site, it is possible to define a static or dynamic solvent-accessible region and thereby correct for such a situation. The term $\Delta E_{int.,lig}$ accounts for the potential increase of the ligand internal energy while bound to the receptor surrogate (relative to a strain-free reference conformation in aqueous solution). This correction is necessary because the internal energy of a ligand molecule may increase while maximizing its interaction with the receptor. $\Delta E_{env.adapt.,lig}$ is associated with the energy uptake upon modifying the averaged receptor envelope to the individual receptor envelope. When using a multiple-conformation, multiple-orientation, or multiple protonation-state representation, the contribution of an individual entity to the total energy is calculated using a normalized Boltzmann distribution:

$$E_{bdg,tot} = \Sigma \, E_{bdg,ind} \cdot \exp \left(-w_i \cdot E_{bdg,ind}/E_{bdg,ind,lowest} \right) \tag{2}$$

where $w_i = (\Sigma \, E_{bdg,ind}/E_{bdg,ind,lowest})^{-1}$ is the normalizing factor

Free energies of ligand binding, ΔG^0_{prd}, are then predicted by means of a linear regression between ΔG^0_{exp} and E_{bdg} using the ligand molecules of the training set:

$$\Delta G^0_{prd} = |\, a \,| \cdot E_{bdg} + b \tag{3}$$

Slope and intercept of equation (3) are inherent to a given receptor model and are subsequently applied to predict the relative binding energy of ligand molecules different from those in the training set. In contrast to other methods, we calibrate each receptor system with a training set [5–6, 11], rather than applying a universal function for the various receptor systems.

(5) Analysis of the model family
A mandatory criterion to validate a family of receptor models is their ability to predict relative free energies of ligand binding for an external set of test ligand molecules, not used during model construction (e.g., its RMS deviation or the predictive r^2 value). A more serious challenge to a model family, however, is the so-called scramble test (cf. [34]). Here, the binding (ΔG^0) data of the training set are randomly scrambled with respect to the true biological values, and the simulation is repeated under otherwise identical conditions. If a solution for the ligands of the training set is nonetheless found, and if the ligands of the test set are predicted similarly correctly compared with the true simulation using unscrambled data, the model is worthless, as it is not sensitive to the biological data used to establish the QSAR. If, on the other hand, the genetic algorithm fails to identify a reasonable model for the scrambled training set, the model family is thought to be robust. Other validation criteria include the cross-validated q^2 value, the lack-of-fit for the ligands of the training set, the variation of ΔG^0_{prd} (cf. equation (3)) over all members of the model family, as well as the uniformity of the distribution of the properties mapped onto the receptor envelope and

the shape of the cavity, if dynamic cavity shaping – allowing for shallow or solvent-accessible binding pockets – had been enabled.

3   Generation and validation of 4D-QSAR models

3.1   Conformational flexibility: the corticosteroid-globulin data set

One of the standard benchmark systems for 3D-QSAR consists of steroids assayed for binding affinity to corticosteroid binding globulin (CBG), a transport protein. This set allows for a comparison with other established QSAR concepts, including receptor-surface models [10], CoMFA [14], Compass [39] and others [30–32]. The original ligand data were kindly provided by Professor Hugo Kubinyi [40]. The 31 ligand molecules were reoptimized in aqueous solution using the AMBER force-field [41] as implemented in Macro-Model [42]. A standard conformational search was then conducted, retaining all structures within 10 kcal/mol of the lowest-energy conformer. From these a small set of 2–8 conformations per molecule was selected for our 4D-QSAR study (Fig. 1). Ligand alignment was obtained using *PrGen* [6]. The atomic partial charge model (MNDO/ESP) was individually determined for all conformers and derived using MOPAC 6.0 [43, 44]. Free energies of ligand solvation were calculated using a semi-analytical approach of Still and co-workers [36]. Corrected experimental binding constants were also obtained from Professor Kubinyi [40].

Based on a training set of 21 ligand molecules (represented by a total of 106 conformers) and an initial population of 200 receptor models, the system was allowed to evolve for 5,000 cross-over cycles (25 generations). With the transcription-error rate set to 0.02, the simulation reached a cross-validated r^2 of 0.926 and a predictive r^2 of 0.928. The RMS deviation for the 10 ligands of the test set (represented by a total of 52 conformers) was 0.329 kcal/mol – a factor of 1.8 in the dissociation constant K. The maximal individual deviation is 0.652 kcal/mol (3.1 in K). A scramble test (predictive $r^2 = -1.47$) demonstrates the sensitivity of the models to the biological data. A stereo representation of the receptor surrogate is shown in Figure 2; experimental and predicted dissociation constants are compared in Figure 3.

An analysis of the individual conformers contributing to the final energy suggests that only the two (out of four included) energetically lowest ring

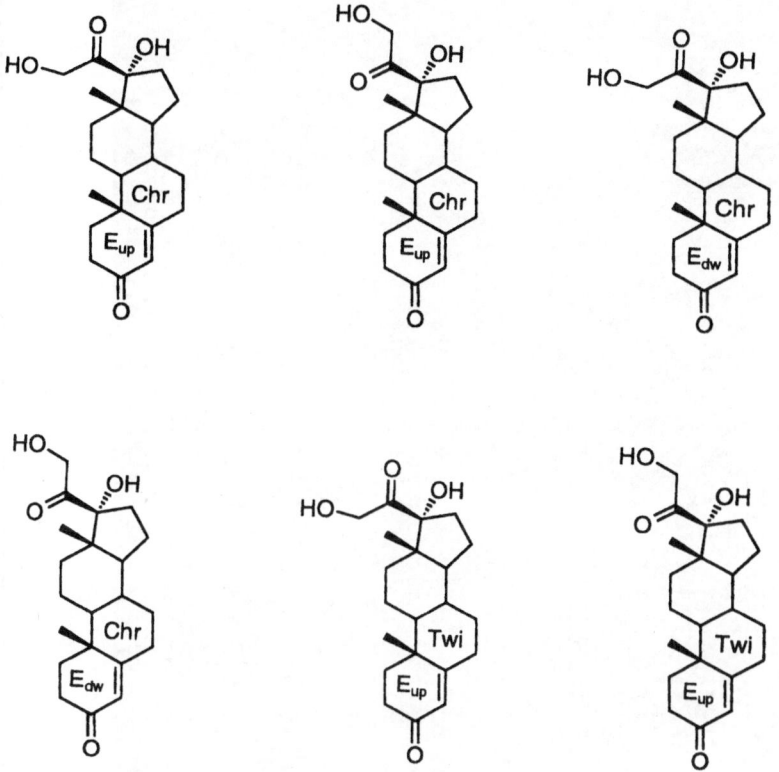

Fig. 1
Conformer selection within the steroid data set. E_{up}, envelope-up conformation; E_{dw}, envelope-down conformation; Chr, chair conformation; Twi, twisted conformation.

puckerings significantly (> 0.05) contribute to the total ligand-receptor interaction (cf. equation 2). This selection protocol demonstrates that the technique is, indeed, capable of identifying a small number of active conformations and does not prefer a larger selection of lesser-contributing entities. The individual standard deviations – averaged over the 200 receptor models – range from 0.11–0.29 kcal/mol (a factor of 1.2–1.6 in K) for the ligands of the training set and from 0.16–0.33 kcal/mol (a factor of 1.3–1.8 in K) for the ligands of the test set.

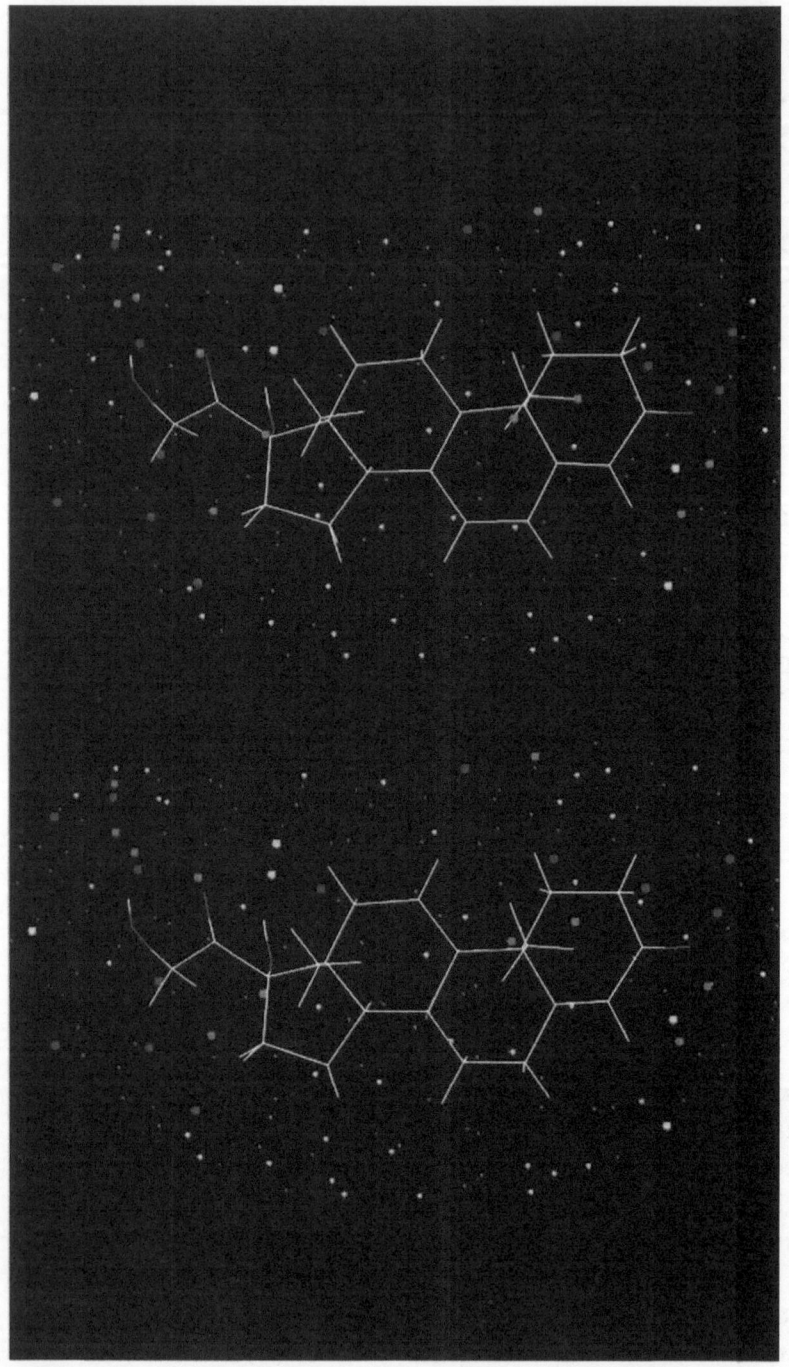

Fig. 2
Stereoscopic view of the surrogate for the steroid receptor. Color-coding scheme: red, positively charged salt bridge; blue, negatively charged salt bridge; yellow, H-bond donor; green, H-bond acceptor; light brown, positively charged hydrophobic; dark brown, positively charged hydrophobic; pink, H-bond flip-flop; grey, neutral hydrophobic.

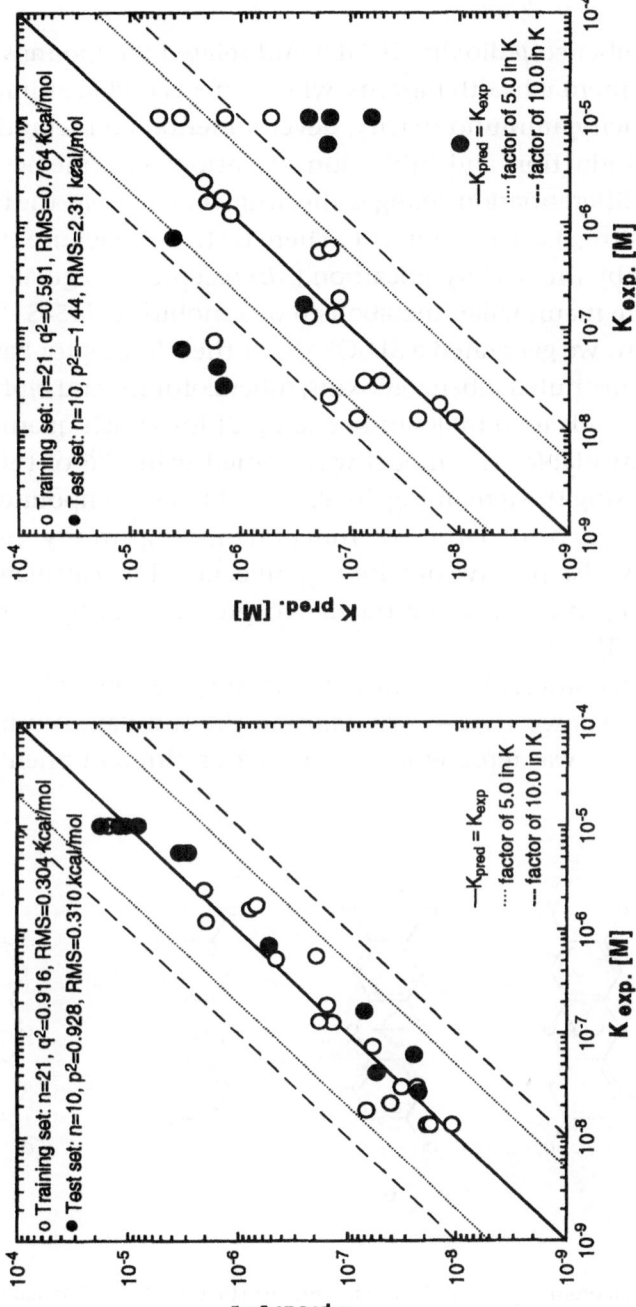

Fig. 3
Graphical comparison of experimental and predicted binding affinities for the steroid receptor: Normal simulation (left), scramble test (right).

3.2 Orientational flexibility: the Aryl hydrocarbon receptor

2,3,7,8-Tetrachlorodibenzo-*p*-dioxin (TCDD) and related compounds represent serious environmental health hazards, whose effects include tumor promotion, dermal toxicity, immunotoxicity, developmental and reproductive toxicity as well as induction and inhibition of various enzyme activities. TCDD also induces differentiation changes affecting, for example, the human epidermis – manifesting itself as chloracne. There is strong evidence that the toxicity is mediated by the Aryl hydrocarbon (*Ah*) receptor, a regulatory element involved in the mammalian metabolism of xenobiotics [45–51].

In an earlier study, we generated a 3D-QSAR for the *Ah* receptor based on a series of 102 polysubstituted dibenzodioxins, dibenzofurans and biphenyls, including all compounds used by Rannug et al. [52] for which quantitative binding data were available. The model was trained using 76 of the compounds and tested using the remaining 26. 92% of the test compounds were predicted within a factor of 10 of the experimental binding affinity. Two toxins were predicted as false-positive or false-negative, i.e., their calculated and experimental binding affinity towards the *Ah* receptor differed by more than a factor of 10 in K [53].

As the relative orientation of the various (quasi-symmetric) toxins cannot unambiguously be assumed (Fig. 4), we repeated the simulation using 4D-QSAR. Here, each toxin was represented by up to four different orientations

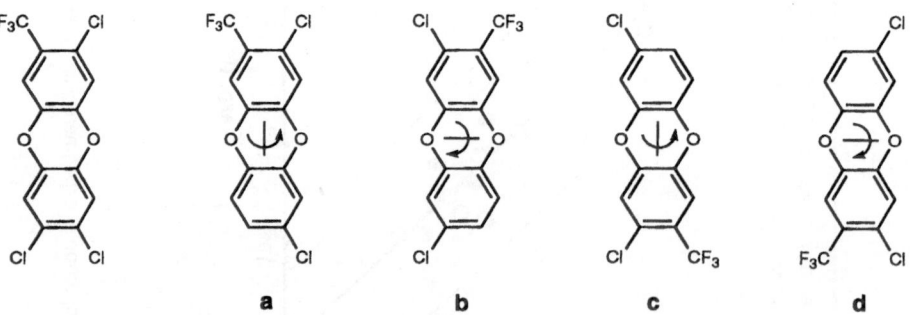

Fig. 4
Possible alignments of 7-trifluoromethyl-2,3-dichlorodibenzodioxin (left) relative to 2-trifluoromethyl-3,7,8-trichlorodibenzodioxin (right: a–d).

and the interaction of this ensemble with the receptor surrogate was calculated according to equation 2 (cf. above). This simulation resulted in a cross-validated r^2 of 0.839 for the 76 training ligands. Of the 26 test compounds, none was predicted as false-positive or false-negative [54]. Finally, we added the class of polyaromatic hydrocarbons (PAHs, a total of 29 compounds) to the data set. Based on 91 training ligands (348 orientations total), we generated a surrogate family comprising 200 receptor models and simulated the evolution for 75 generations, obtaining a cross-validated r^2 of 0.857 and a predictive r^2 of 0.795. Of the 30 test compounds (113 orientations total), none was predicted as false-positive or false-negative (the threshold being a factor of 12.6 in K: a range of 3.2×10^5 in K divided into the five toxicity classes). A negative scramble test (predictive r^2: –0.07) demonstrates the sensitivity of the model family towards the biological data. A stereo representation of the receptor surrogate is shown in Figure 5; experimental and predicted dissociation constants are compared in Figure 6.

An analysis of the individual orientations contributing to the final energy suggests that, indeed, the mutual orientation cannot be trivially derived (from 2-D or 3-D data) and that a multiple representation of each compound significantly reduces the bias associated with the ligand alignment. The fact that better results are also achieved when using 4D-QSAR supports these findings. The fact that 4D-QSAR concepts can successfully be used for predicting the toxicity of known or hypothetical substances – if a receptor-mediated phenomenon can be assumed to underlie the adverse effects – has spawned a new possibility of testing the potential toxicity of any compound by computational approaches (in silico). This most recent research direction is outlined in chapter 3.4.

3.3   Different protonation states: the neurokinin-1 receptor

Substance P (SP), a peptide neurotransmitter, is a member of the tachykinin family of peptides. These peptides bind to a series of three neurokinin receptors, NK-1, NK-2 and NK-3, which have selective affinity for SP, neurokinin A and neurokinin B. A link between transmission of pain, the induction of inflammatory processes as a result of noxious stimuli and the release of SP has been established. These observations suggest that SP-receptor antagonists may be of significant therapeutic use in the treatment of a wide range of clin-

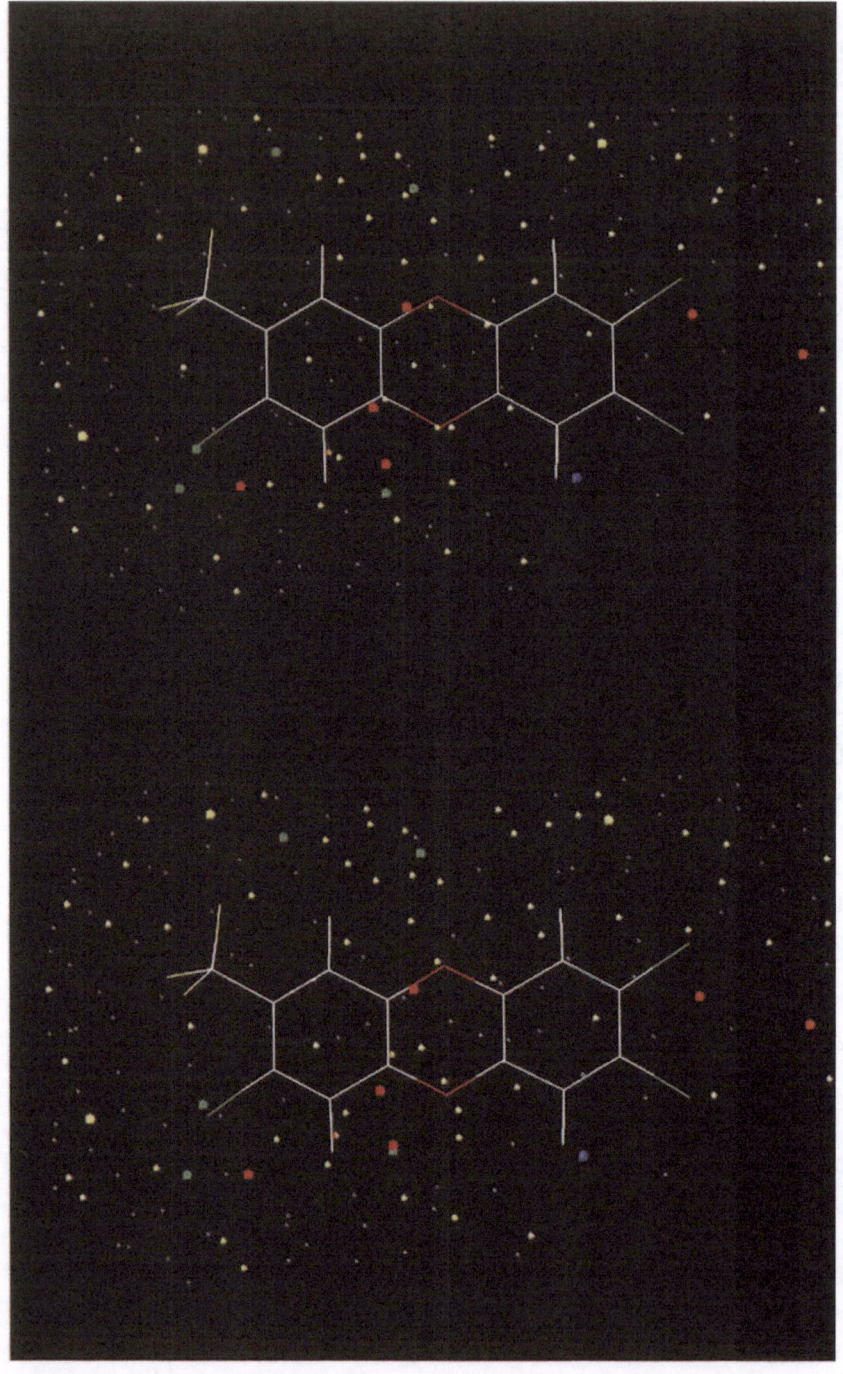

Fig. 5
Stereoscopic view of the surrogate for the aryl hydrocarbon receptor. Color-coding scheme, cf. caption of Figure 2.

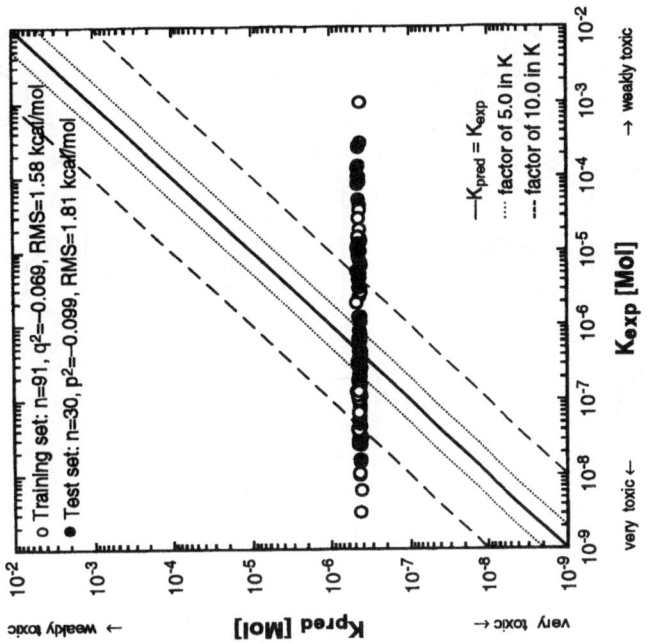

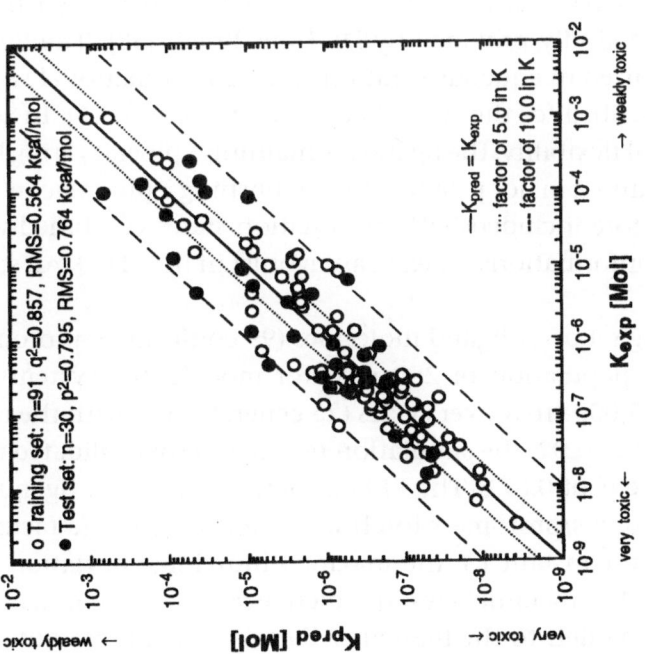

Fig. 6
Graphical comparison of experimental and predicted binding affinities for the aryl hydrocarbon receptor: Normal simulation (left), scramble test (right).

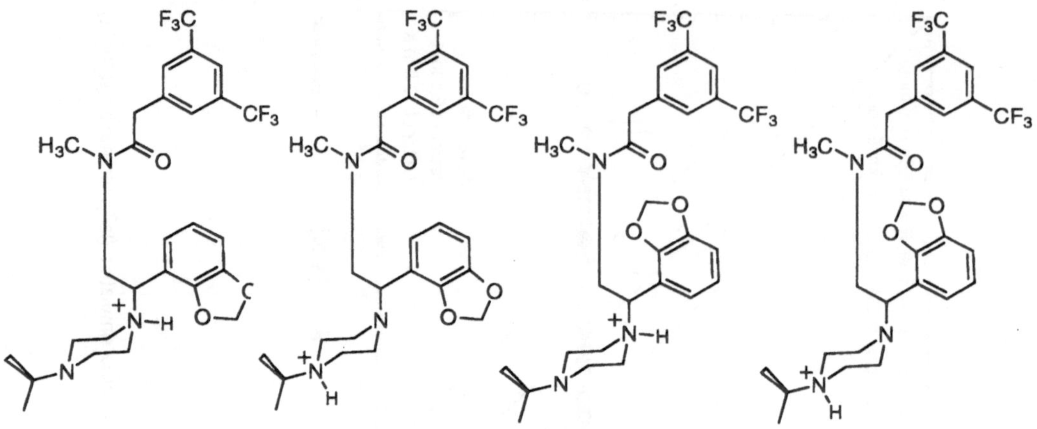

Angelo Vedani and Max Dobler

Fig. 7
Conformer and protomer selection within the neurokinin-1 data set.

ical conditions, ranging from arthritis, migraine and asthma to postoperative pain and nausea [55–57].

The structures of 31 NK-1 antagonists synthesized at Boehringer Ingelheim (Germany) were kindly provided by Dr. Hans Briem [58]. The ligand molecules were optimized in aqueous solution and a conformational search was conducted as described for the steroid data set (cf. section 3.1). In addition to conformational flexibility, the ligands containing a piperazyl ring bear two protonable N atoms – a major problem for establishing a pharmacophore hypothesis. We therefore included both protonation states combined with up to four different conformations for each antagonist in the 4D-QSAR study (Fig. 7).

Based on a training set of 21 ligand molecules (99 conformers/protomers total), and an initial population of 200 receptor models, the system was allowed to evolve for 5,000 cross-over cycles (25 generations). With the transcription-error rate set to 0.02, the simulation reached a cross-validated r^2 of 0.900 and a predictive r^2 of 0.871. The RMS deviation for the 10 ligands of the test set (42 conformers/protomers total) was 0.460 kcal/mol (a factor of 2.2 in the dissociation constant K); the maximal individual deviation was 1.35 kcal/mol (10.0 in K). A scramble test (predictive $r^2 = -0.11$) demonstrates the sensitivity of the models to the biological data. A stereo representation of the receptor surrogate is shown in Figure 8; experimental and predicted dissociation constants are compared in Figure 9.

An analysis of the individual conformers contributing to the final energy suggests that only the central N atom (Fig. 7a) is protonated in all double-protonable species. As this could represent an artifact – three of the 31 compounds feature a single, protonable N atom and, hence, can be unambiguously described – we repeated the simulation, excluding those three antagonist ligands. The result was the same, which underlines the capability of 4D-QSAR to successfully select the correct individuals from an ensemble, consisting of different protonation sites and conformations.

3.4 Virtual laboratory for receptor-mediated toxic phenomena

Toxic agents, particularly those that exert their actions with a great deal of specificity, sometimes act via receptors to which they bind with high affinity. This phenomenon is referred to as receptor-mediated toxicity. Examples of soluble intracellular receptors, which are important in mediating toxic responses, include the glucocorticoid receptor, which can act as a model for other receptors, but is also involved in mediating toxicity-associated effects such as apoptosis of lymphocytes as well as neuronal degeneration as a response to stress, the peroxisome proliferator activated receptor, which is associated with hepatocarcinogenesis in rodents, and the Aryl hydrocarbon receptor ("dioxin receptor") which is involved in a whole range of toxic effects [59].

Our laboratory is currently establishing an internet-based center for receptor-mediated toxicological phenomena. Access to this database will be organized as a virtual laboratory, providing free access to any interested party, but simultaneously ensuring a maximum of data security. At present, the database includes validated models for the Aryl hydrocarbon receptor – data which will be made available immediately. The project will be divided into four distinct sections: (I) setup and solicitation of the virtual laboratory; (II) extension to include all receptors known to mediate toxicity (glucocorticoid receptor, peroxisome proliferator activated receptors); (III) further extension to include all bioregulators possibly susceptible to receptor-mediated toxicity (e.g., NMDA, AMPA, glutamate, cannabinoid receptor as well as newly emerging systems); (IV) extensions to systems involving active or passive

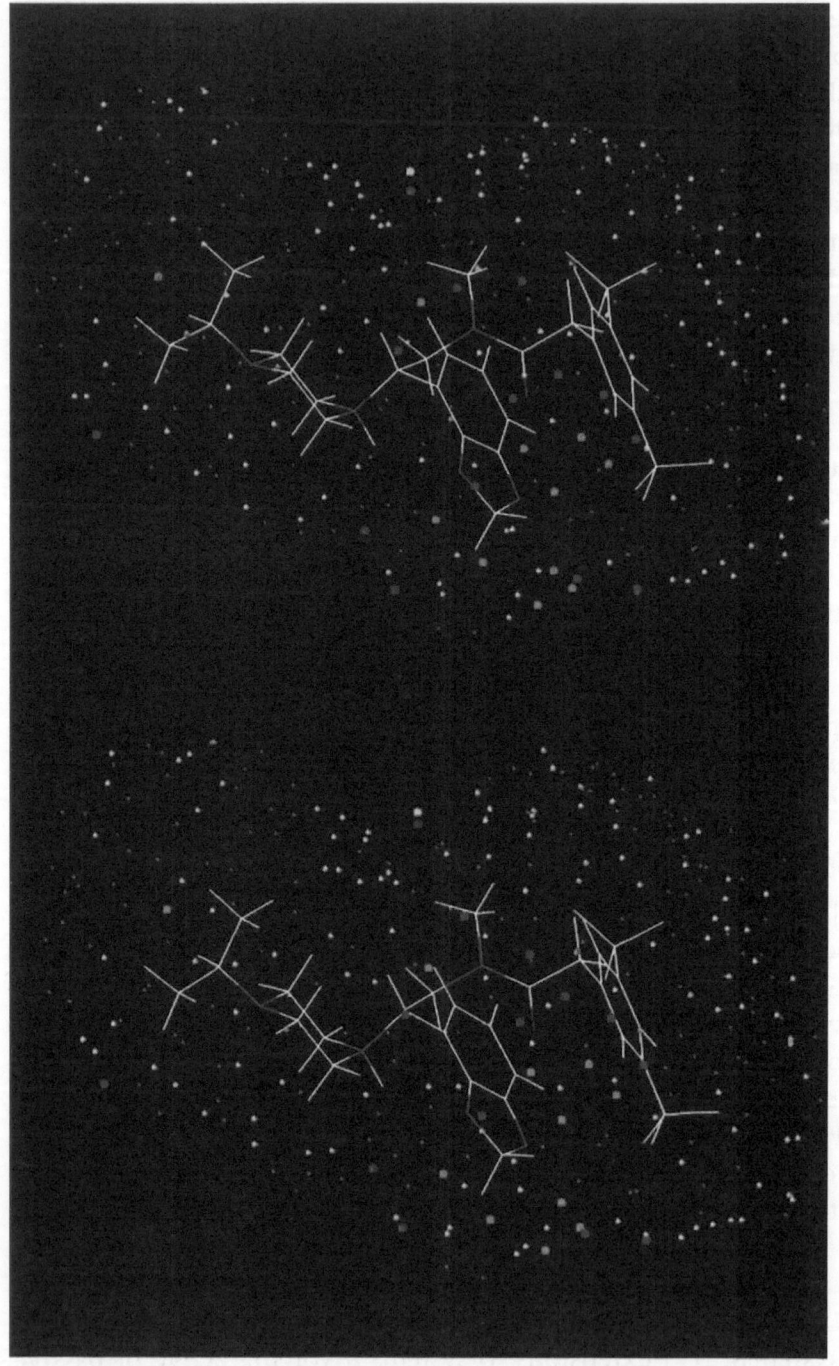

Fig. 8
Stereoscopic view of the surrogate for the neurokinin-1 receptor. Color-coding scheme, cf. caption of Figure 2.

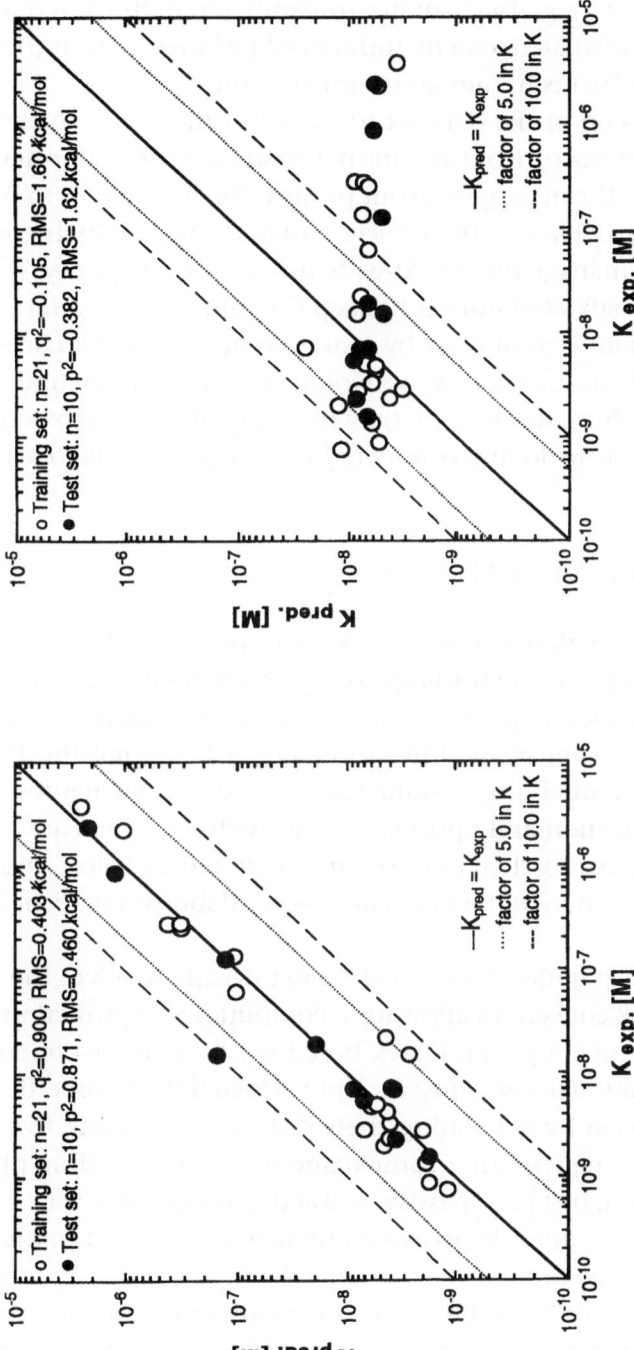

Fig. 9
Graphical comparison of experimental and predicted binding affinities for the neurokinin-1 receptor: Normal simulation (left), scramble test (right).

127

transport phenomena – e.g., the ochratoxin family (cf. [60]) – as a pilot simulation for receptor-mediated toxicity influenced by kinetic effects (here: the binding of the ochratoxins to human serum albumin).

While the extension of the data set for receptor-mediated toxicological phenomena (e.g., glucocorticoid or the peroxisome proliferator activated receptors) represents the main goal of our project, the final idea is to have all interested parties participate in the project and as a community increase its data and efficiently manage this world-wide interactive laboratory. The ethical aim of this (virtual) laboratory is to keep the number of conducted animal tests at an absolute minimum by using computational techniques – where applicable – instead. Thereby, we would comply with the philosophy of the 3Rs (refine, reduce, replace), first, by reducing individual toxicity tests and, second, by omitting doubly-conducted tests at different laboratories.

3.5   Simulating oral bioavailability

Optimization of the distribution of a therapeutic compound between oral or gastrointestinal resorption and the target receptor site is a critical component in the drug-design process. Reliable estimates for these causative factors are essential guides to chemical modifications aimed at optimizing the oral bioavailability of potential drug candidates. Computational methodologies used for the identification and optimization of such molecules are particularly efficient in enhancing their affinity for a given bioregulator; a powerful approach to the prediction of the associated bioavailability, however, has yet to be identified.

A very challenging undertaking for the next decade involves the extension of our 4D-QSAR concept to allow for a computational prediction of the oral bioavailability of drug candidates based on their three-dimensional topology, conformational flexibility and physicochemical properties. This task may be addressed by simulating their distribution among five quasi-atomistic surrogates, representing compartments relevant to drug pharmacokinetics: resorption, first pass, passive and active transport as well as retention in the fatty tissues. In order to avoid any bias with respect to the distribution kinetics, the associated parameters will be governed by a second genetic algorithm: optimizing this set of equations while evolving the family of linked compartment models, each different in size, shape and

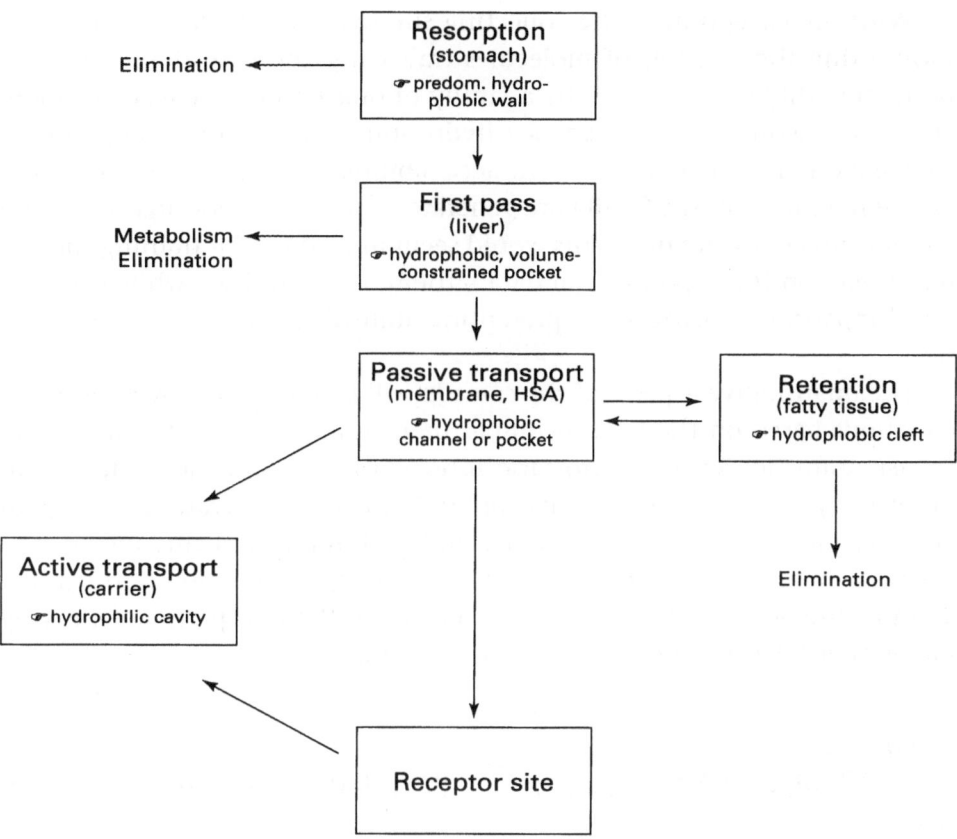

Fig. 10
Surrogate compartments defining the bioavailability-modeling cascade.

hydrophilic/hydrophobic properties. Elimination of the compounds via metabolism or filtration at the various stages will be described by additional parameters, including molecular mass, molecular volume, functional-group distribution and ligand topology. Because the oral bioavailability – a mandatory piece of data for drug approval – can at present only be determined *in vivo*, this computer-based approach has a substantial potential to replace animal tests. Figure 10 represents the possible flow of a target compound through the concatenated compartments defining the bioavailability-modeling cascade.

With the exception of the collecting site (which will solely be used for monitoring the fraction of molecules traversing the cascade), each compartment will be represented by a family of quasi-atomistic receptor models, featuring different sizes, shapes, hydrophilic/hydrophobic properties as well as a different degree of solvent-accessibility. The properties of the individual members of this family are generated using a genetic algorithm and are not subject to any bias. This would seem important for training the system solely on the experimental data – the bioavailability – while evolving the compartment surrogates, representing quite different physiological entities.

The quantitative aspects of the cascade will be controlled by a system of equations based on the ligand-compartment interactions at the molecular (quasi-atomistic) level: electrostatic interactions, polarization effects, salt bridges, hydrogen bonds and hydrophobic forces. Desolvation, change in entropy and internal energy as well as induced fit are explicitly included in the final energy balance (cf. equation (1), above). The fraction of the initial amount (incoming target molecules) traversing the compartment (leaving target molecules) will be determined as follows:

Resorption:

$$f_{Res,i} = Affinity_{Res,i} \, / \, Affinity_{Res,max}; \qquad \{f_{Res,i} \mid 0.0 \le f_{Res,i} \le 1.0\} \qquad (4a)$$

First pass:

$$f_{FP,i} = f_{Res,i} \cdot Affinity_{FP,i} \, / \, Affinity_{FP,max}; \qquad \{f_{FP,i} \mid 0.0 \le f_{FP,i} \le f_{Res,i}\} \qquad (4b)$$

Passive Trsp:

$$f_{PT,i} = f_{FP,i} \cdot Affinity_{PT,i} \, / \, Affinity_{PT,max}; \qquad \{f_{PT,i} \mid 0.0 \le f_{PT,i} \le f_{FP,i}\} \qquad (4c)$$

Active Trsp:

$$f_{AT,i} = f_{PT,i} \cdot Affinity_{AT,i} \, / \, Affinity_{AT,max}; \qquad \{f_{AT,i} \mid 0.0 \le f_{AT,i} \le f_{PT,i}\} \qquad (4d)$$

The fraction of a molecule retained in the fatty-tissue compartment will be assumed to be in a slow equilibrium with the residual system and calculated from the relative affinities in the (hydrophobic) fatty-tissue compartment and aqueous solution, accessible via a quasi-atomistic model characterized solely by solvent particles:

Retention:

$$f_{RT,i} = f_{FP,i} \cdot \text{Affinity}_{RT,i} / \text{Affinity}_{Solvent,i}; \quad \{f_{RT,i} \mid 0.0 \le f_{RT,i} \le f_{FP,i}\} \tag{4e}$$

The fraction of molecules traversing the cascade – the computed bioavailability – will then be determined at a putative receptor site (the properties of which are not of interest for this study and, hence, will not be explicitly modeled) as the sum of molecules shuttled through i) the passive compartment solely and ii) passing through both the passive and active transport compartment:

Bioavailability:

$$f_{BA,i} = (1.0 - f_{RT,i}) \cdot (f_{PT,i} + f_{AT,i}) \tag{5}$$

The esd (estimated standard deviation) of the computed bioavailability is obtained by variation over the *n* models of the surrogate families – one of the main advantages of using a genetic algorithm. Typically, n is defined in the range from 200 to 500. For this complex application, a larger family with up to 5,000 members might, however, be necessary to achieve a successful evolution.

In a final step, the fraction of molecules eliminated by metabolic processes must be accounted for. This fraction may be estimated based on the number and spatial distribution of their functional groups augmented by electrostatic field and dipole information (see for example [61]) or direct methods (cf. [62]). Such information is most efficiently managed within a database storing this 3-D information on a linear code. The use of experimental metabolism data would not seem to be permissible as this information will not be available for true predictions later on. The effect of renal filtration might similarly be addressed, however, including molecular mass, active volume, absorption, solubility and lipophilicity information. Here, we can build on the extensive work of Dearden [62], Palm et al. [63], Camenisch et al. [64–65], Iwatsubo et al. [66] and others. To avoid any bias with respect to the distribution kinetics, the associated constants and boundary conditions will be evolved genetically, optimizing this set of equations (4a–e) while evolving families of linked compartment models, each different in size, shape and atomistic properties mapped onto its surface.

131

4   Conclusions

In the absence of an experimentally determined receptor structure, 3D-QSAR techniques provide an elegant approach to the estimation of free energies of ligand binding. Unfortunately, these concepts would seem to be limited by two approximations: first, the use of a rigid, averaged receptor model to represent the flexible bioregulator in the virtual experiment and, second, the potentially biased determination of the ligand alignment. The 4D-QSAR concept *Quasar* developed at our laboratory not only takes local induced fit and H-bond flip-flop into account but also allows for the representation of the ligand molecules by an ensemble of conformation, orientations, and protonation states. The contribution of a single entity within this ensemble to the total ligand-receptor interaction energy is determined by a Boltzmann criterion.

This new approach was applied to the steroid (conformational flexibility), the aryl hydrocarbon (orientational ambiguity) and the neurokinin-1 receptor (conformational flexibility as well as multiple protonation states). The results indicate that the use of 4D-QSAR is superior to 3D-QSAR and significantly reduces the bias associated with the ligand alignment. Moreover, the selection protocol demonstrates that the technique is capable of identifying a small number of active conformations and does not prefer a larger selection of lesser-contributing entities.

Supplementary material

The three-dimensional coordinates of all receptor models as well as information on the software *Quasar* can be requested at: http://www.biograf.ch. They will be provided along with a Java-based 3D-viewer allowing for real-time 3D transformations (rotation, zooming, scanning) of the models.

Acknowledgments

The authors are indebted to Dr. Daniel McMasters (formerly at the Biographics Laboratory), Professor Felix Althaus (Department of Pharmacology and Toxicology, Veterinary School, University of Zürich), Professor Gerd

Folkers (Department of Pharmacy, ETH Zürich), Professor Peter Maier (Department of Toxicology, ETH Zürich), Dr. Herbert Köppen, Dr. Hans Briem and Dr. Horst Dollinger (Boehringer Ingelheim, Germany) for most valuable discussions. Financial support from the Swiss National Science Foundation (Grant # 3100–052237.97), the Margaret and Francis Fleitmann Foundation (Lucerne, Switzerland) and the Foundation for Animal-free Research (Zürich, Switzerland) is gratefully acknowledged.

References

1   Sali, A., Overington, J.P., Johnson, M.S. and Blundell, T.L.: Trends. Biochem. Sci. *15*, 235 (1990).
2   Snyder, J.P., Rao, S.N., Koehler, K.F. and Vedani, A., in: H. Kubinyi (Ed.): 3D QSAR in Drug Design: Theory, Methods and Applications. ESCOM Science Publishers: Leiden, 1993, 336.
3   Hong, J.-L., Namgoong, S.K., Bernardi, A. and Still, W.C.: J. Am. Chem. Soc. *113*, 5111 (1990).
4   Höltje, H.D. and Anzali, S.; Pharmazie *47*, 691 (1993).
5   Vedani, A., Zbinden, P., Snyder, J.P. and Greenidge, P.A.: J. Am. Chem. Soc. *117*, 4987 (1995).
6   Zbinden, P., Dobler, M., Folkers, G. and Vedani, A.: Quant. Struct.-Act. Relat. *17*, 122 (1998).
7   Hahn, M.: J. Med. Chem. *38*, 2080 (1995).
8   Srivastava, S., Richardson, W.W., Bradley, M.P. and Crippen, G., in H. Kubinyi (Ed.): 3D-QSAR in Drug Design: Theory, Methods and Applications. Escom: Leiden, 1993, 80.
9   Walters, D.E. and Hinds, R.M.: J. Med. Chem. *37*, 2527 (1994).
10   Hahn, M. and Rogers, D.: J. Med. Chem. *38*, 2091 (1995).
11   Vedani, A., Dobler, M. and Zbinden, P.: J. Am. Chem. Soc. *120*, 4471 (1998).
12   Vedani, A., McMasters, D.R. and Dobler, M.: Quant. Struct.-Act. Relat. 19, 149–161 (2000).
13   Cramer, R.D., Patterson, D.E. and Bunce, J.D.: J. Am. Chem. Soc. *110*, 5959 (1988).
14   Cramer, R.D., DePriest, S.A. and Patterson, D.E., in H. Kubinyi (Ed.): 3D QSAR in Drug Design: Theory, Methods and Applications. Escom: Leiden, 1993, 443.
15   Hopfinger, A.J., Wang, S., Tokarski, J.S., Jin, B.Q., Albuquerque, M., Madhav, P.J. and Duraiswami, C.: J. Am. Chem. Soc. *119*, 10509 (1997).
16   So, S.S. and Karplus, M.: J. Med. Chem. *40*, 4347 (1997).
17   Robinson, A.U., Winn, P.J., Lyne, P.D. and Richards, W.G.: J. Med. Chem. *42*, 573 (1999).
18   Momamy, F., Pitha, R., Klimkowsky, V.J. und Venkatachalam, C.M., in: B.A. Hohne and T.H. Pierce (Eds.): Expert Systems Applications in Chemistry. ACS Symp. Ser. *408*, 82 (1989).
19   Snyder, J.P. and Rao, S.N.: Chem. Design Automation News *4*, 13 (1989).
20   Rao, S.N. and Snyder, J.P.: Cray Channels *11*, 4 (1990).

Angelo Vedani and Max Dobler

21   Snyder, J.P., Rao, S.N., Koehler, K.F. and Pellicciari, R., in: P. Angeli, U. Gulini and W. Quaglia (Eds.): Trends in Receptor Research. Amsterdam: Elsevier Science Publishers, 1992, 367.
22   Murray-Rust, P. and Glusker, J.P.: J. Am. Chem. Soc. *106*, 1018 (1984).
23   Taylor, R. and Kennard, O.: Acc. Chem. Res. *17*, 320 (1984).
24   Baker, E.N. and Hubbard, R.E.: Prog. Biophys. Molec. Biol. *44*, 97 (1984).
25   Vedani, A. and Dunitz, J.D.: J. Am. Chem. Soc. *107*, 7653 (1985).
26   Alexander, R.S., Kanyo, Z.F., Chirlian, L.E. and Christianson, D.W.: J. Am. Chem. Soc. *112*, 933 (1990).
27   Vedani, A. and Huhta, D.W.: J. Am. Chem. Soc. *112*, 4759 (1990).
28   Tintelnot, M. and Andrews, P.: J. Computer–Aided Molec. Design *3*, 67 (1989).
29   Montgomery, J.A. and Secrist III, J.A.: Persp. Drug Discov. Design *2*, 205 (1994).
30   Kubinyi, H.: Drug Discovery Today *2*, 457 (1997).
31   Kubinyi, H.: Drug Discovery Today *2*, 538 (1997).
32   Kubinyi, H., Folkers, G. and Martin, Y.C.: Perspectives in Drug Discovery and Design *12*, 3 (1998).
33   The actual force exerted by all atoms of a given ligand on its envelope is determined using a primitive force field using solely van-der Waals forces as – at this point – no atomic properties have been deposited on the surface.
34   Rogers, D. and Hopfinger, A.J.: J. Chem. Inf. Comput. Sci. *34*, 854 (1994).
35   Blaney, J.M., Weiner, P.K., Dearing, A., Kollman, P.A., Jorgensen, E.C., Oatley, S.J., Burridge, J.M. and Blake. J.F.: J. Am. Chem. Soc. *104*, 6424 (1982).
36   Still, W.C., Tempczyk, A., Hawley, R.C. and Hendrickson, T.: J. Am. Chem. Soc. *112*, 6127 (1990).
37   Searle, M.S. and Williams, D.H.: J. Am. Chem. Soc. *114*, 10690 (1992).
38   As a virtual particle (VP) in a quasi-atomistic approach has no bonding partners (i.e., unlike a functional group of a real molecule it bears no lone-pairs), we apply a simplified function to determine the non-electrostatic contribution to the H-bond energy involving a VP. For the constellation Don-H···VP, we correct for non-linearity of the Don-H···VP angle (compulsorily assuming a perfect directionality at the VP). For the arrangement Acc···VP, we correct for the deviation of the virtual hydrogen bond from the closest lone pair at the acceptor fragment (angle LP-Acc···VP) and assume a perfect linearity of the hydrogen bond. Derivation and calibration of the directional function for H-bond interactions are described in [27]; see also [5].
39   Jain, A., Koile, K. and Chapman, D.: J. Med. Chem. *37*, 2315 (1994).
40   Professor Dr. Hugo Kubinyi, Wirkstoffdesign, ZHB/W. A30, BASF AG, D-67056 Ludwigshafen, Germany.
41   Weiner, S.J., Kollmann, P.A., Case, D.A., Singh, U.C., Ghio, C., Alagona,G., Profeta Jr., S. and Weiner, P.: J. Am. Chem. Soc. *106*, 765 (1984).
42   Mohamadi, F., Richards, N.G.J., Guida, W.C., Liskamp, R., Lipton, M., Caufield, C., Chang, G., Hendrickson, T. and Still, W.C.: J. Comput. Chem. *11*, 440 (1990).
43   Stewart, J.J.P.: J. Comp.-Aided Molec. Design *4*, 1 (1990).
44   Distributed by QCPE, University of Indiana, Bloomington, Indiana, USA (Program # 455).
45   Putzrath, R.M.: Reg.Tox. Pharmacol. *25*, 68 (1997).
46   Safe, S. and Krishnan, K., in: D.H. Degen, J.P. Seiler and P. Bentley (Eds.): Archives of Toxicology, Suppl. 17. Springer, Berlin 1995, 116.

47   Okey, A.B., Riddick, D.S. and Harper, P.A.: Toxicol. Lett. *70*, 1 (1994).

48   Swanson, H.I. and Bradfield, C.A.: Pharmacogenetics *3*, 213 (1993).

49   Rappe, C.: Organohalogen Compounds, Dioxin *12*, 163 (1993).

50   Whitlock jr., J.P.: Chem. Res. Toxicol. *6*, 754 (1993).

51   Whitlock jr., J.P.: Annu. Rev. Pharmacol. Toxicol. *30*, 251 (1990).

52   Rannug, U., Sjörgren, M., Rannug, A., Gillner, M., Toftgard, R., Gustafsson, J.-Å., Rosenkranz, H. and Klopman, G.: Carcinogenesis *12*, 20075 (1991).

53   Vedani, A., McMasters, D.R. and Dobler, M.: ALTEX *16*, 9 (1999).

54   Vedani, A., McMasters, D.R. and Dobler, M.: ALTEX *16*, 140 (1999).

55   Takeuchi, Y., Shands, E.F.B., Beusen, D.D. and Marshall, G.R.: J. Med. Chem. *41*, 3609 (1998).

56   Quartera, L. and Maggi, C.A.: Neuropeptides *31*, 537 (1997).

57   Ladduwahetty, T., Baker, R., Cascieri, M.A., Chambers, M.S., Haworth, K., Keown, L. E., MacIntyre, D.E., Metzger, J.M., Owen, S., Rycroft, W. et al.: J. Med. Chem. *39*, 2907 (1996).

58   Dr. Hans Briem, Department of Lead Discovery, Boehringer Ingelheim Pharma, D–55216 Ingelheim, Germany.

59   Gustafsson, J.A.: Toxicol. Lett. *82*, 465 (1995).

60   McMasters, D.R. and Vedani, A.: J. Med. Chem. *42*, 3075 (1999).

61   Bonnabry, P., Sievering, J., Leemann, T and Dayer, P.: Eur. J. Clin. Pharmacol. *55*, 341 (1999).

62   Dearden, J.C.: Compr. Med. Chem. *4*, 375 (1990).

63   Palm, K.: Pharm. Res. *14*, 568 (1997).

64   Camenisch, G., Alsenz, J., van de Waterbeemd, H. and Folkers, G.: Eur. J. Pharm. Sci. *6*, 317–324 (1998).

65   Camenisch, G., Folkers, G. and van de Waterbeemd, H.: Pharm. Acta. Helv. *71*, 309 (1996).

66   Iwatsubo T., Hisaka, A., Suzuki, H. and Sugiyama, Y: J. Pharmacol. Exp. Ther. *286*, 122 (1998)

Progress in Drug Research, Vol. 55 (E. Jucker, Ed.)
©2000 Birkhäuser Verlag, Basel (Switzerland)

NMR spectroscopy in drug discovery: Tools for combinatorial chemistry, natural products, and metabolism research

By Paul A. Keifer

Varian NMR Systems and
NMR Consultant,
6329 South 172nd Street,
Omaha, NE 68135, USA
e-mail: PandKKeifer@att.net

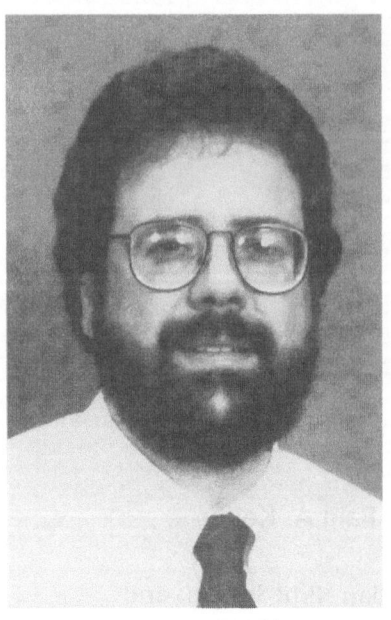

Paul A. Keifer

*is a senior applications chemist at Varian NMR
Instruments. He has spent the last 15 years specializ-
ing in solution-state NMR at high field, for both
organic- and bio-chemicals, and focuses on new hardware, pulse-sequences and software. His path to Varian included a B.S. in Chemistry at the University of
Nebraska (1979, with Norman Cromwell), an M.S.
in Biomedicinal and Pharmaceutical Chemistry at
the University of Nebraska Medical Center (1982,
with Donald Nagel), three years as a synthetic
chemist at the Eppley Institute for Cancer Research, a
Ph.D. in Marine Natural Products at the University of
Illinois (1986, with Kenneth Rinehart), and a two-
year position in spectroscopy, managing the high-field
NMRs in the University of Illinois Chemistry Department (with Vera Mainz). In addition to working at
Varian, he currently holds a teaching appointment as
a Consulting Associate Professor at Stanford University (Chemistry Department).*

Summary

NMR spectroscopy has enjoyed many advances recently, and the pace of
development shows no signs of slowing. This article focuses on advances that
have affected solution-state NMR. These advances fall into three general categories: new experimental techniques (new pulse sequence tools), improved
hardware and more powerful software.

These advances are allowing NMR to help solve important problems in the
field of drug discovery. Their impact is widespread. NMR spectroscopy is now
being used to determine protein structures, to monitor ligand-receptor binding, to study diffusion, to analyze mixtures using LC-NMR, to analyze solid-
phase synthesis resins and to determine the structures of organic small molecules. NMR spectroscopy can provide both qualitative and quantitative
information, and can be used in both routine analytical applications and
demanding research applications. The applications described here can benefit numerous disciplines in drug discovery, including natural products
research, synthetic medicinal chemistry, metabolism studies, drug production, quality control, rational drug design and combinatorial chemistry.

Contents

Paul A. Keifer

Keywords

NMR (nuclear magnetic resonance), natural products, combinatorial chemistry, rational drug design, metabolism, 2D NMR, HR-MAS, flow NMR, LC-NMR, DI-NMR, FIA-NMR, solid-phase-synthesis (SPS) resins.

Glossary of abbreviations

COSY, correlation spectroscopy; DI-NMR, direct injection analysis NMR; DMSO, dimethyl sulfoxide; DOSY, diffusion ordered spectroscopy; DSP, digital signal processing; FDM, filter diagonalization method; FIA-NMR, flow injection analysis NMR; FRED, full reduction of entire datasets; GSQMBC, gradient enhanced single quantum multiple bond correlation; HMBC, heteronuclear multiple bond correlation; HMDS, hexamethyl disiloxane; HMQC, heteronuclear multiple quantum correlation; HR-MAS, high-resolution magic angle spinning; HSQC, heteronuclear single quantum correlation; HT-NMR, high throughput NMR; INADEQUATE, incredible natural abundance double quantum transfer experiment; LC-NMR, liquid chromatography-NMR; MAS, magic angle spinning; MRI, magnetic resonance imaging; NMR, nuclear magnetic resonance; NOESY, nuclear overhauser enhancement spectroscopy; PFG, pulsed field gradient; ppm, parts per million; rf, radiofrequency; ROESY, rotating frame overhauser enhancement spectroscopy; SAR-by-NMR, structure activity relationship by NMR; SPS, solid phase synthesis; TMS, tetramethylsilane; TOCSY, total correlation spectroscopy; TROSY, transverse relaxation-optimized spectroscopy; TSP, 3-(trimethylsilyl)3,3,2,2-tetradeuteropropionic acid, sodium salt; VAST, versatile automated sample transport.

1   Introduction

Nuclear magnetic resonance (NMR) spectroscopy is typically considered to be one of the most powerful analytical techniques available for elucidating molecular structure. Its first application to organic structure determination dates back to 1951 [1]; since then it has become both an essential and a routine tool for organic, medicinal and biomolecular chemists. It can determine both the configuration and conformation of molecules, and can provide information about a variety of molecular motions.

NMR spectroscopy has long played a role in the field of drug discovery. The specifics of that role have changed over the years, because the field of drug discovery itself is continuously evolving. Indeed, many NMR developments have actually been driven by corresponding changes in the pharmaceutical industry.

Most drug discovery research can be classified into one of six different disciplines: (1) natural products research; (2) synthetic medicinal chemistry; (3) metabolism studies; (4) drug production and quality control; (5) rational drug design (protein structure and modeling); and (6) combinatorial chemistry. Many of the advances in NMR technology have occurred when someone tried to address some analytical limitation in one of these disciplines. After that tool has been used for a while it is often recognized that it could also solve a different problem in a different discipline or sometimes the tool spawns a whole new field of NMR. An example of the former is magic-angle spinning, which was first developed to do solid-state NMR, then was adopted for small-volume solution-state NMR (for natural product work), and finally for solid-phase-synthesis-resin NMR (for combinatorial chemistry). An example of the latter is the development of indirect detection, which eventually spawned the use of triple-resonance NMR to determine the structures of isotopically labeled proteins for rational drug-design programs.

In addition to the migration of NMR techniques from one discipline to another, we can often see how various NMR techniques can be combined to yield new techniques whose capabilities are greater than the sum of their parts. A good example is the hyphenated technique of high performance (HP) LC-NMR. In its current implementation it borrows concepts from pulsed field gradient (PFG) experiments (which originally came from medical imaging), shaped pulses, indirect detection, broadband decoupling, PFG shimming, small-sample probe design and automation.

It is the author's contention that there are many "tools" now available to the practicing NMR spectroscopist. To best understand how these tools can be applied to problems in drug research, we will discuss what tools are available, see how they can be combined to create new techniques, and explore how they are being used to solve new kinds of problems.

2   Pulse-sequence tools

To perform an NMR experiment, a pulse sequence is used to control the timing of the actions of the hardware. The pulse sequence is designed to cause the nuclei of interest to exchange information in a controlled manner. Because each pulse sequence is composed of a variety of elements, and there are many ways in which the nuclei can be made to exchange information, it is useful to have many different "tools" available to build these pulse sequences.

2.1   Multidimensional (1D, 2D, 3D, and nD) NMR

Multidimensional NMR was one of the first pulse-sequence tools to be developed. The first NMR spectra to be observed were called "one-dimensional" because they contained only one frequency axis [2, 3]. (Note, however, that what is called a one-dimensional NMR spectrum actually has two dimensions of NMR information: frequency and amplitude.) The early generations of continuous-wave (CW) spectrometers were only capable of one-dimensional (1D) spectroscopy, and a lot of structural information was gained from these 1D NMR spectra [4, 5]. Unfortunately, however, the 1D NMR spectra acquired on some molecules had crowded frequency axes (especially for large molecules like proteins) or had coincidental or overlapping chemical shifts (especially poorly functionalized molecules like some steroids) and it became apparent that methods that could simplify these spectra were needed. The advent of pulsed Fourier transform NMR spectrometers (FT-NMR) in the 1960s [6] led to the development of methods that could obtain additional dimensions of NMR information.

The first papers on two-dimensional NMR (2D NMR) began to appear in the early 1970s [7]. This technique allowed the NMR information to be spread out in two dimensions, and because the two dimensions could encode different kinds of information, almost any kind of overlap present in the first dimension could be resolved. If the first dimension contained chemical shift data, the second dimension usually encoded information about nuclear spin-spin couplings. The kind of coupling could be selected by using different pulse sequences. Different pulse sequences were designed to select information arising from either homonuclear or heteronuclear couplings, through-bond (scalar) or through-space (dipolar) couplings, and single-quantum or multiple-quantum couplings, and were designed to either just detect the presence of, or actually measure the magnitude of, a given kind of coupling. Experiments that exploited all the various combinations of these possibilities were eventually developed and remain in use today. Examples include: homonuclear correlation spectroscopy (COSY), which detects the presence of homonuclear scalar coupling; homonuclear 2D J spectroscopy (HOM2DJ), which measures the magnitude of homonuclear scalar couplings; heteronuclear correlation spectroscopy (HETCOR), which detects the presence of heteronuclear scalar couplings; heteronuclear 2D J spectroscopy (HET2DJ), which measures the magnitude of heteronuclear scalar couplings; nuclear Overhauser effect (NOE) spectroscopy (NOESY), which detects and measures homonuclear dipolar couplings; heteronuclear NOE spectroscopy (HOESY), which detects and measures heteronuclear dipolar couplings; and double-quantum, double-quantum-filtered and multiple-quantum-filtered homonuclear scalar coupling correlation experiments (DQ-, DQF- and MQF-COSYs). Many good books and reviews about 2D NMR and the resulting sequences are available [8–10].

After the basic 2D NMR techniques were developed, it was then recognized that they could be combined to create 3D, 4D and even higher "nD" experiments [11, 12]. The additional dimensions of an nD dataset were created by appending to the pulse sequence a specific pulse-sequence element (one containing an incrementing delay) that generated the desired correlation. A 2D pulse sequence has one incrementing delay and one direct dimension, while 3D and 4D pulse sequences have two and three incrementing delays, respectively. Each dimension of an nD dataset encodes different information, so a 3D HETCOR-COSY has three distinct chemical shift axes (one ^{13}C and two ^{1}H) and three distinct faces. (If the data within the cube of a 3D HETCOR-COSY dataset are projected onto each of the three distinct faces, it displays 2D HETCOR-, 2D COSY- and 2D HETCOR-COSY data, respectively.)

These hyphenated experiments, combined with the power of 3D and 4D NMR, are proving to be very useful for elucidating the structures of large molecules, particularly for large (150–300 residue) proteins [13].

A 2D dataset contains three dimensions of information: two frequency axes and a signal amplitude. The data are plotted on paper as a contour plot. In contrast, a 3D dataset has four dimensions of information, and the data look like a cube in which each point within the cube contains amplitude information. As there is no easy way to represent all of this information on paper at once, spectroscopists usually resort to plotting 3D data as a series of 2D planes (again, usually plotted as contour plots). Four- (and higher) dimensional experiments are easy to acquire (aside from the massive data-storage requirements), but plotting and examining the data become increasingly difficult. For this reason, 3D NMR is often the upper limit for routine NMR. As will be discussed later, the power of multidimensional NMR can be combined with multinuclear NMR to generate truly powerful NMR experiments.

Each of the disciplines within drug discovery tend to use these multidimensional NMR techniques differently. Synthetic medicinal chemistry, drug production and quality control, combinatorial-chemistry groups and, to a lesser extent, metabolism groups, usually only use one-dimensional NMR data to get most of their structural information. This is because medicinal chemists usually only need to confirm a known structure and do not need more information. The drug production and quality control groups will use 2D techniques if they encounter a tough enough problem. Combinatorial chemists might like to have 2D NMR data but they do not have the time to acquire it, while metabolism chemists would like to get 2D NMR data but they often do not have enough sample. In contrast, natural products chemists routinely depend upon 2D NMR techniques to unravel their total unknowns. Finally, there are the rational drug-design groups, which use 2D and 3D NMR techniques routinely and occasionally use 4D NMR.

2.2 Broadband decoupling

Multidimensional NMR was born out of the need to simplify complex NMR spectra. Another way to simplify spectra is to use decoupling [14]. Decoupling collapses the separate frequencies of a coupled multiplet into one single frequency, with an amplitude that is the sum of all the individual components. This both simplifies a spectrum and increases its NMR sensitivity.

Decoupling may be either homonuclear or heteronuclear. Generally, homonuclear decoupling is designed to be very frequency-selective, although sometimes it is designed to be region-selective. Heteronuclear decoupling is generally designed to be broadbanded (i.e., to cover a wide range of frequencies). In addition to spectral simplification, heteronuclear decoupling can have other benefits. In ^{13}C NMR spectra, heteronuclear (^{1}H) decoupling creates further sensitivity increases through nuclear Overhauser enhancements. In other experiments, heteronuclear decoupling can eliminate undesirable relaxation pathways, which also improves sensitivity.

Decoupling is generally desirable, but the first available methods caused too much sample heating to be of routine use [15]. In an effort to improve the effective bandwidth of decoupling for a given amount of power, more efficient decoupling schemes were developed. Starting from CW unmodulated decoupling, wider decoupling bandwidths were obtained with the development of noise-, WALTZ- [16], MLEV- [17], XY32-, TYCKO-, GARP- [18] and DIPSI- [19] decouplings [20, 21]. These modulation schemes allowed decoupling to become quite routine, and allowed new techniques like indirect detection (discussed below) to become practical. As knowledge of shaped pulses improved, ever-more efficient decoupling schemes like MPF1-10 [22], WURST [23] and STUD [24] were developed; the latter two by using advanced pulse shapes called adiabatic pulses [25]. No one form of decoupling is perfect for all applications, or even for all field strengths. Each of these modulation schemes provides a different balance of performance in terms of bandwidth per unit power, minimum linewidth, sideband intensity, complexity of the waveform (what hardware is needed to drive it) and tolerance of mis-set calibrations ("robustness"). What is most important is that now a large set of different decoupling tools is available to be used as needed.

2.3 Spin locks

The many developments in broadband decoupling arose because of better theories of spin physics. These theories also allowed better spin locks to be developed. Although spin locks were initially designed for experiments on solid-state samples, it was shown during the 1980s that experiments using spin locks were also useful for solution-state samples. Bothner-By and co-workers used a CW spinlock to develop the CAMELSPIN experiment (later known as ROESY) to get dipolar coupling (ROE; through-space) information [26]. Subsequent reports from other groups used both lower rf field strengths [27] and pulsed spinlocks [28] to improve the quality of the ROESY data. Braunschweiler and Ernst used a spinlock to develop the Homonuclear Hart-mann-Hahn experiment (HOHAHA; later known as TOCSY) which provided a total scalar-coupling correlation map [29]. Bax and Davis showed that the quality of TOCSY data could be improved by using the MLEV-16 modulation scheme (which was originally used for broadband decoupling) [30]. Kupce and co-workers, who had used adiabatic pulses to improve decoupling schemes, have recently developed adiabatic-pulse spinlocks [31]. It will be discussed later how adiabatic spinlocks are proving useful in obtaining TOCSY data under magic angle spinning (MAS) conditions and on solid-phase-synthesis (SPS) resin NMR. Generally, although experiments that use spinlocks often require the use of more sophisticated hardware, they often provide better (more complete or more powerful) data than corresponding experiments that do not use spinlocks.

The most common use of spinlocks is as mixing schemes to allow spins to exchange information. Examples include the TOCSY and ROESY experiments. Spinlocks have also been used to destroy unwanted magnetization. In some applications the spinlock is designed to destroy unwanted resonances over the entire spectral width [32]. This use of a spinlock as a general purge pulse is a viable alternative to the use of homospoil pulses [33] and is in routine use in our laboratories. In other instances, the spinlocks are combined with frequency-selective pulses (discussed below) to only affect resonances at a specific frequency. This technique has been used for the suppression of solvent resonances [34]. In its simplest sense, the presaturation experiment [35] can be thought of as the use of a CW spinlock to destroy the solvent resonance. (Solvent suppression is important when data is to be acquired on samples dissolved in protonated solvents, like H_2O, as is discussed below).

The spin physics of decoupling and spinlock sequences are related, and any given modulation scheme can often serve both purposes. In general, however, sequences are usually optimized for only one of the two applications. Hence, MLEV-16, MLEV-17 [17] and DIPSI [19] are usually used as spinlock sequences. WALTZ [16], GARP [18], WURST [23] and STUD [24] are usually used as decoupling schemes.

2.4 Shaped pulses

All of the rf pulses discussed in this section change either the amplitude, phase, or frequency of the rf (or some combination) as a function of time. This can change the bandwidth of the pulse (making it either more selective or more broadbanded in frequency), make it more tolerant of mis-set calibrations, or make it capable of either off-resonance or multi-frequency excitation.

2.4.1 Shaped selective pulses

If an rf pulse becomes longer in duration, its bandwidth becomes narrower [36]. Further, if the rf pulse is shaped, its excitation profile can become even more selective in frequency [37]. Selective rf pulses have allowed a whole variety of new applications to be developed. One application is what is called "dimensionality reduction". This is where a selective (n-1)D experiment is used instead of an nD experiment (e.g., where a 1D experiment is used instead of a 2D experiment, or a selective 2D experiment is used instead of a 3D experiment). If you already know what chemical information you are looking for, selective experiments will often acquire selected bits of NMR information faster (and with higher signal-to-noise) than non-selective higher-dimensionality experiments. This is often used to study smaller samples or more dilute samples, as is often required for natural products or metabolism studies. Examples include the use of 1D NOE [38], 1D COSY and 1D TOCSY [39], DPFGSE-NOE (also called GOESY) [40, 41], 1D HMQC (called SELINCOR) [42, 43], 1D HMBC (called SIMBA) [44] and 1D INADEQUATE [45].

Another use of selective pulses is for frequency-selective solvent suppression. (Presaturation experiments are a very simple example of the use of a frequency-selective pulse; however, they typically do not use shaped pulses.) Examples of the use of shaped selective pulses for solvent suppression include S and SS pulses [46], Node-1 [47] and WET [48]. Historically, solvent suppression was used primarily only when obtaining spectra of biomolecules (proteins, RNA, etc.) dissolved in $H_2O:D_2O$ mixtures. More recent work is showing that obtaining NMR spectra of organic samples dissolved in fully protonated solvents (e.g., DMSO-h_6, $CHCl_3$, and aqueous mixtures of CH_3CN and CH_3OH) has become important. As discussed below, this is playing a big role in direct-injection NMR, which is being used to analyze combinatorial-chemistry libraries [49], as well as for LC-NMR applications.

Frequency-selective pulses can also be used to accomplish narrow-band selective decoupling. They are usually placed in evolution periods to help simplify spectra [50].

There are many diverse examples of the use of shaped selective pulses in the primary literature, and a large number of different shaped pulses (each with different properties) have been investigated. Many good reviews already exist on these subjects [37, 51].

2.4.2 Shaped broadband pulses

Although shaped pulses were first developed to be narrow-band (frequency-selective), they can also be either band-selective or broadbanded. Band-selective pulses are sometimes used as excitation pulses, but more typically are incorporated into decoupling schemes that are designed to hit a selected and controlled – but moderately wide – region. The most well-known application of band-selective rf is probably the use of either pulses [52] or decoupling schemes [53, 54] to affect carbonyl-carbon resonances differently from aliphatic-carbon resonances in triple-resonance biomolecular experiments (discussed below). In these applications, the band-selective pulses have bandwidths of between one and four KHz. Adiabatic pulses with region-selective profiles have also been described [55, 56].

It has also become popular to use shaped pulses to affect very wide (broadband) regions. Adiabatic pulses are commonly used for this purpose [25]. There are three advantages to the use of adiabatic pulses. First, they are uniquely capable of creating a good frequency profile over a wide region. Second, for a given bandwidth they deposit less power into a sample than most other pulses and so they cause less sample heating. Third, they are quite tolerant of mis-set calibrations. This advantage was originally exploited in surface coil applications where the adiabatic pulses could compensate for the bad B_1 homogeneity [57], but some groups are attempting to exploit this feature to simply make routine solution-state NMR spectroscopy more robust and less sensitive to operator errors. Adiabatic pulses are being used as excitation pulses in experiments like heteronuclear single-quantum correlation (HSQC) to achieve wider and more uniform excitation over the wide ^{13}C spectral width [23, 58]. Adiabatic pulses have also been heavily used to create more efficient and wider-bandwidth decoupling schemes (see the decoupling section above). Both of these applications are being driven by modern biomolecular NMR spectroscopy, which uses higher magnetic fields to simplify the NMR spectra of large biomolecules, yet the rf requirements become much more demanding as the field strength increases. The electronic difficulties of exciting and decoupling the entire ^{13}C spectral width of a protein in an 800 MHz (18.8 T) magnet are daunting, so research has turned towards using the existing power more efficiently rather than continually boosting the power applied to the sample.

2.4.3 Off-resonance (SLP; phase-ramped) pulses

A third kind of shaped pulse is the off-resonance pulse, also known as a shifted-laminar pulse (SLP) or a phase-ramped pulse [59]. This is a pulse whose effects are delivered off-resonance without a change of the transmitter frequency. (It is undesirable to change the frequency of a transmitter during a pulse sequence because this affects its phase.) If an SLP pulse that affects only one off-resonance frequency is created, its phase will be ramped as a function of time, hence the alternative name of phase-ramped pulses. When a pulse that will affect two (or more) off-resonance frequencies is created, however, the resulting pulse will contain both phase- and amplitude-modulation due to the interaction of the two different phase ramps.

SLP pulses can be created to affect any number of frequencies. They can also be created using any shape or duration (or combination) of pulse. This means, for example, that an SLP pulse can be made to hit three different frequencies, each with a different pulse width, and each with a different pulse shape or phase if desired. This allows one pulse to be capable of suppressing multiple solvent resonances within one spectrum. This is proving especially useful in LC-NMR, DI-NMR and FIA-NMR, as will be discussed below.

2.5 Indirect detection

Indirect detection has probably had a bigger impact on all stages of drug discovery than any other NMR technique yet developed. Indirect detection is a technique (as well as a class of experiments) that correlates the chemical shifts of two heteronuclei (e.g., ^{1}H and ^{13}C). It complements direct-detection techniques discussed above (like HETCOR) that acquire a series of ^{13}C spectra and extracts the frequencies of the coupled protons by using a Fourier transform in the t_1 dimension. Indirect detection reverses the process by acquiring a series of ^{1}H spectra and Fourier transforms the t_1 dimension of this dataset to "indirectly" obtain the ^{13}C frequencies [60]. The major benefit of indirect detection over direct-detection methods is improved sensitivity. Indirect-detection methods can be up to 30-fold more sensitive than direct-detection methods, depending upon which X nucleus is indirectly observed.

The concept of indirect detection was first published in 1979 [61]. Although in hindsight the concept and the ensuing experiments may seem like obvious developments, the experiments were so much more demanding upon hardware that the commercial instruments of that time could not adequately run them. This delayed their widespread acceptance for almost a decade. Indirect-detection methods do not completely replace direct-detection methods (which afford better ^{13}C-nucleus resolution) but they are now the default for most users. Whenever sensitivity is important the indirect-detection version of an experiment should be used.

The three classic indirect-detection experiments are heteronuclear multiple-quantum correlation, heteronuclear multiple-bond correlation and heteronuclear single-quantum correlation: HMQC, HMBC and HSQC, respectively. One-bond H–X correlations are detected by using HMQC and HSQC, while HMBC detects long-range H–X scalar couplings. HMQC uses a multiple-quantum coherence pathway, while HSQC uses single-quantum coherence. The initial applications of indirect detection all used HMQC because it is technically easier to run, but HSQC is now the preferred tool because of the improved B_1 homogeneity of most NMR probes. Virtually all modern biomolecular experiments, and many natural-product experiments, currently use HSQC-style coherence pathways [62, 63]. HMBC is an important tool for the *de novo* structure elucidations of small molecules, particularly for natural products [64–68].

Although indirect-detection experiments have higher sensitivity than direct-detection experiments, the conventional (phase-cycled) versions of the experiments also have higher amounts of artifactual t_1 noise. This occurs because only the 1.1% abundant ^{13}C satellites of a ^1H resonance are detected in a $^1H\{^{13}C\}$ HSQC experiment; the rest of the ^1H signal (98.9%) must be removed. In datasets acquired with conventional pulse sequences, this is accomplished with a two-step phase cycle in which the ^{13}C satellites are cycled differently from the central ^1H-^{12}C resonance. Unfortunately, many (especially older) spectrometers are not stable enough to provide clean cancellation and the poorly cancelled central-resonance signal ends up creating excessive (t_1) noise in the spectrum. This is only a minor problem when isotopically enriched molecules (like ^{13}C-labeled proteins) are being used, but it can be a significant problem when studying compounds that have natural abundance levels of ^{13}C (or ^{15}N). It is most problematic for experiments that detect weaker long-range couplings (like HMBC), because then the t_1 noise is often larger than the signals of interest, and the majority of the experiment time is actually spent just trying to decrease the t_1 noise through further signal averaging. This often takes more time than is needed to simply detect the signals of interest above the thermal noise. One potential solution is to acquire the data using PFG techniques.

2.6   Pulsed-field gradients (PFG)

A chemist, Paul Lauterbur, discovered in 1973 that NMR experiments that used linear gradients of the main magnetic field (B_0) could be used to generate spatial information about what was located in the magnet [69]. This was the birth of NMR imaging. The technique was originally known as zeugmatography but it eventually became known as Magnetic Resonance Imaging (MRI). As NMR technology developed, it soon became possible to generate pulses of linear B_0 gradients, of different strengths, in a controlled fashion. Barker and Freeman were the first to demonstrate that these pulsed magnetic-field gradients could be used to acquire 2D NMR data [70]. This capability was expanded and popularized by Hurd and coworkers in the early 1990s, who showed that this tool could be used in a number of different NMR experiments to select the desired coherence pathways [71–73]. This capability caused a rapid and significant shift in how NMR spectra were acquired.

151

The first applications of PFG for imaging were in the field of medical imaging (MRI) for clinical diagnostics. Many of these techniques were then adopted in the field of drug discovery, primarily to study animal metabolism of drugs [74]. Since that time, PFG has also developed into a primary tool in high-resolution solution-state NMR experiments [75].

There are three benefits to using PFG techniques. The first is that PFG allows some experiments to be acquired without phase cycling. Phase cycling is a process in which the data acquired on different scans contain different information (by phase-shifting the transmitters and the receiver in certain patterns). The data from the different scans are co-added to select only the desired information. This requires two, four, or eight scans (or more) per t_1 increment. Phase cycling is essential for conventional indirect-detection experiments, but it is also used in homonuclear correlation experiments (like COSY). Pulsed field gradients, however, are able to select the desired information in one scan. They can reduce the minimum time required to acquire a dataset – as long as the quantity of sample (or the signal-to-noise) is sufficient. Hence the elimination of phase cycling allows PFG experiments to often acquire the data faster.

Another limitation of phase cycling is that it often generates t_1 noise. These t_1-noise artifacts can be reduced in PFG experiments that are used to acquire the data. This is best illustrated with indirect detection. Conventional indirect detection uses a two-step phase cycle to cancel the large signals from protons not bound to ^{13}C (or ^{15}N) nuclei, which in unlabeled samples is 98.9% of the signal. The residual signals left by imperfect cancellation cause troublesome t_1-noise artifacts, which significantly degrade the quality of the data. In HMBC, which detects the long-range (low sensitivity) multiple-bond correlations, this t_1 noise may be bigger than some of the desirable signals [76]. Because the PFG versions of HMBC select the desired signals (coherences) within a single scan, better quality data can be obtained (and usually in less time). This is especially useful for elucidating the structures of natural products because the structures are usually unknown and the sample sizes are often quite small, so every sensitivity improvement that can be made in HMBC is welcomed [64–68].

The third advantage of PFG experiments is that they often help suppress unwanted solvent resonances without any extra setup effort by the operator. In addition, the quality of this suppression is usually less dependent upon having a narrow NMR lineshape than with other solvent-suppression experiments. (Presaturation of an H_2O resonance is a classic example of a situation in which the NMR spectral quality heavily depends upon how well the lineshape of the water resonance can be shimmed to have a narrow base. The corresponding PFG experiments typically do not have this constraint.) The solvent-suppression capabilities of PFG experiments have become quite important because of the large number of NMR studies of biomolecules dissolved in $H_2O:D_2O$ mixtures [77]. Another interesting use of PFG has been to eliminate the solvent resonances (and unattached molecules) in slurries of SPS resins [78, 79].

These three advantages – potentially faster experiments, reduced amounts of t_1 noise and "free" solvent suppression – are obtained with many pulse-field gradient (PFG) experiments. PFG experiments further serve three other purposes: they allow old experiments to be run in different ways, they have allowed entirely new pulse sequences to be developed, and they are changing how users "shim" samples (i.e., to optimize and minimize the resonance line widths).

2.6.1 PFG: new variations of old sequences

PFG experiments have become popular because of the advantages listed above. Most indirect-detection data are now acquired by using PFG versions of the experiments [80–82]. The advantage of using the PFG version of HMBC is now well recognized and this experiment is now routinely used in natural products programs [76, 83]. Other variations such as ACCORD-HMBC [84, 85], EXSIDE [86], GSQMBC [87], constant-time HMBC [88], IMPEACH-MBC [89], psge-HMBC [83] and ADEQUATE [90, 91] have also been developed. PFG-HSQC [92] has become a standard experiment for biomolecular NMR in rational drug-design programs as well as in SAR-by-NMR (discussed later). There are also benefits to the use of the PFG version of COSY [93], so the PFG versions of homonuclear correlation experiments are also now routine [71, 94, 95]; PFG versions of selective 1D TOCSY and 1D NOESY experiments have also been developed [96].

2.6.2 PFG: new sequences

PFG have also allowed new pulse sequences and NMR techniques to be developed. One of the most dramatic examples are the diffusion experiments. First developed in 1965 [97], diffusion techniques are not only being used to measure the physical properties of molecules, but they are also being used to study ligand binding and to evaluate library mixtures for compounds which bind to receptors in rational drug-design programs [98–100]. Diffusion experiments are also being used for solvent suppression [101] and to eliminate the solvent resonances (and unattached molecules) in slurries of SPS resins [78, 79]. Another water suppression sequence is a spin-echo sequence called WATERGATE [102]. It suffers from a number of limitations due to the spin echo; limitations that are not present in the solvent-suppression technique called WET [48]. WET combines the use of PFG, shaped pulses and SLP pulses to make a self-compensating sequence. Although derived from an imaging sequence called CHESS, WET solvent suppression has become a standard tool in LC-NMR [103], a technique that is becoming a popular tool for metabolism studies [104]. WET is also being used in the NMR analysis of combinatorial libraries dissolved in non-deuterated solvents [49].

2.6.3 PFG: gradient shimming

PFG have also been shown to be useful in automating the process of shimming samples [105, 106]. The gradient pulses can be delivered by either the PFG coils or from the room-temperature shim coils. Gradient shimming is easier to learn, the results are less subjective, and the process is usually faster and more reliable than alternative forms of shimming. In our laboratories, both ^{1}H and ^{2}H gradient shimming are in routine use, both for research samples and for samples being analyzed by routine automation [49]. Gradient shimming is now commonly used to run the walkup spectrometers used in medicinal chemistry programs.

2.7 Water suppression (and solvent suppression)

Many important NMR studies are performed on molecules of biological interest. Many molecules of interest (like proteins and nucleic acids) contain nitrogen-bound protons, whose NMR signals are critical to the structure-determination process. Unfortunately, these protons also readily exchange with water. This means that biomolecular samples cannot be dissolved in D_2O

(because the proton signals would be exchanged away), so the samples are dissolved in a predominantly H_2O environment. (A small amount of D_2O is desired for a ^2H lock, however, so biomolecules are typically dissolved in a solution composed of $H_2O:D_2O$ in a ratio of 90:10 or 95:5.) Because the H_2O signal in these samples is 100,000 times larger than the signal from a single proton in a 1-mM protein, techniques have had to be developed for working with these kinds of samples.

There are three major techniques available. The first is to suppress the water signal, the second is to not excite it in the first place, and the last is to just live with it. None of these strategies is perfect, and a wide range of various techniques have been developed to try to exploit at least the first two strategies. Many good reviews of water suppression techniques exist elsewhere [107–109]. It is of interest, however, to note two things. First, virtually all of the common water suppression techniques are composed of some combination of shaped pulses, PFG and indirect-detection methods, all of which have been discussed above. Second, virtually all of the techniques are designed for the particular needs of suppressing only water, and are not necessarily capable of solving the more general problem of suppressing any solvent signal. This latter problem is more difficult than water suppression because the ^1H signal of most common solvents contains ^{13}C satellites in addition to the central resonance. The suppression of signals from organic solvents is becoming a more important issue, and will be discussed in the section on flow NMR.

2.8   NMR of biomolecules

In the 1980s, NMR started to be used to support rational drug-design programs. In rational drug design, the complete three-dimensional structure of a protein target (one which serves as a receptor) is determined. Once the protein's structure is known, molecular modeling can be used to design small molecules to fit into its receptor site. Protein structures were originally determined using X-ray crystallography, although NMR spectroscopy has developed enough that it can now also be used. NMR spectroscopy has since become the best tool for verifying the structure of the protein in solution.

The determination of a protein structure by NMR consists of three steps: determining the amino acid sequence (the primary structure), making chemical-shift assignments and determining the secondary and tertiary structure of the protein [110–112]. This last step can be accomplished by measuring either NOEs or coupling constants. The ^{1}H-^{1}H NOEs provide information about through-space distances. (If two protons located in different parts of the peptide chain show an NOE, the resulting intra-strand structural constraint requires these two protons to be close in the final 3D structure of the protein.) Homonuclear or heteronuclear coupling constants give information about bond angles. The 3D structure of the protein can be determined if enough bond angles can be known.

These three steps can be very difficult for proteins larger than 10 KDa, even if the primary sequence is determined by other means. The chemical-shift assignments become more difficult as the spectral complexity increases, and it becomes harder to obtain coupling-constant information because the linewidths become broader as the molecules become larger.

2.8.1 Multiple-resonance (multiple RF channel) NMR

The field of biomolecular NMR spectroscopy was given a significant boost when three things happened. First, methods were developed for incorporating NMR-active isotopic labels (namely ^{13}C and ^{15}N) into proteins. Second, indirect-detection techniques were developed that facilitated the chemical-shift assignments of these labeled proteins [113, 114]. Third, 3D and 4D NMR techniques were developed to simplify and sort the vast amount of information needed to determine the structure of these large molecules [115]. These three developments greatly simplified the interpretation of protein NMR data and made the determination of protein structures both more routine and more powerful. Although the techniques for acquiring indirect-detection NMR data on small molecules were well developed by the late 1980s, the experimental requirements of performing these experiments on proteins are a bit different. There were also opportunities to obtain new kinds of information. Many of these issues were worked out in the early 1990s, and this resulted in a significant burst of development that led to the field of multiple-resonance protein NMR [12, 52, 116]. The resulting experiments (described below) are certainly powerful, and initially required new NMR hardware, but conceptually one can think of them as simply being composed of combinations of the fundamental techniques that had already been developed (and which have already been described above).

There are four different aspects of pulse-sequence methodology that prove important in biomolecular NMR spectroscopy. The first is the one-step heteronuclear coherence transfers used in HMQC and HSQC. When HMQC and HSQC are performed on unlabeled compounds, only one transfer step can be performed per experiment because the ^{13}C and ^{15}N nuclei are only about 1% abundant and these isotopes are rarely adjacent. Because labeled proteins contain abundant amounts of three kinds of NMR-active nuclei (^1H, ^{13}C and ^{15}N), and so the chances of several of these isotopes being adjacent are much higher, the one-step transfers can be concatenated to form a multiple-step process. A common multi-step pathway in a protein is for magnetization to be transferred from ^1H to ^{13}C to ^{15}N, where it evolves, and then is sent back through ^{13}C to ^1H for detection. Second, indirect-detection experiments allow the t_1 dimension's evolution time to be used for any X nucleus. Third, three- and four-dimensional experiments allow multiple evolution times to be used. Fourth, the range of homonuclear and heteronuclear scalar coupling constants (J) found in a protein allow 1/2J evolution delays to be fine-tuned to select virtually any spin system in the molecule. These four capabilities, combined with the use of either partial or complete isotopic labeling within a protein, allows experiments to be designed which can correlate virtually any two kinds of spins.

In biomolecular NMR, the starting point for many of these correlation experiments are often the protons on the amide-bond nitrogens. The identity of the second spin depends upon the goals of the experiment. When making chemical-shift assignments of all the nuclei within a protein, one option is for the second nucleus be a carbonyl carbon. If so, then an experiment called HN(CA)CO finds intra-residue correlations. A different experiment, called HNCO, finds inter-residue correlations to the adjacent carbonyl carbon. In HN(CA)CO, the magnetization starts on the NH proton, is transferred to the directly bonded ^{15}N (where there is an evolution time), is transferred to the C-alpha ^{13}C (no evolution), and then is transferred to the carbonyl ^{13}C where it has its second evolution (Fig. 1). It then reverses its path (CO to CA to N to H) for detection of ^1H. The parentheses around the CA in HN(CA)CO indicate that the CA nuclei are used in the transfer, but they enjoy no evolution time so they are not actually detected. To find correlations to the C-alpha carbons instead of the carbonyl carbons, the corresponding experiments would be HNCA (for intra-residue assignments) and HN(CO)CA (for inter-residue assignments to the previous C-alpha carbon).

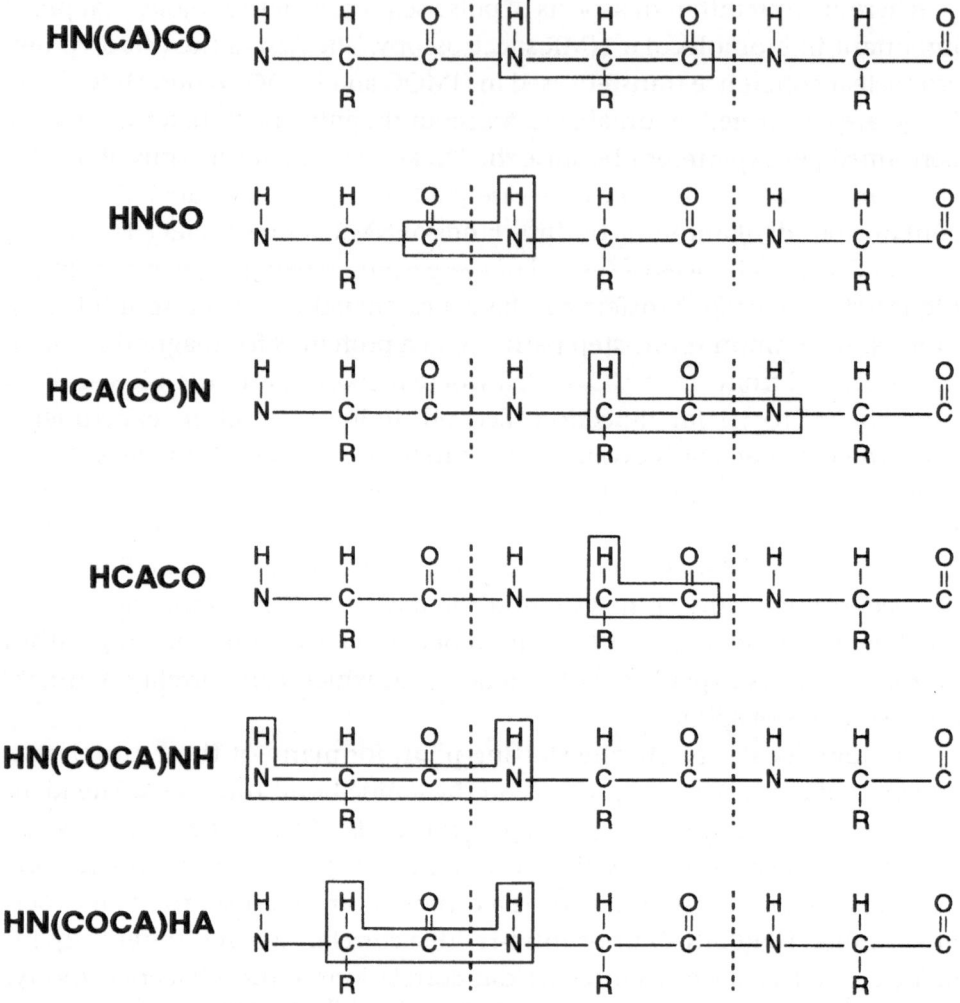

Fig. 1
Examples of biomolecular multiple-resonance experiments. This figure shows six triple-resonance experiments that can be used to find inter- and intra-residue correlations in isotopically (^{13}C, ^{15}N) labeled proteins. The nuclei involved in each correlation experiment are indicated with solid-outline boxes. The location of the peptide bonds are indicated with dotted vertical lines. The "i–1", "i" and "i+1" amino acids are displayed left-to-right. The names of the experiments are listed on the left.

In a similar manner, a variety of other correlation experiments can be constructed. Examples such as HCA(CO)N, HCACO, HN(COCA)NH, and HN(COCA)HA are shown in Figure 1.

2.8.2 New and alternative biomolecular experiments

Large molecules have different relaxation properties than small molecules, and this affects the usefulness of some NMR experiments. One example is that the usefulness of DQFCOSY decreases as molecules get bigger. DQFCOSY generates antiphase signals whose frequency separation can be measured to find scalar coupling constants. Unfortunately, as a molecule gets larger, its T_2 relaxation becomes faster, which broadens its NMR linewidths, and this results in increased errors in the measured coupling constants. As a consequence, the determination of 3D structures by measuring bond angles becomes harder and less accurate as the size of a protein increases. Experiments have been designed to try to overcome this limitation, principally through the use of combined hetero- and homonuclear scalar couplings [117, 118].

Another limitation of faster T_2 relaxation is that NMR signals can decay before they can pass through evolution times or 1/2J filters. This has had several effects. First, this has caused HSQC experiments to become more popular than HMQC experiments. This is because transverse magnetization in a multiple quantum state (HMQC) relaxes even more quickly than transverse magnetization in a single-quantum state (HSQC) [119]. Second, some pulse sequences now use a variety of heteronuclear and/or homonuclear decoupling schemes during evolution times to reduce T_2 decay rates [120]. Third, some groups have resorted to perdeuteration of those large proteins which have very fast relaxation; this reduces the decay rate of signals in the transverse plane [121–123]. Fourth, an experiment called TROSY (transverse relaxation-optimized spectroscopy) has been introduced, which manipulates spins so as to maintain those signals that have longer relaxation times [124–127]. TROSY is allowing much larger proteins to be studied by NMR.

NMR is also useful for studying ligand-receptor binding. The classic way of doing this is to look for intermolecular NOEs between the ligand and the receptor, which can only occur when they are bound. The problem is that the NMR spectrum of a protein-ligand complex is quite complicated, and small NOEs are hard to detect. The spectra can be simplified if isotopically labeled ligands are mixed with unlabeled proteins, and isotope filtered experiments used to selectively observe the labeled resonances [128]. As more complex ligands and receptors are studied, techniques for selectively observing the resonances from the unlabeled molecule were needed and therefore developed [129].

It was recently discovered that NMR can sometimes observe correlations arising from scalar couplings across hydrogen bonds. This indicates that these hydrogen bonds have a measurable amount of covalent character. This class of bonds is now called "hydrogen bond J couplings". Among the correlations that have been observed are one-bond 1hJHN correlations [130], two-bond 2hJNN correlations [131] and three-bond 3hJC'N correlations [132, 133], all of which have now been placed upon a solid theoretical foundation [134]. This will undoubtedly facilitate the structure elucidation of biomolecules.

Another way to determine structures in biomolecular NMR is to use internuclear dipolar couplings [135]. Normally these couplings are averaged to zero because molecules in solution are tumbling freely. However, if the molecules are aligned with the magnetic field even slightly, these couplings will become nonzero and measurable. If these one-bond ^{15}N-^1H and ^{13}C-^1H dipolar couplings are measured, and if the internuclear distances are known (which they are), then the orientation of the vectors of these bonds (with respect to the magnetic susceptibility tensor of the molecule) can be determined. This gives direct information about the torsion angles of the bonds, and this leads to the structure of the biomolecule. The resulting structural information complements the information that can be obtained from an analysis of NOEs and J couplings.

Some molecules naturally exhibit weak alignments with the magnetic fields, but a recent trend has been to use different kinds of liquid crystals and bicelles to not only create more alignment, but to also control the degree of alignment [136]. Once aligned, measurement of the changes of either the one-bond coupling constants (typically ^1JNH) or the ^{15}N chemical shifts, measured at a variety of magnetic field strengths, gives the dipolar couplings [137]. An alternative that is just beginning to be explored is to measure the differences in both the chemical shift and the coupling constants for data acquired both in a 5-mm probe and in a MAS nanoprobe (see the discussion below). In contrast to other methods, this technique requires only one set of measurements to be obtained on only one sample.

2.9 Combination experiments – Part 1

Many of the techniques discussed above are being combined in an ever-increasing number of ways. As an example, the resolution and sensitivity of the HMBC experiment for poorly resolved multiplets was improved significantly by using semi-selective pulses [138]. The 3D version of HMBC has been advocated for the elucidation of natural-product structures [139]. Selective excitation has been combined with a PFG version of a 3D triple-resonance experiment to make a 2D version (SELTRIP) for the study of small biomolecules [140].

PFG and selective excitation have been combined into a powerful tool called the "double pulse field gradient spin echo" (DPFGSE), also known as "excitation sculpting" [41]. This tool offers a lot of flexibility in selecting desirable NMR signals – or discriminating against undesirable signals – to produce both cleaner and more sensitive NMR data. It has been used in a number of applications. One example is the DPFGSE-NOE experiment [41], which produces significantly cleaner data than the conventional 1D-difference NOE experiment. Another example is the HETGOESY indirect-detection experiment used for detecting heteronuclear NOEs [141]. DPFGSE sequences have been used to perform isotopic filtering to select only ^{13}C-bound protons [142] and for removing t_1 noise in 2D experiments [143]. It has also been used in band-selective homonuclear-decoupled (BASHD) TOCSY [144] and ROESY [145] experiments.

3   Hardware tools

The NMR technique developments discussed above have forced the hardware and software of NMR spectroscopy to undergo corresponding improvements. All aspects of an NMR spectrometer – magnets, consoles and probes – have been affected.

3.1   High-field magnets

Multidimensional NMR was born out of the need to simplify complex NMR spectra. Another way to simplify complex or overlapped NMR spectra is to generate more dispersion along the observed (chemical-shift) axis. One way to accomplish this is to use magnets with higher field strengths. This helps resolve overlapping signals, simplifies second-order multiplets and increases the NMR sensitivity.

The ever-higher magnetic fields that are used to simplify complex spectra have required improvements in both superconducting magnet materials and magnet designs. Magnets having proton resonance frequencies of 800 MHz (18.8 Tesla) are now routinely available, and 900 MHz (21.15 Tesla) magnets are being built. Other improvements in magnet and shim coil technologies have increased magnetic field homogeneity. This has been complemented by improved spectrometer installation methods that now "map" the inhomogeneities of each magnet and adjust them for maximum homogeneity. This has allowed lineshape specifications to be cut in half over the last decade, and is allowing NMR spectra of samples dissolved in fully protonated solvents to be more readily acquired. Field strengths of 14.1 Tesla (600 MHz) and above are routinely used in rational drug-design programs, and occasionally in metabolism programs (due to limited sample sizes). Natural products groups, and some drug production and quality control groups, routinely use 400-600 MHz systems, while combinatorial chemistry and especially synthetic medicinal chemistry groups use 300–500 MHz systems.

3.2 Console developments

Advances in pulse sequences usually are followed by corresponding improvements in the spectrometer console. Originally this meant improvements only in the rf circuitry; for example, FT NMR required the development of pulsed rf. Later developments, however, like 2D NMR, required the development of rf hardware and pulse-sequence-control software that could work together to perform both more flexible phase cycling and power-level control. Indirect detection – which was a technique that required extensive signal cancellation *via* phase cycling of the rf when it was initially developed – required the design of both more stable rf and magnet anti-vibration hardware. Spinlock sequences (e.g., TOCSY) required phase-coherent rf to be developed. PFG experiments required the development of noise-free amplifiers with rapid recovery. More recently, improvements in the digital control of the rf and the receiver chain have taken priority. Modern systems have considerably better receivers and analog-to-digital converters (ADCs) that sample a wider range of signals and provide better sensitivities than ever before.

A previous section discussed how multiple-resonance NMR experiments on biomolecules use increasingly complex pulse sequences that require multiple rf channels (sometimes as many as five). Each of these rf channels is required to deliver not only more – but also a wider variety – of different pulses per sequence. For example, any one rf channel may be called upon to deliver high-power uniform-excitation broadband pulses, lower-power region-selective pulses, broadband or region-selective decoupling, broadband or region-selective spinlocks, or very-low-power frequency-selective pulses. These rf requirements have driven the development of faster and more flexible rf control, including more powerful pulse-shaping hardware and software. PFG pulses of a variety of amplitudes are now freely intermixed with rf pulses, and stronger gradients with ever-faster recoveries are always being sought.

Another trend in console developments has been the availability of higher powers. This comes about for several reasons. First, higher-field magnets spread resonances over a wider frequency range, and so require shorter pulses to maintain uniform excitation. These shorter pulses are often accomplished with higher power rf. Second, more advanced experiments often require more uniform excitation. Third, probes have improved to the point where they can now handle these higher powers. And fourth, the popularity of solid-state-style experiments has increased the use of (and need for) shorter pulses and higher decoupling powers.

3.3 Probe developments

Advanced NMR experiments have led not only to hardware improvements in the spectrometer console and magnet, but also to continual improvements in probe designs. These improvements usually arise from better probe designs, better circuitry, more precise assembly techniques and the use of better electronic components and coil materials.

The emphasis on water and solvent suppression (and the acquisition of NMR spectra on other samples with a large dynamic range of signal intensities) has created an emphasis on lineshape specifications, especially for nonspinning samples. NMR nonspin lineshape specifications – defined as the width of the NMR peak at 0.55% and 0.11% of the height of the peak – have improved and are only half as wide as they were a decade ago. Proton NMR linewidths of 4/6 Hz (nonspin) are achievable. This improved specification does not guarantee good water suppression, but is often considered to be an essential element. The improved specifications arise partly from better probe design and partly from better magnet designs, better shim set designs and better installation (field mapping) procedures. NMR resolution (the width of the NMR peak at 50% of the height of the peak) for spinning samples has not improved, but like the lineshape, the resolution of nonspinning samples for all high field NMR spectrometers is now much better than it has been in the past. This is now considered an important specification because most nD and water suppression experiments are run non-spinning.

Another important probe development has been ever-increasing probe sensitivities. The ^{1}H sensitivity specifications of modern probes are several-fold better than they were a decade ago. It is important to remember that a 3.2-fold increase in signal-to-noise can reduce the total time of an NMR experiment by a factor of ten.

The emphasis on multiple-pulse NMR experiments (such as HSQC and multiple-resonance experiments) has led to improvements in the rf homogeneities of probes. Every probe produces rf pulses that are non-uniform to different extents. This non-uniformity means that NMR experiments that use many pulses can suffer from a sensitivity degradation, with the degradation directly proportional to the non-uniformity (inhomogeneity) of each pulse and the number of pulses. Five 90° pulses in a sequence may generate only 80–95% of the sensitivity of a single 90° pulse. The specification is often quoted as the ratio of signal intensities for a 450° versus a 90° pulse (the 450°/90° ratio) or, on better probes, as the 810°/90° ratio. The homogeneities of both the observe (inner) and decoupler (outer) coils must be taken into account for multiple-channel experiments. All else being equal, higher rf homogeneity numbers are better, and these numbers have increased significantly over the last decade, largely because of the needs of multiple-resonance experiments.

The emphasis on higher-field NMR means that spectral widths – as measured in hertz – are wider. This requires the rf pulses to become shorter to maintain the same effective bandwidth of excitation (as measured in ppm). One way to accomplish this is to use higher-power rf amplifiers, so probes are always being redesigned to handle ever-increasing powers. Unfortunately, the power-handling problem becomes harder as the frequency increases, so an 800-MHz probe is actually harder to make than a 500-MHz probe.

Another probe-design factor is driven by the emphasis on studying biomolecular samples dissolved in aqueous ionic buffers. As the sample become more conductive two things happen. The first is that the NMR sensitivity drops. A sample dissolved in a 1M buffer may have only 75% of the sensitivity of a sample dissolved in plain water. This factor, often referred to as the "salt tolerance" of a probe, means that a probe optimized to provide high sensitivity for organic samples may not be optimal for samples dissolved in aqueous buffers. Signal-to-noise losses due to salt increase as the filling factor of the probe increases, as the probe volume increases as the Q of the probe increases and as the salt concentration increases. Large volume (8 or 10 mm) ^{1}H probes, or superconducting probes, are particularly prone to this problem, and care must be taken when using them to study aqueous samples.

The second problem with performing NMR spectroscopy on conductive samples is that they heat up as power is applied to the sample. For a given amount of power, the more conductive the sample is, the hotter it gets. This is only a minor problem when running experiments containing spinlocks (like TOCSY), but it is a significant problem with indirect-detection experiments. The X-nucleus decoupling used in indirect detection tends to use a relatively high power to increase its bandwidth. The resulting temperature increase can change solute chemical shifts (because the frequency of water changes with temperature and this moves the frequency of the ^{2}H lock on D_2O) and can also change lineshapes and cause sample degradation. This has required probes to have better variable-temperature performance: partly to maintain water samples at a more accurate and stable temperature, and partly to dissipate any heat generated within the sample by rf heating.

3.4 Probes for larger- and smaller-volume samples

Conventional NMR techniques sometimes produce NMR spectra with unacceptably low signal-to-noise on some samples. Sometimes this is due to limited sample quantities, and sometimes it is due to limited sample solubilities. For solution-state samples there are two ways to address this problem. The first is to use a larger volume of a solution of the same concentration (and hence more solute). The second is to use the same quantity of solute but to dissolve it in a smaller volume of solvent and place it in a more efficient small-volume probe. In the latter case, this will not only increase the size of the NMR signal, but it will decrease the size of the extraneous signals arising from excess solvent or solvent impurities.

The default probe for obtaining NMR data on solution-state samples is a probe whose geometry has been optimized for 5-mm (O.D.) sample tubes (Fig. 2a). If the volume of the sample solution is large enough, probes designed for 8- and 10-mm sample tubes are also available. (Probes that use sample tubes larger than 10 mm in diameter have existed in the past, but are rarely used anymore.) Probes that are optimized for detecting X (i.e., ^{13}C) nuclei have been available in 10-mm sizes for years, while 8- and 10-mm diameter probes that are optimized for ^1H detection (and indirect detection) have only been available since about 1993 (when advanced shim sets improved magnet homogeneities). If samples in 5-mm tubes are placed in larger-diameter (8- or 10-mm) probes, data can still be acquired, but the NMR sensitivity decreases because of the decrease in "filling factor". The converse is not true, and 10-mm sample tubes physically will not fit within 5-mm probes.

Large-diameter sample tubes are especially useful if samples have limited solubility, or if the NMR signal-to-noise is low, and if plenty of solute exists. This is classically encountered when acquiring X-nucleus NMR spectra on inorganic complexes of limited solubility, but is also now common when studying biomolecules (e.g., for rational drug design) where dilute solutions are often used to minimize solute aggregation.

3.4.1 Microcells, microprobes, submicroprobes and flow probes

The opposite situation is encountered when the quantity of solute is limited but the solubility is not. This is common in small-molecule studies, especially in pharmaceutical studies of natural products and metabolites. In this case, better NMR sensitivity can be obtained by concentrating the solution into a smaller volume. Optimal NMR sensitivity can then be obtained using one of several options. One option is to use 5-mm-diameter sample tubes equipped with "susceptibility plugs" (Fig. 2b) (or certain types of microcells), of which a variety of types are available, to reduce the depth (length) of the sample. This gives high sensitivity, although the lineshape usually suffers a bit and sample preparation can be significantly more difficult, largely because all air bubbles must be removed from the sample. A second option is to use a smaller-diameter sample tube in a probe with a smaller-diameter rf coil (Fig. 2c). This usually gives a better lineshape than can be obtained with suscep-

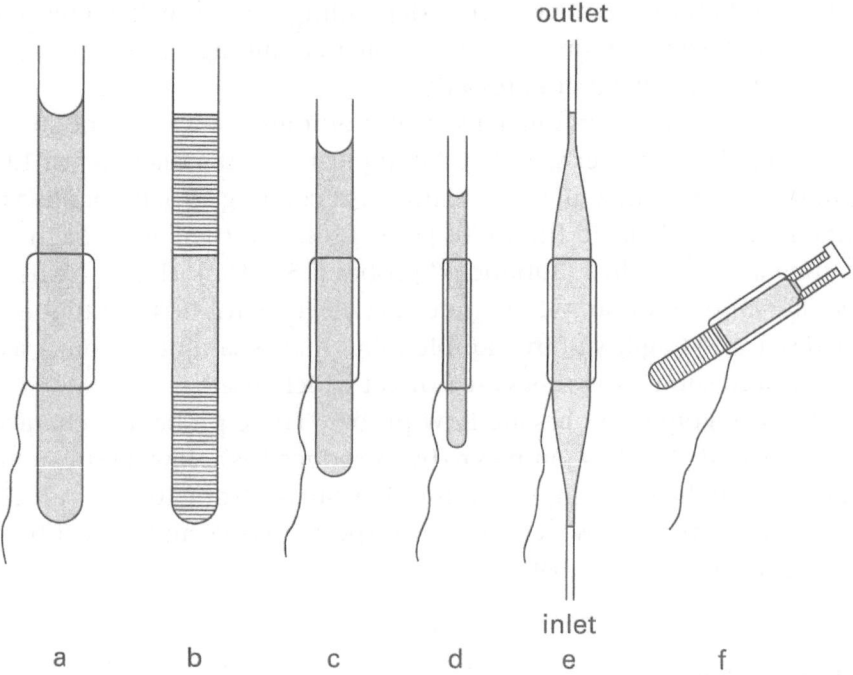

Fig. 2
This figure shows the different types of sample-tube and probe geometries that are available for acquiring solution-state NMR data. The dark gray areas indicate the sample solution. The cross-hatched areas indicate inert space-filling polymers or glass. The rf coils are indicated by outlines to illustrate their active volumes. Shown in order from left-to-right are: (a) a standard 5-mm tube in a 5-mm probe; (b) a 5-mm tube with susceptibility-matched restrictive inserts; (c) a 3-mm tube in a microprobe; (d) a 1.7-mm tube in a submicroprobe; (e) a flow probe; (f) a nanoprobe sample. A 5-mm probe has an (approximately) 220 µl active volume, while this flow probe has a 60 µl active volume. A nanoprobe sample tube has a 40 µl active (and total) volume. All figures are drawn to the same scale.

tibility plugs; partly because it uses a smaller cross-section of the magnet, and partly because the susceptibility plugs are never a perfect susceptibility match to every sample. The use of this geometry places fewer nuclei in the rf coil, and may produce a lower filling factor, but both of these factors are often offset by the better lineshape, and other factors may actually result in higher effective sensitivities. Probes designed to use these smaller tubes are called "microprobes" [146–148]. The sample tubes in microprobes typically range from 2.5 to 3 mm in diameter. The sample volume is much smaller – ranging from about 80 to 150 microliters – depending upon the diameter of the probe's rf coil. Like 5-mm probes, the sample in a microprobe is still aligned along the Z (vertical; magnet-bore) axis.

Probes designed for even smaller sample volumes now exist. One strategy is to use a smaller-diameter sample tube, typically with a diameter of 1.0 or 1.7 mm, in a probe with a matched diameter rf coil (Fig. 2d). Probes like this were first made available in the 1970s [149, 150], and then again in the late 1990s; they are now called "submicro" probes [151, 152]. Higher NMR sensitivities per amount of sample are indeed achieved with this technique, but the small size and fragility of the sample tubes makes sample handling a difficult issue, and submicro probes are not yet widely used.

Another category of probes are flow probes. These probes are characterized by their ability to allow samples to be introduced as a flowing stream (Fig. 2e). They usually have a sample volume that ranges from 100–200 µl. They have spawned entirely new fields of NMR spectroscopy, and so will be discussed in a separate section below.

3.4.2 Nanoprobes

A revolutionary new way to obtain NMR spectra on small-volume solution-state samples was introduced by Jim Shoolery (Varian) in the early 1990s. It uses a hybrid of MAS technology and traditional high-resolution probe technology. The resulting product, called a Nanoprobe, has had a large impact upon pharmaceutical research, not only for its ability to obtain NMR on very small-volume samples, but also on heterogeneous samples such as SPS resins and tissues [153, 154].

All previous sample geometries for solution-state samples were long relative to the rf coil (the "infinite cylinder" approximation) because this is a reliable and convenient way to obtain good lineshapes. This geometry moves all magnetic-susceptibility discontinuities (like liquid-air and liquid-glass interfaces) far away from the active region of the rf coil. The closer the discontinuities (interfaces) are to the rf coil and the nuclei being observed, the more NMR linebroadening they can introduce. Interfaces that have a perfectly cylindrical geometry do not cause lineshape problems. As a result, sample tubes are usually made to be cylindrical, and the samples themselves need to be made "infinitely long" relative to the rf coil in order to get good NMR lineshapes (Figs. 2a, 2c and 2d). Susceptibility plugs (Fig. 2b) attempt to mimic this infinitely long geometry, to greater-or-lesser degrees of success. (According to theory, spherical sample geometries should also give good lineshapes, and so microcells having a spherical geometry are also available. In practice, however, these sample tubes usually produce substandard lineshapes, presumably due to imperfections in the sphere, such as the hole used to introduce the sample.)

Unfortunately, in this infinite-cylinder-approximation sample geometry, only a minority of the sample can contribute to the NMR sensitivity. The fraction that can be utilized depends upon the diameter of the rf coil, but in a 5-mm probe most of the signal comes from the central 35% of the sample, and even a 3-mm probe uses only about 50%. Susceptibility plugs, discussed above, can constrict the entire sample to within the active region of the rf coil, but usually the lineshape degrades as the percentage approaches 100%. (This is because the plugs are never a perfect match to the magnetic susceptibility of the sample.) Sample handling also becomes more difficult when susceptibility plugs are used.

Nanoprobes, however, work on an entirely different principle [153–155]. To maximize sensitivity, 100% of the solution-state sample is placed within the rf coil of the probe. Although this would normally result in severe broadening of the NMR lines (because of the various liquid-air and liquid-glass interfaces – the magnetic-susceptibility discontinuities – close to the rf coil), these linebroadenings can be removed if the samples are spun about the magic angle (54.7° relative to the Z axis; Fig. 2f) [156, 157]. Solution-state quality lineshapes can then be obtained if the rf coil is built using magnetic-susceptibility compensated materials and designs (discussed below).

This MAS also allows samples that are smaller than the volume of the rf coil (40 µl in the case of a standard Nanoprobe) to be properly studied by NMR, because MAS completely eliminates the linebroadening that would otherwise be introduced by the large air bubbles. The author has obtained good NMR data on samples dissolved in less than 2 µl of solvent, and found that the linewidths and lineshapes are good, the water suppression is outstanding, and a stable ^{2}H lock can be maintained, even on this volume of solvent (unpublished observations).

The initial purpose of the design of the Nanoprobes was to allow NMR spectra to be obtained on small-volume (≤ 40 µl) solution-state samples (Fig. 3) [153, 154]. That this was accomplished is illustrated by five classes of

Paul A. Keifer

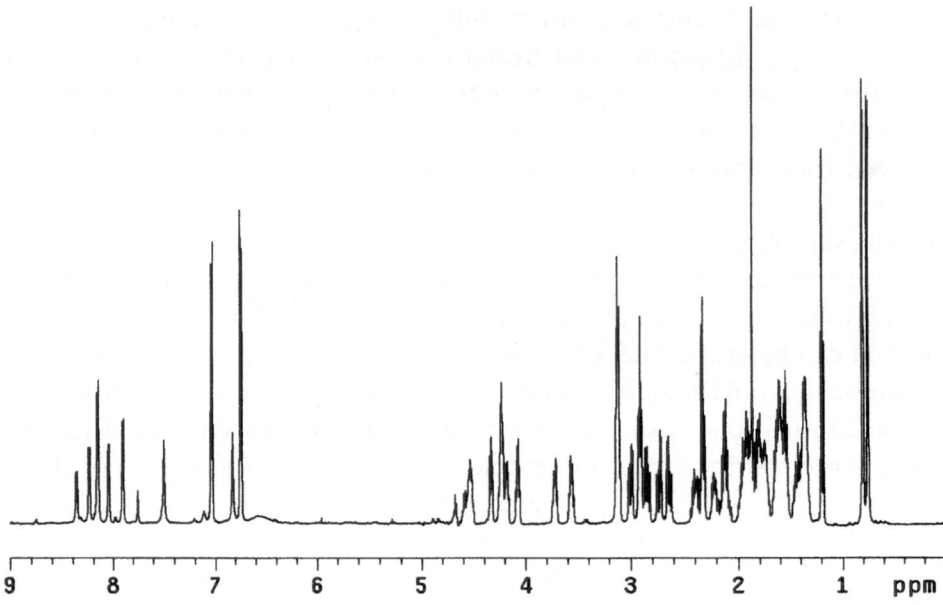

Fig. 3
A ^{1}H NMR water-suppression spectrum acquired using a PFG indirect-detection nanoprobe. The sample consisted of 750 nanomoles of a peptide dissolved in $H_2O:D_2O$ (90:10). The sample was spun about the magic angle at 2.0 KHz; the data were acquired in 8 scans using presaturation to saturate the water resonance (at 4.6 ppm). The combination of good lineshape specifications plus magic angle spinning allows the residual water resonance to be characteristically very small and narrow in all water-suppression Nanoprobe spectra regardless of the sample volume. Because of the good lineshape, this spectrum was also processed with a digital signal processing (DSP) notch filter at the water frequency, which allows the residual water resonance to be virtually gone in this spectrum.

applications. First, Nanoprobes capable of [1]H-only detection have solved the structures of several unknowns using the data from a variety of 1D and 2D ^{1}H NMR experiments [158, 159]. Second, Nanoprobes capable of acquiring ^{13}C{^{1}H} NMR data have used conventional ^{13}C data to solve the structures of unknowns [146, 160]. Third, these ^{13}C-detect Nanoprobes have also been used to generate high-sensitivity INADEQUATE data to obtain the complete carbon skeleton of the unknown molecule in a manner more rigorous than any indirect-detection methods (like HMBC) could [95, 161, 162]. Fourth, Nanoprobes have been used to acquire solvent-suppressed ^{1}H NMR spectra on samples dissolved in 90:10 $H_2O:D_2O$ to solve structures using 1D and 2D NMR (homonuclear) techniques [163–166]. Fifth, Nanoprobes capable of generating indirect-detection and PFG data are now available as well [167, 168]. These kinds of applications are primarily of benefit to natural-product and metabolism chemists, both of which typically suffer from limited amounts of sample, but there is also an unrecognized potential for rational drug-design programs that is currently beginning to be explored (especially for the removal of dipolar couplings in large oriented molecules).

The advantages of the Nanoprobes are that they are the highest-sensitivity-per-nucleus NMR probes commercially available, they shim equally easily for 40 and 4 μl samples, and they have the unique capability of producing lineshapes for samples in H_2O that are very narrow at the base (which facilitates water suppression) (Fig. 3). There are some limitations, however, to acquiring solution-state data while using MAS. First, because the sample is spinning during the entire experiment, spinning sidebands may be present in all spectra (even multidimensional spectra). Second, the sample spinning also diminishes the stability of the NMR signal and produces increased levels of t_1 noise. Although this is a problem for experiments that utilize phase-cycled cancellation of large signals (like phase-cycled indirect detection), this has been largely addressed by the recent availability of Nanoprobes capable of running PFG experiments (Fig. 4).

Nanoprobes have only been available for the last decade, but MAS itself was first described in 1958 as a way to obtain narrow linewidths in solid-state samples [169]. MAS alone was never used before for fully solution-state samples, however, for two reasons. First, MAS was initially developed for removing the much larger linebroadenings that occur only in solid-state samples (i.e., those that arise from molecular interactions such as dipolar coupling and chemical-shift anisotropy). The ability of MAS to eliminate the much smaller linebroadenings that arise from magnetic-susceptibility discontinuities was not considered nearly as important, although its utility was recognized early on by several groups [153, 154, 170, 171]. Second, to obtain high-quality solution-state lineshapes (< 1, 10 and 20 Hz at the 50%, 0.55% and 0.11% levels, respectively) NMR probes also must be built using susceptibility-matched designs and materials. While this has long been a criterion in the design of vertical-spinning solution-state probes [172, 173], it was never considered important in the design of solid-state MAS probes until after the utility of Nanoprobes became apparent [174]. The Nanoprobe was the first MAS probe designed to incorporate this magnetic-susceptibility-matched probe-design technology, and as such it was the first MAS probe that was

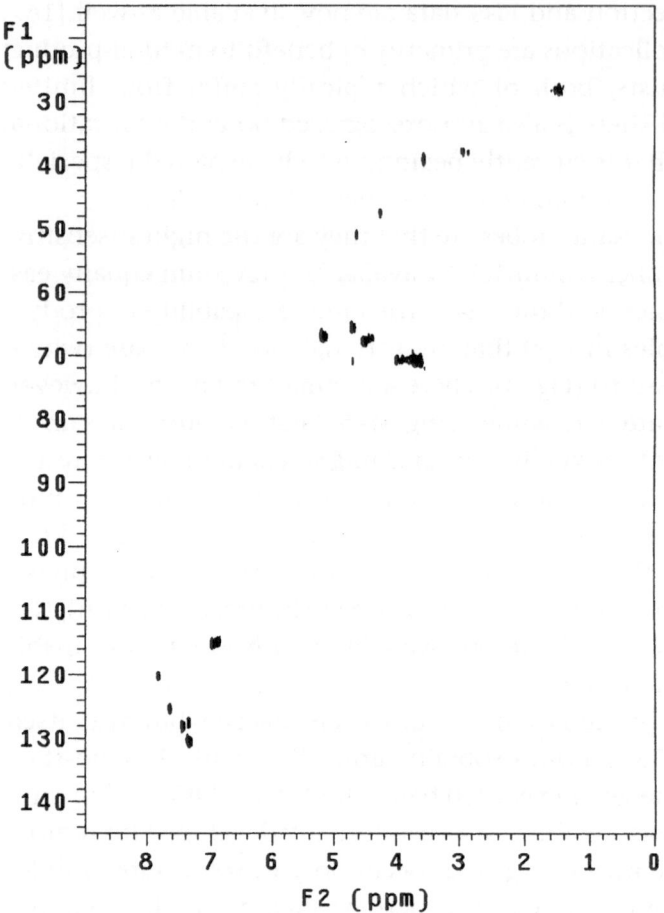

Fig. 4
A 2D PFG-HSQC $^1H\{^{13}C\}$ spectrum of a solid-phase-synthesis (SPS) resin acquired using a PFG Indirect-Detection Nanoprobe. The sample contained approximately 3 mg of FMOC-Asp(OtBu)-NovaSyn TGA resin slurried in CD_2Cl_2. The sample was spun about the magic angle at approximately 2.0 KHz. These data were acquired in 32 scans per increment in 1.5 h using a gradient-selected PFG HSQC.

really designed to handle solution-state samples. (Solid-state samples often have ^1H linewidths of 100 Hz or more, so an additional linebroadening of 5–20 Hz coming from the probe design was previously considered insignificant. This additional linebroadening is large, however, when compared to the natural linewidths of solution-state samples that may well be under 1 Hz.) Conventional MAS probes are built to emphasize both very high-speed spinning and the ability to handle high rf powers. Although these characteristics are needed for solid-state NMR, they are unnecessary for (and often conflict with the needs of) solution-state NMR.

3.5 NMR of solid-phase synthesis (SPS) resins

The use of SPS resins for organic synthesis has grown significantly since 1963 when the technique of SPS was first published [175]. It has become a key technology in the growing field of combinatorial chemistry. As such, techniques for obtaining NMR data on samples still bound to insoluble SPS resins have been a topic of considerable importance during the last few years [153, 154]. It has been shown that there are three main types of NMR probes that can be used to get meaningful NMR data on SPS resins: conventional solution-state probes, MAS probes and Nanoprobes [155]. (HR-MAS probes will be discussed below.) To compare the performances of these probes, and the techniques for using them, requires a consideration of both magnetic susceptibilities and molecular motions [154, 155, 176]. Most chemists who want to obtain NMR spectra from resin-bound materials normally mean they want solution-state-style NMR spectra with narrow lineshapes (Figs. 4 and 5).

Swelling the resins with solvent is the most important way to narrow the NMR linewidths. In general, solid-state samples tend to exhibit much broader NMR resonances than those of solution-state samples. (This is because of several parameters, including faster relaxation caused by less molecular mobility, chemical shift anisotropy, sample heterogeneity and homonuclear dipolar couplings.) Although NMR data can be obtained on SPS resins in the solid state (by using traditional solid-state tools like CP-MAS), most chemists prefer to swell the SPS resins to make them as liquid-like as possible, primarily to obtain the narrowest possible resonances. Because the SPS resin itself does not dissolve, the compounds bound to the resin can be solvated by swelling the resin to a slurry with an excess of solvent.

3.5.1 SPS resin NMR: the influence of the observe nucleus

The second-most important parameter that controls the NMR linewidths is the NMR nucleus that is to be observed [155]. This is because the magnetic-

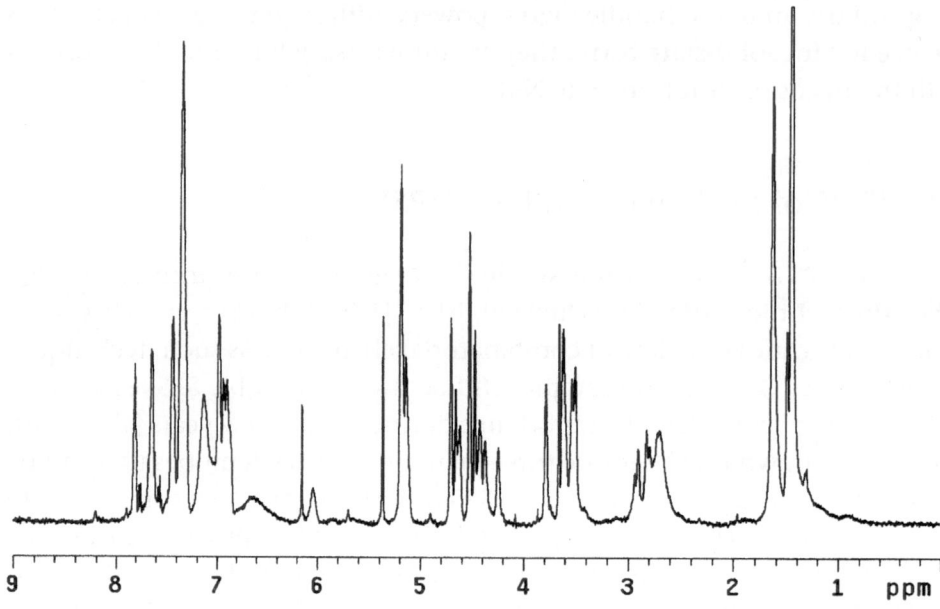

Fig. 5

A ^{1}H NMR spectrum of a solid-phase-synthesis (SPS) resin acquired using a PFG indirect-detection nanoprobe. The sample contained approximately 3 mg of FMOC-Asp(OtBu)-NovaSyn TGA resin slurried in CD_2Cl_2. The sample was spun about the magic angle at approximately 2.0 KHz; the data were acquired in 4 scans using presaturation to saturate a large polyethylene glycol (PEG) resonance at 3.6 ppm. Probes capable of magic angle spinning are the only way to acquire ^{1}H NMR spectra having narrow lineshapes for compounds still bound to resin beads [155].

susceptibility linebroadening is directly proportional to the frequency of NMR resonance. As an example, the ^{13}C resonances of a SPS resin will have narrower NMR linewidths than the ^{1}H resonances because of this field dependence.

One way to think about this effect is that a slurry of SPS resin is a physically heterogeneous mixture. It contains regions of free solvent, bound solvent, cross-linked polymer, bound samples and possibly even long tethers, and each of these regions possesses its own unique magnetic susceptibility. This mix of magnetic-susceptibility discontinuities broadens the NMR resonances of any nearby nuclei. The field dependence of this effect means that protons suffer four times as much magnetic-susceptibility linebroadening as ^{13}C nuclei, because protons resonate at four times the frequency of ^{13}C nuclei. (If ^{13}C nuclei resonate at 125 MHz, ^{1}H nuclei will resonate at 500 MHz.) This also means that resin spectra obtained on a 600 MHz NMR spectrometer will have linewidths that are twice as broad in hertz as those obtained on a 300 MHz system, although the linewidths in ppm will be the same. Not all linebroadenings in a given spectrum arise from magnetic-susceptibility discontinuities (the resonances from the cross-linked polymer, for example, suffer from other broadening mechanisms), but it is largely true for those nuclei bound to the surface of the resin.

3.5.2 SPS resin NMR: the influence of resin and solvent

The choice of the resin used and the solvent used to swell the resin are the third- and fourth-most important parameters that control the resonance linewidths of resin samples [176, 177]. NMR resonances become narrower as the corresponding nuclei of interest obtain more mobility, so anything that increases that mobility will produce narrower resonances. Many SPS resins used today contain long "tethers" made up of flexible chains of atoms that allow bound solutes to be located a significant distance from the more rigid cross-linked-polymer portions of the resin bead and allow them to enjoy considerable freedom of motion. This facilitates organic synthesis because it allows ready diffusion of reagents to the solute, and it is desirable for NMR because the additional freedom of motion decreases the T_2 relaxation and produces narrower NMR resonances. This means that the NMR spectra of resins with either short or no tethers (like the original Merrifield resins) contain NMR linewidths that are broad compared to the linewidths obtained on resins with long tethers (like Tentagel or Argogel resins).

In addition to the resin structure, proper solvation is needed to increase molecular mobility. Solvents which swell and properly solvate the resin are the most likely solvents to produce narrow NMR linewidths. This requires solvation not only of the bound solute itself, but also of those portions of the resin that are around the bound solute. If any part of the resin is not properly solvated, the reduced molecular motion will increase the NMR linewidths. In summary, this means that, to acquire a NMR spectrum with narrow linewidths, you need both a proper resin and a proper solvent; a poor choice of either will produce a low-quality NMR spectrum (i.e., one with only broad NMR resonances).

3.5.3 SPS resin NMR: the influence of the NMR probe

The fifth and final parameter is the choice of which NMR probe is to be used [155]. Conventional solution-state probes can generate high-resolution spectra for homogeneous liquids (because they use magnetic-susceptibility-matched probe design technology as discussed above) but they cannot eliminate the magnetic-susceptibility linebroadenings caused by heterogeneous samples (like SPS resin slurries). Conventional MAS probes can remove magnetic-susceptibility linebroadening caused by heterogeneous SPS resin slurries, but, because they do not use magnetic-susceptibility-matched probe design technology, the probe introduces additional linebroadening of its own (ca. 3–30 Hz, depending upon the resonance frequency and the design of the probe). This is one reason why conventional MAS probes cannot acquire good NMR data on homogeneous liquids. Nanoprobes (and to a lesser extent the other HR-MAS probes discussed below) use both MAS and magnetic-susceptibility-matched probe design technology, and so they can acquire high-quality NMR spectra on both homogeneous liquids and heterogeneous resin slurries (Fig. 5). For some SPS resin spectra, however, a Nanoprobe is not required. A conventional solution-state probe produces acceptable ^{13}C NMR data, and this technique is even common enough to have acquired the name of "gel-phase NMR" [154, 178, 179], but the linewidths of ^{1}H NMR spectra acquired this way are usually considered unacceptably broad. Conventional MAS probes are the best choice for unswelled resins, and also produce acceptable ^{13}C NMR data on swollen resins, but are usually considered to be a poor choice for generating ^{1}H NMR data (although the data are better than if a conventional solution-state probe were used). A Nanoprobe produces the best ^{1}H NMR data, and the highest resolution ^{13}C NMR spectra, but often the additional resolution in the ^{13}C spectrum is not needed, and data from either of the other two probes would have been acceptable [155]. Most people agree that Nanoprobes (or HR-MAS probes) are the only way to generate ^{1}H NMR data on SPS resins [153, 154, 180–182]. Nanoprobes can also be used to acquire high-quality multidimensional spectra on resins (Fig. 4). Nanoprobes were the first probes capable of acquiring high-resolution ^{1}H NMR spectra of compounds still bound to SPS resins [183], and are still the only probes capable of acquiring NMR data on single beads of 100-micron resin [184].

Nanoprobes are also unnecessary if you are acquiring ^{1}H NMR data on resins with no tether or if you have chosen a poor solvent – in these cases your spectra will have broad linewidths regardless of which probe you use. (A Nanoprobe may allow the resonances to be 50 Hz narrower, but if the lines are already 200 Hz wide that will not help much.) These conclusions can also all be extended to acquiring NMR data on any other kind of semi-solid, slurry, emulsion, or membrane-bound compound – they are all examples of physically heterogeneous samples that contain enough localized mobility to allow NMR resonances to be narrow if the data are acquired properly. Biological tissues are another kind of semi-solid. Methods for using NMR to study mammalian tissues are an area of considerable interest to the pharmaceutical community [168], and investigations into the use of MAS and HR-MAS probes (see below) to acquire NMR spectra of tissues and intact cells are in progress [185–189]. Nanoprobes have also been used to analyze the oils in seeds for nutritional studies [190].

3.5.4 HR-MAS probes

After the (Varian) Nanoprobe demonstrated the virtues of using MAS on both solution-state and semi-solid samples, a variety of related MAS probes became available from other NMR probe vendors (including Bruker, Doty Scientific and possibly JEOL). This spawned a class of probes – and a field of NMR – that has come to be known as "high-resolution MAS" (HR-MAS) [189, 191]. The different available probes, however, exhibit a variety of performances, usually arrived at by striking a different balance between the differing needs of solution-state NMR versus solid-state NMR. This indirectly influences the quality of magnetic-susceptibility matching. The result is that the biggest differences among the various HR-MAS probe designs are in their lineshape specifications (not simply the resolution) and their filling factors (the sensitivity efficiencies). Less important differences include the maximum spin rate, the leakproofness of the sample container, the cost of the sample container, the cost and ease of automation, and the ease of changing between MAS and non-MAS probes. The reliability of sample spinning is usually not an issue with solution-state (or semi-solid) samples. In general, the performance of the Nanoprobes is biased towards high-resolution applications, while the HR-MAS probes are biased towards more solid or semi-solid applications. To date, all of the published solution-state applications appear to have been run only on Nanoprobes.

Paul A. Keifer

There is one very big difference between MAS probes and non-MAS probes. As discussed above, non-MAS probes (those that orient samples along the vertical Z axis of the magnet) use cylindrical (and spherical) sample geometries to eliminate linebroadenings arising from magnetic-susceptibility discontinuities surrounding the sample, but this has no effect on magnetic-susceptibility discontinuities within the sample itself. Only MAS can eliminate linebroadenings that arise from the latter (the magnetic-susceptibility discontinuities that are within the sample). This is a crucial and critical difference. A homogeneous (filterable) solution-state sample has a uniform magnetic susceptibility (as long as there are no air bubbles in the sample). If any heterogeneity is introduced anywhere near the rf coil, either accidentally or purposefully – and this can be an air bubble, a flocculent precipitate, or any form of suspension or slurry – the sample is physically heterogeneous as far as NMR is concerned, and only MAS can be used to regenerate narrow lineshapes. This means that cylindrical (or spherical) microcells must be filled completely, with no air bubbles, or the NMR resonances will be broadened, whereas an MAS microcell will generate the same lineshape regardless of how completely the microcell is filled. It should also be pointed out that the use of MAS does not necessarily guarantee that all resonances will be narrow. Although MAS removes some (not all) linebroadening effects, some parameters (e.g., rapid T_2 relaxation) can still cause broad linewidths.

One final note about high-resolution MAS NMR: not all solution-state experiments translate directly into the realm of MAS. We have found, and the author has recently helped document, that spinlock experiments (like 2D TOCSY and ROESY) cannot always be run the same way that they are run on conventional solution-state probes [166]. The rf inhomogeneities of solenoidal coils, combined with sample spinning during the experiment, cause destructive interferences during the spinlocks that lead to signal intensities that are a function of the sample spinning rate. The solution is to use either different spinlocks [31] or different sample geometries (unpublished observations).

3.6   Flow NMR

An entirely new field of NMR spectroscopy has grown up around the flow probes discussed above. Because any number of devices can be attached to the inlet and outlet of the probe (Fig. 2e), many entirely different approaches to introducing samples into the NMR spectrometer have been developed, especially by groups in the pharmaceutical industry. All of these techniques are now often grouped into a category called "flow NMR" [192] even though the samples may or may not be flowing at the time of NMR acquisition. The first and prototypical illustration of this approach is HPLC-NMR, more commonly called just LC-NMR. More recently, direct-injection NMR (DI-NMR) [49] and flow-injection-analysis NMR (FIA-NMR) [193] have also been used as ways to acquire NMR data without the use of the traditional precision-glass sample tubes. By interfacing robotic autosamplers and liquid handlers to NMR spectrometers, samples in disposable vials and 96-well microtiter plates are now routinely being analyzed by NMR.

3.6.1 LC-NMR

LC-NMR is an analysis technique that can separate complex mixtures and examine their individual components one at a time. The traditional way of accomplishing this is to perform the separation off-line, collect the individual fractions, evaporate them to dryness (to remove the mobile phase), redissolve them in a deuterated solvent, and examine them by conventional NMR, using microcells and microprobes if needed. LC-NMR, however, offers both on-line separation and an immediate analysis, and this is especially useful if the solutes are volatile, unstable, or air-sensitive [194]. Because of these advantages, the use of LC-NMR has become much more popular during the last few years.

LC-NMR was first developed in 1978 [195], but for the first 10–15 years it was regarded more as an academic curiosity rather than as a robust analytical tool. A number of reviews of LC-NMR exist, both of the early work [196, 197] as well as of the later applications [198, 199]. More recently, the technique has evolved rapidly as probe sensitivities increased and as techniques for working with non-deuterated solvents were developed [48]. LC-NMR has now become almost a routine technique for metabolism groups [104, 200] and is proving useful for drug production and quality control groups [201, 202], for combinatorial chemistry groups [203] and for natural products groups [204–206].The hardware for LC-NMR consists of an LC-pump, an injector port, a chromatography column, some sort of in-line detector (usually a sin-

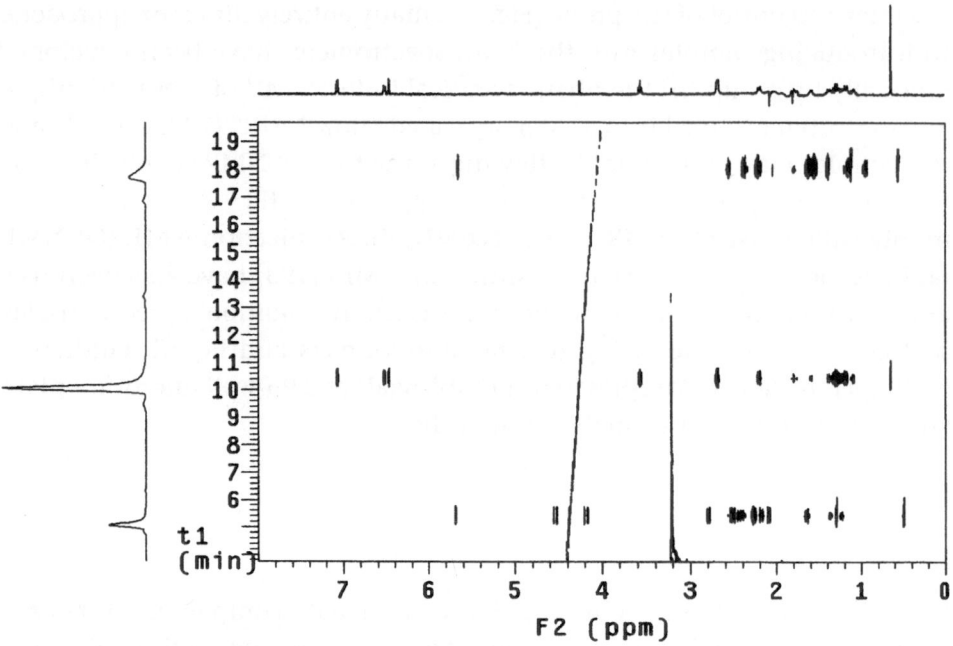

Fig. 6
On-flow LC-NMR data acquired using a solvent gradient. Three steroids (cortisone, estradiol and prog-esterone – 100 μg of each on-column) were separated using a $CH_3CN:D_2O$ mobile phase whose com-position was ramped during the experiment. The ^1H chemical-shift axis runs horizontal; the chro-matographic time axis runs vertical. Plotted on the left is the corresponding UV chromatogram (290 nm). Plotted on the top is the 1D spectrum (the "trace") of the compound that eluted at 10.5 min (estradiol). The data were acquired while the sample flowed continuously through the probe by using two-frequency WET solvent suppression (at 1.95 and 4.4–4.1 ppm). The resonance that is moving from 4.4 ppm (at 4 min) to 4.1 ppm (at 19 mins) is the water resonance – which moved as the sol-vent composition changed during the solvent gradient run. To compensate for this, the solvent-sup-pression frequencies were automatically determined during the experiment by using the SCOUT-scan technique. The sample was dissolved in CH_3OH; the resonance from the tailing chromatographic peak can be seen at 3.2 ppm.

gle-wavelength or photodiode array UV detector or two detectors in series) and an NMR flow probe. The experiments can be run in either an on-flow mode, in which the mobile phase moves continuously (Fig. 6), or in a stopped-flow mode, in which peaks of interest are stopped in the NMR flow probe for as long as needed for NMR data acquisition (Fig. 7). Onflow data are useful for preliminary or survey-mode analyses, while stopped-flow data are useful for careful examinations of individual components. In the stopped-

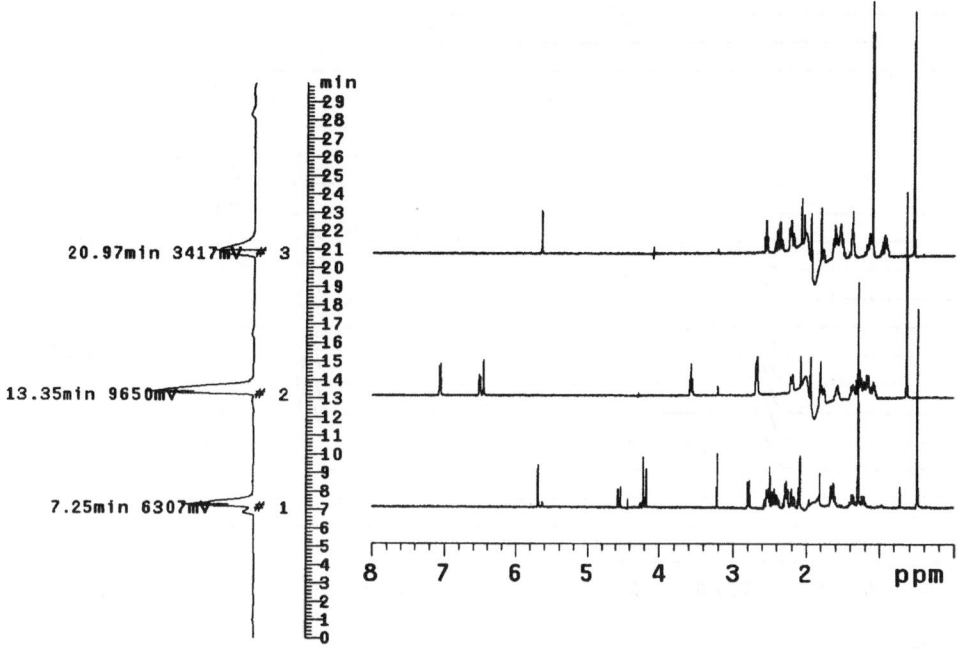

Fig. 7
Stopped-flow LC-NMR data acquired using a solvent gradient. Three steroids (cortisone, estradiol and progesterone – 100 μg of each on-column) were separated using a $CH_3CN:D_2O$ mobile phase whose composition was ramped during the experiment (starting at 30% CH_3CN and increasing at 2% per minute). The ^{1}H chemical-shift axis runs horizontal; the chromatographic time axis runs vertical. On the left is the HPLC chromatogram; the corresponding ^{1}H NMR spectra are aligned with each peak. This is the default (and automatic) output display for stopped-flow LC-NMR data. The data were acquired by using two-frequency WET solvent suppression (at 1.95 and 4.4–4.1 ppm) and a two-frequency DSP notch filter; suppression and filter frequencies were automatically determined using the SCOUT-scan experiment.

flow mode, either 1D or 2D NMR data can be acquired, although the limited amounts of sample usually injected onto an HPLC column makes the acquisition of extensive 2D heteronuclear correlation data sometimes difficult. Stopped-flow runs can also use any one of three different kinds of sample handling. First, the samples may be analyzed, one chromatographic peak at a time, directly as they elute from the chromatography column. This is often the default mode of operation. Second, the LC pump may be programmed to "time slice" through a chromatographic peak, stopping every few seconds to acquire a new spectrum. This is useful for resolving multiple components (by

Paul A. Keifer

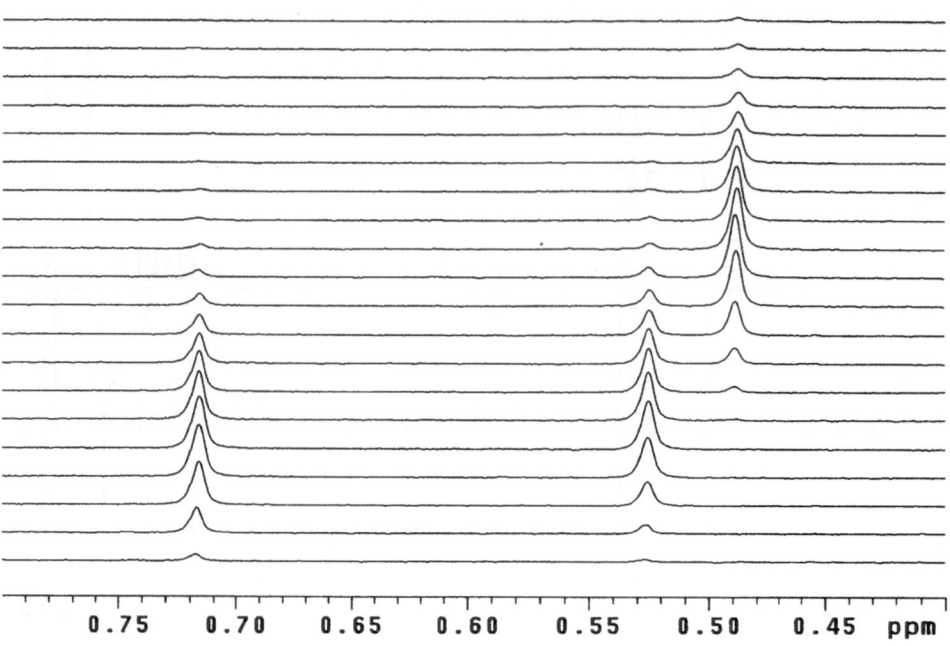

Fig. 8
Time-slice LC-NMR data. Three steroids (cortisone, estradiol and progesterone – 100 µg of each on-column) were barely separated using a $CH_3CN:D_2O$ solvent gradient. The ^1H chemical-shift axis of the resulting LC-NMR data runs horizontal; the chromatographic time axis (not labeled) runs vertical and time increases from bottom-to-top. The chromatographic (UV) detector only detected two signals, but the LC-NMR time-slice data, expanded to show the three methyl signals between 0.4 and 0.8 ppm, demonstrate that there are actually three compounds. This can be verified by noting that the ratios of the peak heights of the two highest-frequency methyl resonances (0.72 and 0.53 ppm) are different in different increments (see the third and tenth spectra from the bottom). This indicates that the first UV peak contains two different compounds. The second UV peak contains a compound that has a methyl resonance at 0.49 ppm. The NMR data show that this third compound (containing the 0.49 ppm resonance) is chromatographically more well-resolved from compounds 1 and 2 (which contain the 0.72 and 0.53 ppm resonances). These data were acquired by using two-frequency WET solvent suppression (at 1.95 and 4.4-4.1 ppm) that was optimized on-the-fly for each spectrum by using an automated SCOUT-scan experiment.

NMR) from within a peak that is not fully resolved chromatographically, or for verifying the purity of a chromatographic peak (Fig. 8). (Alternatively, on-flow acquisition with a very slow flow rate has been used for similar purposes [207]). The third method is to collect the chromatographic peaks of interest into loops of tubing (off-line) and then flush the intact fractions into the NMR flow probe one at a time as needed. A variation of this technique is to trap the eluted peaks onto another chromatographic column and then re-elute them with a stronger solvent into the flow probe [208]. This process increases the solute concentration and allows the NMR signal-to-noise to be increased.

The acquisition of LC-NMR data can be challenging for several reasons. The first is that the mobile phases in LC-NMR are usually mixtures, and the solvents are rarely fully deuterated, so there are usually one or more solvent resonances to be suppressed. Second, the resonances of the organic solvents contain ^{13}C satellites that complicate the NMR spectrum and these also need to be suppressed. Third, the pulse sequences of many solvent suppression schemes (like presaturation) take so much time that they don't work well on samples that are flowing through the probe. All of these problems were solved when the WET solvent suppression experiment was developed [48]. WET uses a combination of shaped-pulse selective excitation, multifrequency SLP pulses, PFG and indirect-detection-style ^{13}C decoupling during the shaped pulses (all described above) to quickly and efficiently suppress multiple resonances using only a simple two-channel spectrometer (Fig. 9).

The LC-NMR data acquisition is also challenging because, during gradient HPLC, which is the most common mode of chromatography, the solvent resonances that need to be suppressed are constantly moving. This occurs because, by definition, the solvent composition changes during the experiment. Gradient LC-NMR is also usually performed in a reversed-phase mode, which means that one of the co-solvents is water, and unfortunately the chemical shift of water changes up to three ppm as the solvent composition changes. (The author has also observed that the resonances of several other solvents and modifiers also change, but to a much lesser extent.) In addition, if the mobile phase is fully protonated (non-deuterated) there will be no ^{2}H lock to keep the frequencies constant.

To compensate for these changing frequencies, and to allow the solvent-suppression frequencies to be automatically optimized, the SCOUT-scan technique was developed [48]. This technique takes a single-scan, small-tip-angle, non-suppressed ^{1}H spectrum, moves the transmitter to the constant resonance (this serves as an active ^{1}H lock), measures where the other resonances to be suppressed have moved to, and creates an SLP pulse that suppresses all of these resonances (Fig. 9). This whole process take only a few seconds. It can be used in an interleaved fashion during an on-flow solvent-gradient run (Fig. 6), as well as a precursor to stopped-flow data acquisitions (Fig. 7). We

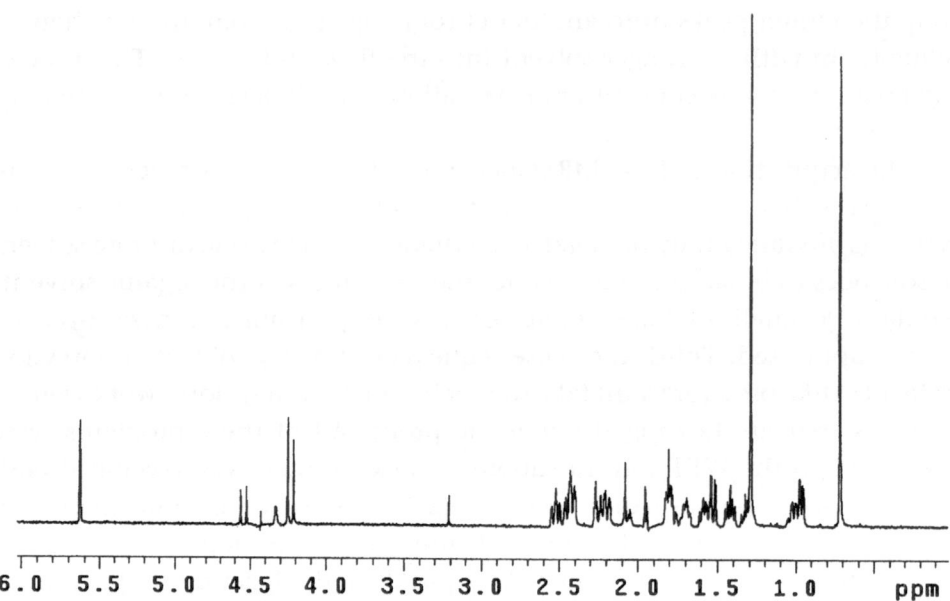

Fig. 9
An example of two-frequency WET solvent suppression in LC-NMR. The sample contained 100 micrograms of cortisone dissolved in 10 microliters of $CH_3CN:D_2O$ (50:50). The sample also contained other components, but they were separated from the cortisone by the HPLC column. The UV absorption signal from the HPLC detector was used to stop the flow of solvent (trapping the sample in the flow cell in the NMR probe) and then signal the NMR spectrometer to start the acquisition. This spectrum was acquired in 256 transients using two-frequency WET solvent suppression (at 1.95 and 4.43 ppm). The WET solvent suppression was automatically set up using a SCOUT-scan automated experiment. Exponential weighting (0.5 Hz) was applied.

will see later how it forms an integral part of the DI-NMR and FIA-NMR techniques.

The presentation of the resulting LC-NMR data depends upon the type of experiment being run. On-flow LC-NMR data are usually displayed as a contour map like a conventional 2D dataset, although the Fourier transform is only applied along one axis (the F_2 axis) to give a frequency-versus-elution time plot. The 1D data plotted along the "pseudo-t_1" axis may either be the LC detection output, or a projection of the NMR data (Fig. 6). Stopped-flow LC-NMR data on the other hand are usually presented as a series of individual 1D spectra, plotted one spectrum per page, although stacked-plot presentations are also possible (Fig. 7).

3.6.2 LC-NMR-MS

LC-NMR is usually considered a very powerful (although usually not a fast) technique. One way to exploit its power is to hyphenate it farther by adding mass spectrometry to produce LC-NMR-MS. This is usually done by splitting a fraction of the chromatographic effluent to the mass spectrometer, usually prior to the NMR flow cell. Although it is still in its infancy, LC-NMR-MS appears to be the ultimate tool for pharmaceutical analysis and it is proving its worth by analyzing in only one step those compounds that are either sample-limited or proving to be tough structural problems [103, 104, 209, 210].

3.6.3 Flow-injection-analysis NMR (FIA-NMR)

Although LC-NMR and LC-NMR-MS both exploit the analytical power of flow NMR, neither technique can be regarded as particularly fast. In contrast, the two techniques of FIA-NMR and DI-NMR (discussed below) are techniques that exploit the speed and robustness of flow NMR, even though they are not regarded as particularly powerful in the traditional analytical sense. Because neither FIA-NMR nor DI-NMR uses chromatography, they are not particularly well suited to the analysis of mixtures. In one sense, both techniques are essentially just automated sample changers. FIA-NMR appears to be more useful as a tool for repetitive analyses or to perform quality control (Fig. 10), whereas DI-NMR is particularly well suited to the analysis of libraries of combinatorial-chemistry samples (Fig. 13). It is interesting to note that LC-NMR is most popular at 500 MHz and above (primarily due to sensitivity limitations) while DI-NMR is more popular at 500 MHz and below. FIA-NMR, which is not yet a commercial product from any vendor, will undoubtedly resemble DI-NMR in being more popular at 500 MHz and below.

The hardware for FIA-NMR is similar to LC-NMR except there is no chromatography column. The technique has sometimes been referred to as "columnless LC-NMR" [153, 154, 193]. No additional detectors (other than the NMR) are needed, nor is a pump capable of running solvent-gradient methods. The technique uses the mobile phase as a hydraulic push solvent, like a conveyor belt, to carry the injected plug of sample from the injector port to the NMR flow cell. After the pump stops, the spectrometer can acquire

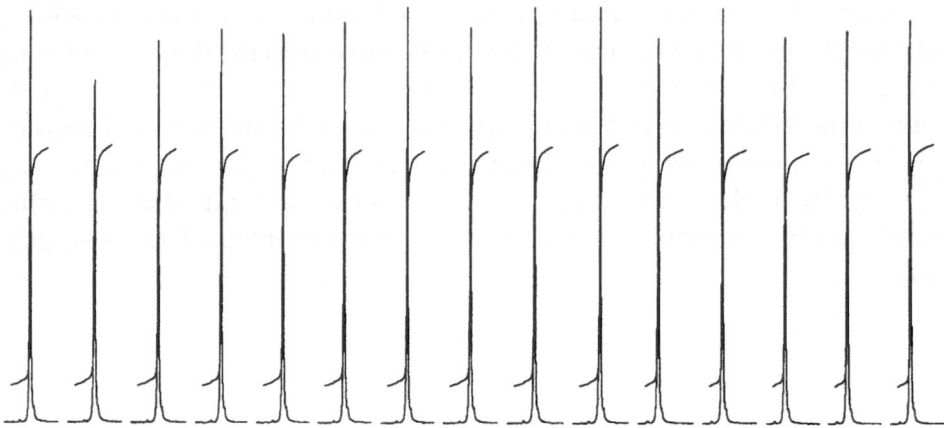

Fig. 10
These spectra illustrate the performance of repetitive analysis by FIA-NMR. The 15 spectra were acquired on 15 separate injections of a caffeine standard solution (200 µl of a 1 mg/ml caffeine solution dissolved in 50:50 $CH_3CN:D_2O$). Only the caffeine's N-methyl resonance at 3.22 ppm is displayed. Each spectrum was acquired with 32 scans and two steady-state scans and was processed using 1 Hz linebroadening, a one-frequency DSP notch filter, and two zerofilling steps. The vertical scales and integral scales were identical for all spectra. As expected, the integral areas were constant in all spectra with a standard deviation percent for the 15 spectra of 1.4%. The data were acquired without re-shimming, and the variable linewidths resulted in the peak heights being less consistent, however, a quick round of ^1H gradient shimming prior to each acquisition was shown to generate more uniform peak heights.

the SCOUT scan, analyze it and acquire the signal-averaged data (again using WET solvent suppression) (Fig. 11). When finished, the NMR sends a start signal to the solvent pump to flush the sample out of the NMR flow cell and bring in the next sample. In classic FIA-NMR, as in LC-NMR, the sample always flows in only one direction, and enters and exits the NMR flow cell through different ports. Also, the flow cell is always full of solvent in FIA-NMR (and LC-NMR), and because this can dilute incoming samples, neither technique produces the maximum NMR sensitivity from any given sample. The first (and so far the only) published applications of FIA-NMR originated from our laboratories [153, 154, 193].

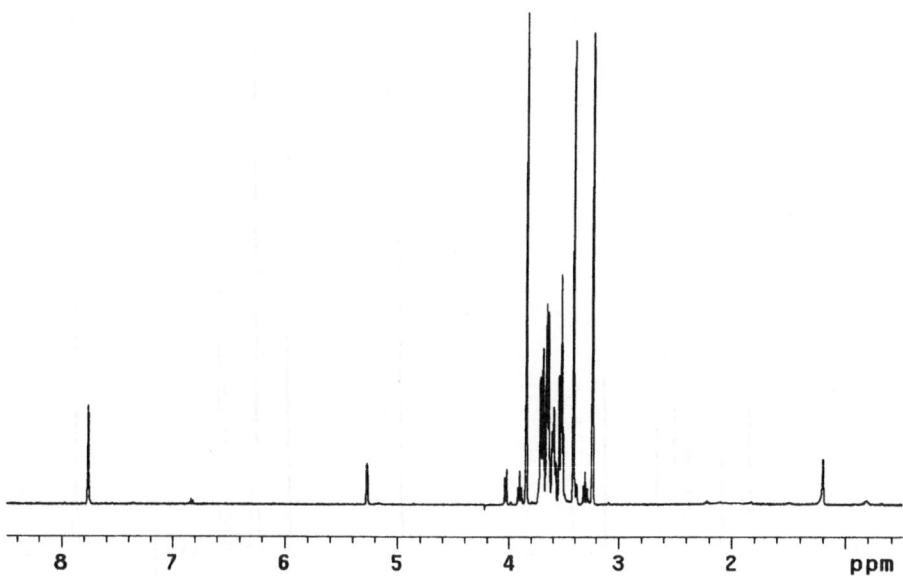

Fig. 11
An example of two-frequency WET solvent suppression in FIA-NMR. The sample consisted of 200 µl of a solution made by dissolving a No-Doz™ tablet in 20 milliliters of $CH_3CN:D_2O$ (50:50) and injected into an FIA-NMR system. This spectrum was acquired in 4 scans using automated ^1H gradient shimming and two-frequency WET solvent suppression (at 1.95 and 4.2 ppm). The WET solvent suppression was automatically set up using a SCOUT-scan automated experiment. Exponential weighting (0.2 Hz) was applied.

3.6.4. Direct-injection NMR (DI-NMR)

DI-NMR, which was also first developed in our laboratory [49, 153, 154], uses a significantly different plumbing scheme. Unlike LC-NMR and FIA-NMR, DI-NMR starts off with an empty flow cell. This yields the maximum NMR sensitivity per sample.

In DI-NMR, a plug of sample solution is injected directly into the NMR flow cell. When finished, the spectrometer is triggered to acquire the SCOUT scan, analyze it and acquire the WET-suppressed signal-averaged NMR spectrum (Fig. 12). When this is finished, the sample is pulled back out the inlet port, and is returned to either the original or an alternate sample container. After the flow cell is emptied, clean solvent can be injected into the flow cell

187

Paul A. Keifer

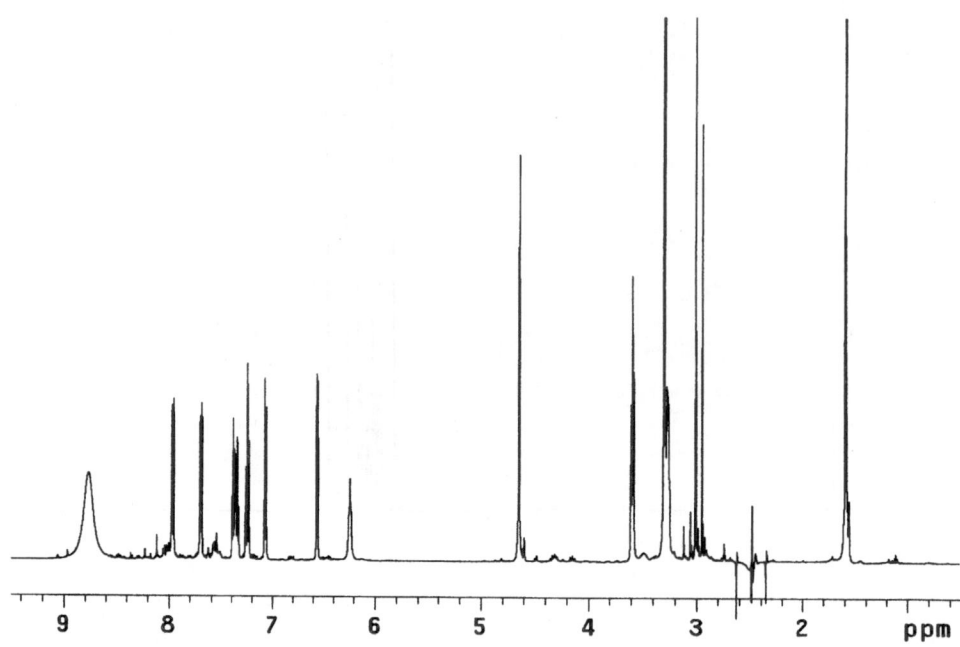

Fig. 12
A ^{1}H DI-NMR spectrum acquired on a combinatorial-chemistry library sample dissolved in DMSO-h_6 using WET suppression and VAST automation. This spectrum was acquired in one minute (32 scans) on a 25 mM solution using single-frequency WET solvent suppression and a single-frequency DSP notch filter (both at 2.5 ppm). These are the data from just one compound from the library used for Figures 13, 14 and 15 [49].

to rinse it. The solvents used for both the sample and the rinse must be at least miscible, and should preferably be identical, to avoid either lineshape degradations caused by magnetic susceptibility discontinuities (arising from liquid-liquid emulsions or precipitation of solutes in the flow cell) or avoid plugged transfer lines (because of precipitation of solutes).

The hardware used for DI-NMR is also very different than what is used in FIA-NMR or LC-NMR. Varian uses a standard Gilson 215 Liquids Handler, containing a syringe pump and a Rheodyne injector port, to deliver samples to the NMR flow probe. The injector valve is never actually switched, and the samples are injected directly through the injector port into the bottom of the NMR flow cell. This liquids handler is capable of accepting a variety of sample containers, including both vials and microtiter plates.

188

One of the rationales for developing DI-NMR was to improve the robustness and speed of automated NMR. The improvement in robustness has occurred, partly through the elimination of locking, spinning, gain adjustment and cumbersome shimming routines. PFG shimming is used instead of simplex shimming. Although the other techniques can be automated, operation is more robust if they can just be eliminated. This has allowed batches of samples to be run at a time without error, even multiple 96-well plates full of samples, and some installations have used this to run tens of thousands of samples in a highly automated fashion. Although DI-NMR can be robust, there is no way to guarantee that it can run faster than a conventional sample-changing robot for 5-mm tubes, because the speed at which DI-NMR can be run greatly depends upon the viscosity of the solvent being used. Although most solvents can be pumped in and out of the probe quite rapidly, DMSO, which is one of the most popular DI-NMR solvents, is viscous enough that sample flow rates are decreased, and the resulting analysis may not be much faster than traditional robotic sample changers.

DI-NMR and FIA-NMR were designed for different purposes, and as such they offer different advantages and disadvantages. The advantages of DI-NMR over FIA-NMR are that it generates a higher signal-to-noise per sample, and consumes less solvent. The advantages of FIA-NMR over DI-NMR are that it has no minimum sample volume (since the flow cell is always full), it can filter samples (with an in-line filter), and it can rinse the NMR probe better in a shorter period of time (albeit by consuming more solvent). The big disadvantages of DI-NMR are that it has a minimum sample volume (if the sample volume is smaller than the NMR flow cell the lineshape rapidly degrades), and no sample filtration is possible. Both techniques will always have some degree of carryover (although it may be < 0.1%) and are subject to blockages from solid particles. Conventional robotic sample changers that use glass tubes suffer from none of these problems. In terms of applications, FIA-NMR is more valuable for repetitive analyses or quality control functions, especially when there is plenty of sample and the samples are to be discarded [193]. In contrast, DI-NMR is proving to be more valuable when there is a limited amount of sample and the samples need to be recovered. DI-NMR, as implemented by Varian in the product called VAST, has become well regarded as a tool for the analysis of single-compound combinatorial-chemistry libraries [49, 168, 211], biofluids [212], biomolecules [213] and for SAR-by-NMR studies (described below).

3.6.5 DI-NMR (HT-NMR) data processing and analysis

The DI-NMR (VAST) tools discussed above have allowed the acquisition of NMR spectra every few minutes to become routine, even with protonated solvents (Fig. 12). However, this creates another challenge – the presentation and interpretation of the resulting mass of data. We have recently examined a number of different ways to display the spectral data acquired on samples in a 96-well microtiter plate [49]. Combinatorial-chemistry samples present a unique challenge because there will be relationships between samples located in the rows and columns of each plate, and we may chose to examine subsets of the data based upon these relationships.

One way to present the data is as a stack of 96 spectra, plotted one spectrum per piece of paper. This is the most traditional presentation, but once the novelty of running so many spectra so easily wears off, this option tends to prove less popular, especially with the chemist responsible for interpreting all these data. Another option is to display all 96 spectra (and/or their integrals) at once on one piece of paper (Fig. 13). This provides a good printed record of the data, but the data analysis can be difficult unless only part of the chemical shift range is plotted. An alternative presentation is to display the data as a contour (or stacked) plot with the ^{1}H frequency axis along F_2 (Fig. 14). This is similar to a display used for LC-NMR data (Fig. 6); however, in DI-NMR the t_1 axis corresponds to individual wells. Another option is to display the spectral data from a subset of the wells (either from one row, one column, or from a discrete list of well locations) as a stacked plot (Fig. 15).

It is also possible to display the integral information in one of three ways. First, one can extract integral intensities for many regions across the chemical shift range, for each of the 96 spectra, and list them serially in a text file. Second (and more usefully), one can take this text file and extract just one integral value per spectrum (all from the same region) and display it in a spreadsheet database. Third, one can display this same information as a color map, with color intensity representing integral intensity (or peak height or any other quantitative information). Each of these options has been examined in detail [49].

Without question, it would be useful to be able to interpret DI-NMR data through the use of automated computer software. Although software does not yet exist to determine the structure of an unknown compound *de novo* from its 1D ^{1}H spectrum, software does exist that can do this with 1D ^{13}C

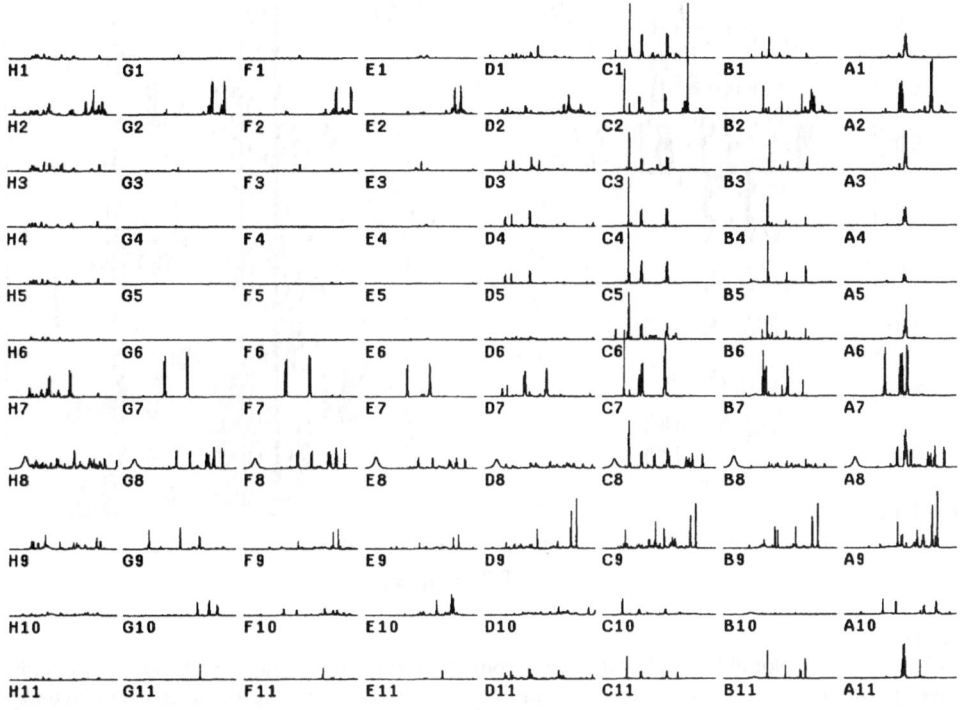

Fig. 13
A contour plot of the ^{1}H DI-NMR data from 88 combinatorial-chemistry library samples dissolved in DMSO-h_6 (25 mM). The 0.5 to 9.5 ppm region is shown. This represents one way to plot the data from an entire titer plate on one page. Each spectrum was acquired, processed and plotted with identical parameters (using one-minute acquisitions). Data from the same library were used for Figures 12, 14 and 15 [49].

NMR data. The automated interpretation of ^{1}H NMR data is harder due to the presence of homonuclear couplings (especially second-order couplings), although software is getting better at handling this [214]. Current technology, however, does allow software to determine if a given NMR spectrum is consistent with a suspected structure. This capability is expected to be of great interest in combinatorial chemistry. This is because the expected structure usually already exists in an electronic database somewhere, and can easily be submitted to the analysis software along with the experimental NMR spectral data.

191

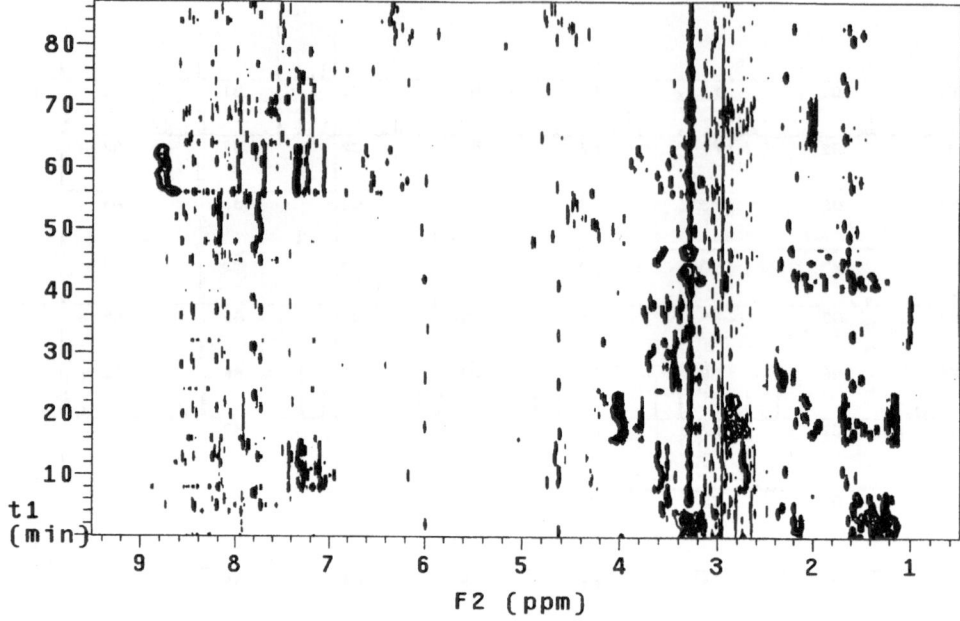

Fig. 14
An 8 × 11 matrix plot of the ^{1}H DI-NMR data from 88 combinatorial-chemistry library samples dissolved in DMSO-h_6 (25 mM). The 6.8 to 9.0 ppm region is shown. This represents an alternative way to plot the data from an entire titer plate on one page. The position of each spectrum represents the corresponding position of each sample in the microtiter plate; each spectrum is also labeled with its alphanumeric position coordinates. Each spectrum was acquired, processed and plotted with identical parameters (using one-minute acquisitions). Data from the same library were used for Figures 12, 13 and 15 [49].

3.7   Other hardware

Three other probe developments should also be mentioned. Two arise from efforts to extract more signal-to-noise from a given sample. The third arises from efforts to make probe repairs easier in flow NMR.

3.7.1 Superconducting and supercooled probes

To improve the signal-to-noise ratio of a probe, one can either increase the signal or decrease the noise. Although the former technique is the most common, the latter can be accomplished by designing probes to use low-temperature rf

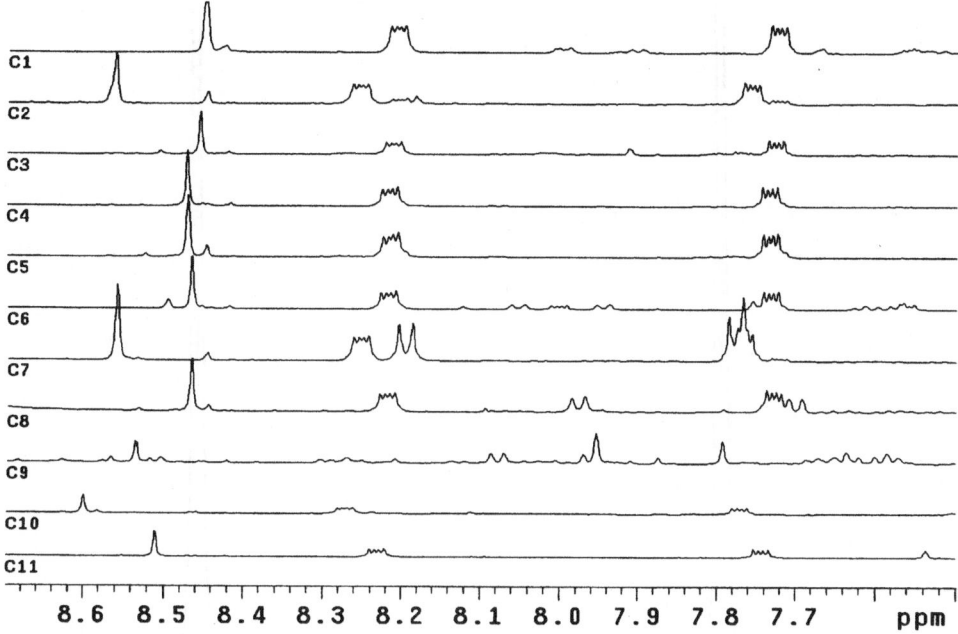

Fig. 15

A stacked plot of the ¹H DI-NMR data from a portion of an 88-member combinatorial library. Although VAST was used to acquire data on every sample, only the data from one column of wells were selected to be displayed. The 7.5 to 8.7 ppm region is shown. Each spectrum was acquired, processed and plotted with identical parameters (using one-minute acquisitions). Data from the same library were used for Figures 12, 13 and 14; this figure contains only a subset of the data shown in Figures 13 and 14 [49].

coils to reduce the noise level. The rf coils are typically maintained at 20–25° K while the samples are left at room temperature. Probes have been made that use rf coils made of either supercooled normal metal [215] or superconducting metal [216, 217]. A ¹H superconducting probe was used to study natural products [218]. A ¹⁹F superconducting probe was used to study the kinetics of protein folding [219]. The protein-folding studies required higher sensitivity because the reaction rate was so fast that signal averaging was not possible, so high-sensitivity single-scan 1D spectra were needed to follow the reaction. Probes equipped with full PFG and indirect-detection capabilities are now available with coils built of supercooled normal metal, but are not yet readily available for superconducting metal coils. These supercooled normal-metal probes have already been used as tools in SAR-by-NMR applications [220].

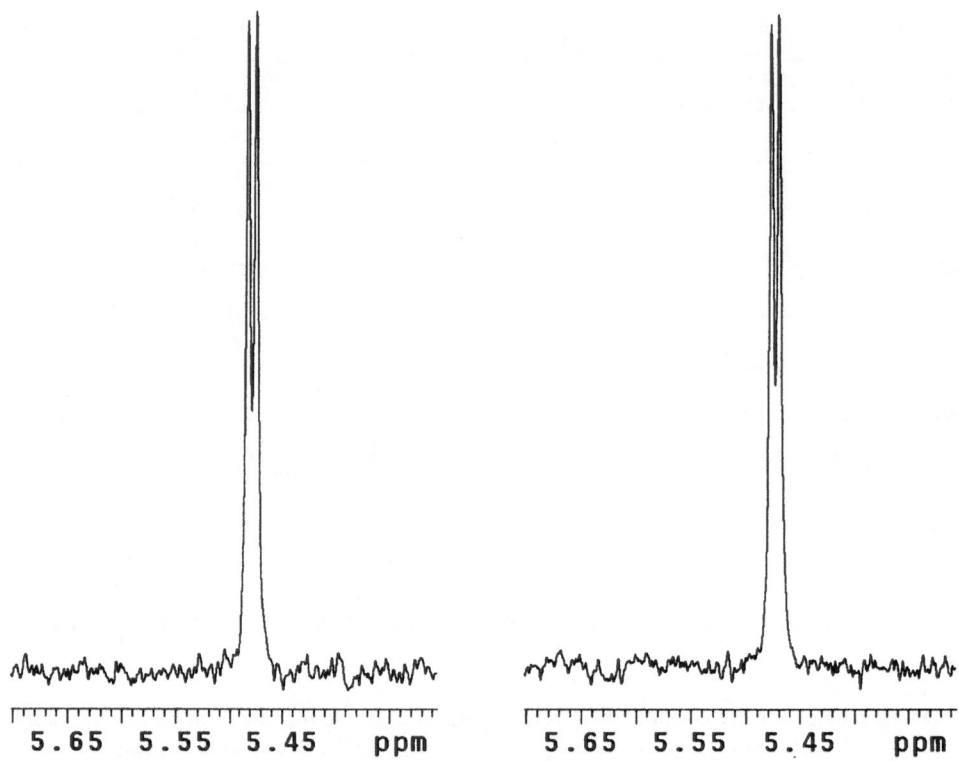

Fig. 16
Interchangeable flow cell (IFC) probe data. Both spectra were acquired in one scan each on 2 mM sucrose in D_2O using a 60 µl H{C,N} PFG IFC probe. In the left-hand spectrum the sucrose solution was contained in a standard flow cell. In the right-hand spectrum the sucrose solution was contained in a 3-mm tube. (The 3-mm tube was placed in the same IFC probe, but only after the flow cell was removed. The flow cell was later put back in for other flow-cell applications.) Both spectra were acquired under otherwise identical conditions (both nonspin) and plotted with identical vertical scales.

3.7.2 Microcoils

Another probe development is the use of small-scale microcoils for data acquisition on very small-scale samples. Pioneered by Sweedler and Webb at the University of Illinois starting in 1994 [221], microcoil NMR spectroscopy allows data to be acquired on samples ranging in size from approximately one microliter down to one nanoliter [222–224]. The primary justification is to support flow-NMR applications such as the NMR analysis of capillary HPLC and capillary electrophoresis effluents [225]. The biggest problem in using microcoils is dealing with the magnetic susceptibility interfaces [223], although probes capable of acquiring two-dimensional indirect-detection data have recently been generated [226]. Other groups have also worked on capillary-scale NMR [227].

3.7.3 IFC – interchangeable-flow-cell probes

One common problem with flow NMR is that after the probe has been used for thousands of samples, the sample cell can become contaminated. One of the first symptoms of a contaminated sample cell is that the quality of solvent suppression becomes degraded. This presumably occurs because the contaminants create a magnetic-susceptibility distortion that degrades the NMR lineshape. Efforts to rigorously wash the cell are sometimes successful, but not always. In these situations it is advantageous to allow a user to change the flow cell themselves. This capability has now become available with Varian's new interchangeable flow cell (IFC) probes.

An IFC probe design allows users to change the flow cell by themselves, as well as to acquire NMR data without the flow cell in place. In the latter situation (when the flow cell is removed) the probe behaves as a microprobe. (The standard 60-µl flow-cell probe can be configured to be a 3-mm microprobe. The 120-µl flow-cell probe can be configured to be a 4-mm microprobe.) This dual-purpose nature of the IFC probes not only allows a user to service their own flow probe, but allows the probe to still be a fully functional high-resolution probe, even if a new clean flow cell is not available (Fig. 16).

4   Software tools

The last decade has seen the introduction of a number of powerful software tools to massage and analyze data. One of the most well-known is digital signal processing (DSP). There are actually a number of DSP techniques, some of which use additional (embedded) hardware processors, but all of them use low-pass filters to enhance spectral signal-to-noise (through oversampling) and to reduce data sizes [228]. In a related DSP technique, software containing high-pass DSP filters (or notch filters) are now being used to eliminate unwanted solvent resonances [46, 229]. Another tool is linear prediction, which is now routinely available and is commonly used to flatten baselines and remove broad resonances [230].

A number of more specialized software tools have also become available. Bayesian analysis software is facilitating quantitative analyses by providing a more powerful and statistically meaningful form of spectral deconvolution [231, 232]. FRED analysis software is providing automated interpretation of a number of kinds of homonuclear and heteronuclear datasets [162, 233]. As an example, FRED has helped analyze INADEQUATE data to provide the complete carbon skeletons of unknown molecules both automatically and with higher effective signal-to-noise [161]. ACD software [234] is not only generating organic structures from 1D ^{1}H and ^{13}C data, but is also helping analyze NMR data acquired on combinatorial-chemistry libraries [214]. The filter diagonalization method (FDM) shows promise for very rapid 2D data acquisition and improved spectral resolution (and possibly reduced data storage requirements) [235, 236]. This too should prove useful for combinatorial chemistry.

5   Other techniques and applications

5.1   SAR-by-NMR

Rational-drug-design programs have also been exploring other new techniques [237]. In 1996, a group at Abbott Laboratories published the first in a series of articles about a technique called "SAR-by-NMR" [238]. SAR, or structure activity relationship mapping, has been an integral part of drug discovery for years, but SAR-by-NMR uses NMR chemical-shift changes to map ligand binding. This is accomplished by first acquiring a ^{1}H{^{15}N} 2D HSQC correlation dataset on an ^{15}N-labeled receptor (a protein) and assigning the correlations. The experiment is then repeated on a series of samples made by adding different ligands (small molecules) to aliquots of this receptor solution. If the ligand does not bind to the receptor, the HSQC spectrum will remain unchanged. If the ligand does bind to the receptor, individual ^{1}H-^{15}N correlations within the spectrum will change positions, with the largest changes usually occurring for those nuclei that are closest to the active site of the receptor. (The ligand is not ^{15}N labeled and thus will not appear in a ^{1}H{^{15}N} HSQC spectrum.) A map of the active site of the receptor is obtained by correlating the resonances that change position with the structures of the ligands. A number of reports have appeared documenting the use of this technique [220, 239, 240]. One of the drawbacks of this technique, however, is that it requires the use of a significant amount of purified ^{15}N-labeled protein to study a number of ligand:receptor complexes.

The SAR-by-NMR technique requires the acquisition of a large number of essentially identical 2D NMR spectra. Because it is such a repetitive technique, it is desirable to employ automated techniques for handling the samples and acquiring the data. Both conventional automated NMR sample changers and DI-NMR systems have been used. The advantages of a DI-NMR system are that it can be programmed to prepare the samples, and it uses less sample than is required by a 5-mm tube. The advantages of using a robot based upon 5-mm tubes are that it will not be affected by sample precipitation and it has no carryover from sample-to-sample.

5.2 The analysis of mixtures: diffusion-ordered and relaxation-ordered experiments

NMR spectroscopy is not usually thought of as a tool for studying mixtures. From a historical point of view, solution-state NMR has always focused on the bulk properties of the solution. Few attempts were ever made to resolve the individual components of mixtures, except for LC-NMR. The following methods show that this is changing.

5.2.1 Mixtures: diffusion-ordered spectroscopy (DOSY)

Diffusion-ordered spectroscopy, or DOSY, is the most well-known method for analyzing mixtures intact. DOSY uses PFG to separate compounds based upon their diffusion rates. Diffusion rates have been measured for years by using PFG [97], but Johnson and coworkers showed in a series of articles starting in 1992 how the diffusion rates could also be used as a separations tool

[241, 242]. Their developments stimulated similar research by a number of other groups [243–245]. DOSY data are usually presented as a 2D dataset where F_2 is the ^1H chemical-shift axis and F_1 is the diffusion-rate axis. Compounds having different diffusion rates are separated along F_1. Multiple components within a 5-mm tube have been separated [246]. The technique can also be combined with other experiments, and extended to multiple dimensions, to create COSY-DOSY [247], DOSY-TOCSY [248], DOSY-NOESY [249], ^{13}C-detected INEPT-DOSY and DEPT-DOSY [250] and DOSY-HMQC [251], among others [242].

5.2.2 Mixtures: affinity NMR

A number of closely related techniques have been published by Shapiro and co-workers. They combined a PFG diffusion sequence (the standard longitudinal encode and decode (LED) sequence [252]) with 2D TOCSY to create what they call "diffusion encoded spectroscopy" (DECODES) [98–100]. This technique resolves mixtures that suffer from either extensive chemical-shift overlap (which is resolved using the diffusion filter) or from similar diffusion coefficients for each component (which is resolved using TOCSY) but not both simultaneously. Multiple 2D TOCSY datasets are acquired, each with a different diffusion delay. The peak intensities of the TOCSY-resolved resonances are plotted against the diffusion delay to identify different chemical species in solution.

This group also developed a variation of this technique called "affinity NMR". In affinity NMR an unlabeled receptor is added to a mixture of ligands and a 1D or 2D DECODES spectrum is acquired [253]. If the diffusion delay is set long enough, only the resonances of the receptor and the bound ligands are visible. The TOCSY component then helps to resolve the chemical shifts of the detected (actively bound) individual components. A NOESY-based version of this diffusion-filtered technique has also been developed [254]. It is claimed that an advantage of this method over SAR-by-NMR is that binding is detected by the observation of the ligand resonances and not by changes in the receptor resonances [100]. More recently, isotope-editing sequence elements were added to suppress the NMR signals from the receptor and to eliminate signals from the nonbinding ligands [255].

5.2.3 Mixtures: relaxation-ordered experiments

A third method for analyzing mixtures is relaxation-edited, relaxation-resolved, or relaxation-ordered NMR spectroscopy. Large molecules have longer rotational correlation times than small molecules, and this results in shorter T_2 relaxation times (and larger NMR linewidths). These differences in T_2 relaxation can be used to edit the NMR spectrum of a mixture, based upon the different relaxation rates of the individual components, in a manner analogous to diffusion ordering or diffusion editing [256–259]. A combined "diffusion and relaxation edited experiment" (DIRE) has been used to analyze biofluids [258].

5.3 Combination experiments – Part 2

The strength of LC-NMR is that it uses a chromatography column to separate mixtures into individual chromatographic peaks. The limitation of this technique is that no single combination of mobile phase and column can completely resolve all compounds, and a single chromatographic peak may still contain multiple components. This overlap can still be resolved by time-slicing if the individual components have even slightly different chemical shifts (Fig. 8), but only if the compounds and their chemical-shift assignments are already known in advance [207]. The hyphenated technique LC-DOSY-NMR would be a powerful way to analyze a mixture using as many as three different physical characteristics (retention time, diffusion rate and chemical shift). This experiment has not yet been performed, and the limited sample quantities used in LC-NMR may preclude its success, but it remains an intriguing idea. Similarly, DI-NMR and FIA-NMR currently have no easy way to resolve a mixture, yet it would be nice to be able to use NMR to determine if a sample is a mixture or not. The DOSY or DECODES techniques may prove quite useful in this regard.

Another interesting application is saturation-transfer-difference (STD) NMR. A target receptor protein is bound to a SPS resin, which is swollen in solvent. A mixture of ligands is added to the resin slurry. A normal spectrum of the slurry is acquired. A second spectrum is acquired during which the resonances of the protein are saturated. This second spectrum only shows unbound ligands, since the bound ligands are saturated by saturation transfer from the protein. A difference spectrum of the two spectra will now show only the bound ligands. Because the resin slurry is a heterogeneous sample, the use of MAS is required. The combined technique is called HR-MAS STD NMR [260].

5.4   Quantification

Sometimes NMR information is used simply for qualitative analyses, but the desire to obtain quantitative information from NMR is growing rapidly, especially for high-throughput techniques like combinatorial chemistry. This seems to arise in part from the difficulties encountered in performing accurate quantification with mass spectrometric techniques, especially for samples still bound to SPS resin beads [261]. NMR data can be very quantitative as long as certain precautions are observed [262, 263]. The biggest precaution is to ensure that complete relaxation has taken place, but other important precautions include the need to use broadbanded excitation, to generate flat baselines, to minimize spectral overlap and to minimize NOE interferences [264].

Internal standards are also an important aspect of quantification. There appears to be no one perfect internal standard. Some standards are too volatile to give reliable signals (for example, TMS) while some standards are too involatile to be removed from the sample after measurement (like TSP). Standards have been shown to sometimes interact with the glass sample container [265]. A good standard should exhibit minimal spectral overlap with the signals of interest. This has prompted the use of signals that are sharp singlet resonances (like TMS, TSP, HMDS, or CHCl3), yet such resonances often exhibit painfully long T_1 relaxation rates. The compound 2,5-dimethylfuran has been proposed as an internal standard because the integral ratio of the two resonances can be used to verify complete relaxation [266]. We demonstrated the utility of using HMDS (hexamethyl disiloxane) as an internal standard for DI-NMR, both for quantification and for verifying the reliability of an injection (Fig. 17) [49]. Others have demonstrated recently the use of incorporating an ^{19}F nucleus into a SPS resin to serve as an internal quantification standard for ^{19}F Nanoprobe NMR [267].

200

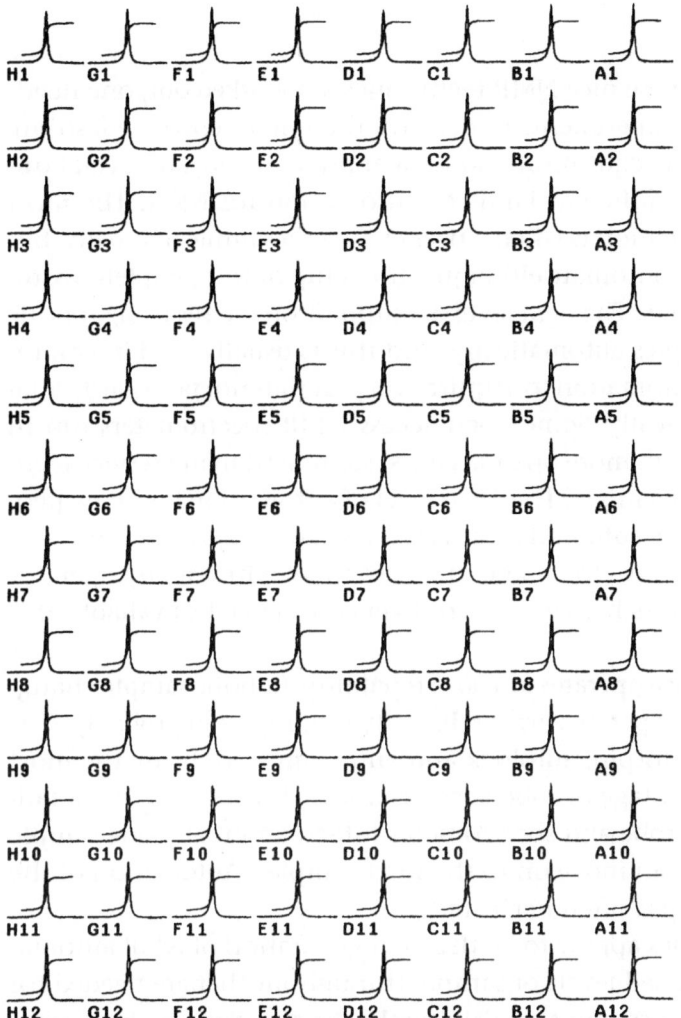

Fig. 17
VAST reproducibility data. This figure shows one way to document the reproducibility of peak height, lineshape and peak area during DI-NMR automation. Each of the 96 spectra is a plot of one resonance from an internal standard placed in each of 96 different samples stored in a 96-well (8 × 12) microtiter plate. The concentration of the internal standard was constant across the plate, as were the NMR acquisition, processing and plotting parameters. The well-to-well consistency of the data is a measure of the consistency of automated sample injection, gradient shimming and NMR acquisition using VAST. The alphanumeric label for each well is also plotted. (Each spectrum is a 75-Hz wide plot of the olefinic resonance of caffeine (at 7.9 ppm) dissolved in DMSO-h_6. Each spectrum was acquired with VAST automation using ^{1}H gradient shimming and 32-scan acquisitions and was plotted in an absolute intensity mode.)

5.5 Automation

Of course, once all of these nice NMR techniques are worked out, one needs a way to automate the experiments to perform them in a repetitive fashion. This includes both data acquisition and data analysis. There are several different levels and many different kinds of automation for NMR. The most primitive level of automation is when a user changes a sample manually, but uses software macros to automate either just the setup or the complete acquisition of multiple datasets. The next level of automation entails using robotic devices to change samples automatically, and this is usually used in combination with software automation to acquire and plot (but not necessarily analyze) the data automatically. Some open-access NMR spectrometers run in this latter mode, although more open-access systems and many service facilities run in a very manual mode. The ideal level of automation for many people, however, is complete automation; this is a system that prepares the sample, acquires the data, stores them and analyzes them without any operator intervention. Although such a system is not yet commercially available, it is a goal for many users.

No automation device operates at 100% reliability. Robotic sample changers that use 5-mm tubes operate with a reliability ranging from probably 75% up to 99%, with the autospin, autolock and autoshim steps being the most failure-prone. The advantage of tube-based robotics, however, is that a failure always leaves the probe and spectrometer intact, and if any one sample fails, the spectrometer can move on to the next sample. (Automation of the sample-preparation step is often neglected.)

Flow NMR techniques appear to be the next generation of NMR automation devices. The increased levels of sample throughput that are needed for modern drug-discovery programs are driving the development of these more robust methods of NMR automation. Flow NMR techniques (Varian's DI-NMR VAST system in particular) are designed to avoid the failure-probe steps of 5-mm operation. This has pushed reliability up to at least 99.9%, and this is important when thousands of samples are being analyzed. One advantage of DI-NMR is that sample preparation is minimal. An often-forgotten limitation of DI-NMR, however, is that dirty samples (those that contain precipitates, solids, emulsions, or immiscible mixtures) can clog up flow cells and degrade NMR lineshapes and solvent-suppression performance. Because of this limitation, DI-NMR is probably not optimized for use in open-access environments. Tube-based NMR spectrometers – or FIA-NMR – are more appropriate for open-access applications, or for the automated analysis of samples that have not undergone basic preparation such as filtration.

6 Conclusion

In conclusion, it seems appropriate to reflect upon the dual nature of NMR spectroscopy. NMR can be used for both research and analytical applications. It started off as a research tool, and it continues to serve in that role; however, there is a growing emphasis on its role as an analytical tool. Many aspects of drug discovery are depending more heavily upon repetitive analyses, and the current desire to develop more automation and increase the level of high-throughput will probably only intensify. The high cost of NMR instrumentation, and the expertise required to operate it, have previously precluded NMR from being used as a routine analytical tool. Many NMR spectroscopists hope, however, that one day benchtop NMR spectrometers will be readily available to all chemists.

Acknowledgements

I would like to thank Jim Shoolery, Steve Smallcombe, Karen Salomon and Evan Williams for their guidance and technical assistance, and Layne Howard, Ron Haner, Justine Lee, Chris Kellogg, and Igor Goljer (all of Varian Associates) for their contributions. I am indebted to Vera Mainz for the opportunities she provided, and to both Kellie and Kayla Keifer for their invaluable assistance.

References

1   J.T. Arnold, S.S. Dharmatti and M.E. Packard: J. Chem. Phys. *19*, 507 (1951).
2   E.M. Purcell, H.C. Torrey and R.V. Pound: Phys. Rev. *69*, 37 (1946).
3   F. Bloch, W.W. Hansen and M. Packard: Phys. Rev. *69*, 127 (1946).
4   I.H. Sadler: Natural Products Reports *101* (1988).
5   C.J. Turner: Prog. Nucl. Magn. Reson. Spectrosc. *16*, 311 (1984).
6   R.R. Ernst and W.A. Anderson: Rev. Sci. Instrum. *37*, 93 (1966).

7   R. Freeman and G.A. Morris: Bull. Magn. Reson. *1*, 5 (1979).
8   G.E. Martin and A.S. Zektzer: Two-dimensional NMR methods for establishing molecular connectivity, VCH, New York, NY 1988.
9   D.L. Turner: In: J.W. Emsley, J. Feeney and L.H. Sutcliffe (eds.): Progress in nuclear magnetic resonance spectroscopy, Pergamon Press Inc., Elmsford, NY 1985, 281–358.
10   J.N. Shoolery: J. Nat. Prod. *47*, 226 (1984).
11   C. Griesinger, O.W. Soerensen and R.R. Ernst: J. Magn. Reson. *84*, 14 (1989).
12   H. Oschkinat, T. Mueller and T. Dieckmann: Angew. Chem. Int. Ed. Engl. *33*, 277 (1994).
13   G.M. Clore and A.M. Gronenborn: Science *252*, 1390 (1991).
14   A.J. Shaka: In: D.M. Grant and R.K. Harris (eds.): Encyclopedia of nuclear magnetic resonance, John Wiley & Sons, Ltd., West Sussex, England 1996, 1558–1564.
15   D.D. Traficante: Concepts Magn. Reson. *3*, 13 (1991).
16   A.J. Shaka, J. Keeler, T. Frenkiel and R. Freeman: J. Magn. Reson. *52*, 335 (1983).
17   M.H. Levitt and R. Freeman: J. Magn. Reson. *43*, 502 (1981).
18   A.J. Shaka, P.B. Barker and R. Freeman: J. Magn. Reson. *64*, 547 (1985).
19   A.J. Shaka, C.J. Lee and A. Pines: J. Magn. Reson. *77*, 274 (1988).
20   A.J. Shaka and J. Keeler: Prog. Nucl. Magn. Reson. Spectrosc. *19*, 47 (1987).
21   M.H. Levitt, R. Freeman and T. Frenkiel: Adv. Magn. Reson. *11*, 47 (1983).
22   T. Fujiwara, T. Anai, N. Kurihara and K. Nagayama: J. Magn. Reson. A *104*, 103 (1993).
23   E. Kupce and R. Freeman: J. Magn. Reson. A *115*, 273 (1995).
24   M.R. Bendall: J. Magn. Reson. A *112*, 126 (1995).
25   M.S. Silver, R.I. Joseph and D.I. Hoult: J. Magn. Reson. *59*, 347 (1984).
26   A.A. Bothner-By, R.L. Stephens, J.M. Lee, C.D. Warren and R.W. Jeanloz: J. Am. Chem. Soc. *106*, 811 (1984).
27   A. Bax and D.G. Davis: J. Magn. Reson. *63*, 207 (1985).
28   H. Kessler, C. Griesinger, R. Kerssebaum, K. Wagner and R.R. Ernst: J. Am. Chem. Soc. *109*, 607 (1987).
29   L. Braunschweiler and R.R. Ernst: J. Magn. Reson. *53*, 521 (1983).
30   A. Bax and D.G. Davis: J. Magn. Reson. *65*, 355 (1985).
31   E. Kupce, P. Schmidt, M. Rance and G. Wagner: J. Magn. Reson. *135*, 361 (1998).
32   S. Mattila, A.M.P. Koskinen and G. Otting: J. Magn. Reson. *109*, 326 (1995).
33   G.G. McDonald and J.S. Leigh, Jr.: J. Magn. Reson. *9*, 358 (1973).
34   B.A. Messerle, G. Wider, G. Otting, C. Weber and K. Wuethrich: J. Magn. Reson. *85*, 608 (1989).
35   G. Wider, R.V. Hosur and K. Wuthrich: J. Magn. Reson. *52*, 130 (1983).
36   L. Emsley: In: D.M. Grant and R.K. Harris (eds.): Encyclopedia of nuclear magnetic resonance, John Wiley & Sons, Ltd., West Sussex, England 1996, 4228–4236.
37   W.S. Warren and S.M. Mayr: In: D.M. Grant and R.K. Harris (eds.): Encyclopedia of nuclear magnetic resonance, John Wiley & Sons, Ltd., West Sussex, England 1996, 4275–4283.
38   F.A.L. Anet and A.J.R. Bourn: J. Am. Chem. Soc. *87*, 5250 (1965).
39   H. Kessler, H. Oschkinat, C. Griesinger and W. Bermel: J. Magn. Reson. *70*, 106 (1986).
40   K. Stott, J. Keeler, Q.N. Van and A.J. Shaka: J. Magn. Reson. *125*, 302 (1997).
41   K. Stott, J. Stonehouse, J. Keeler, T-L. Hwang and A.J. Shaka: J. Am. Chem. Soc. *117*, 4199 (1995).
42   T. Facke and S. Berger: Magn. Reson. Chem. *33*, 144 (1995).
43   S. Berger: J. Magn. Reson. *81*, 561 (1989).

44   R.C. Crouch and G.E. Martin: J. Magn. Reson. *92*, 189 (1991).
45   S. Berger: Angew. Chem. *100*, 1198 (1988).
46   S.H. Smallcombe: J. Am. Chem. Soc. *115*, 4776 (1993).
47   H. Liu, K. Weisz and T.L. James: J. Magn. Reson. A *105*, 184 (1993).
48   S.H. Smallcombe, S.L. Patt and P.A. Keifer: J. Magn. Reson. A *117*, 295 (1995).
49   P.A. Keifer, S.H. Smallcombe, E.H. Williams, K.E. Salomon, G. Mendez, J.L. Belletire and C.D. Moore: J. Comb. Chem. *2*, 151 (2000).
50   D.H. Live and K. Greene: J. Magn. Reson. *85*, 604 (1989).
51   R. Freeman: Chem. Rev. *91*, 1397 (1991).
52   A.C. Wang, S. Grzesiek, R. Tschudin, P.J. Lodi and A. Bax: J. Biomol. NMR *5*, 376 (1995).
53   M.A. McCoy and L. Mueller: J. Magn. Reson. A *101*, 122 (1993).
54   M.A. McCoy and L. Mueller: J. Am. Chem. Soc. *114*, 2108 (1992).
55   M.R. Bendall: J. Magn. Reson. A *116*, 46 (1995).
56   T.-L. Hwang, P.C.M. Van Zijl and M. Garwood: J. Magn. Reson. *138*, 173 (1999).
57   M. Garwood and Y. Ke: J. Magn. Reson. *94*, 511 (1991).
58   T-L. Hwang, P.C.M. Van Zijl and M. Garwood: J. Magn. Reson. *133*, 200 (1998).
59   S.L. Patt: J. Magn. Reson. *96*, 94 (1992).
60   G.E. Martin and R.C. Crouch: J. Nat. Prod. *54*, 1 (1991).
61   L. Mueller: J. Am. Chem. Soc. *101*, 4481 (1979).
62   A. Bax, M. Ikura, L.E. Kay, D.A. Torchia and R. Tschudin: J. Magn. Reson. *86*, 304 (1990).
63   W.F. Reynolds, S. McLean, L-L. Tay, M. Yu, R.G. Enriquez, D.M. Estwick and K.O. Pascoe: Magn. Reson. Chem. *35*, 455 (1997).
64   K.L. Rinehart, T.G. Holt, N.L. Fregeau, J.G. Stroh, P.A. Keifer, F. Sun, L.H. Li and D.G. Martin: J. Org. Chem. *55*, 4512 (1990).
65   R. Mukherjee, B.A. Da Silva, B.C. Das, P.A. Keifer and J.N. Shoolery: Heterocycles *32*, 985 (1991).
66   R. Mukherjee, B.C. Das, P.A. Keifer and J.N. Shoolery: Heterocycles *38*, 1965 (1994).
67   P. Crews, J.J. Farias, R. Emrich and P.A. Keifer: J. Org. Chem. *59*, 2932 (1994).
68   H.C. Vervoort, W. Fenical and P.A. Keifer: J. Nat. Prod. *62*, 389 (1999).
69   P.C. Lauterbur: Nature (London) *242*, 190 (1973).
70   P. Barker and R. Freeman: J. Magn. Reson. *64*, 334 (1985).
71   R.E. Hurd: J. Magn. Reson. *87*, 422 (1990).
72   R.E. Hurd, B.K. John and H.D. Plant: J. Magn. Reson. *93*, 666 (1991).
73   J. Boyd, N. Soffe, B.K. John, D. Plant and R.E. Hurd: J. Magn. Reson. *98*, 660 (1992).
74   S.K. Sarkar: Curr. Sci. *61*, 331 (1991).
75   W.S. Price: In: G.A. Webb (ed.): Annual reports on NMR spectroscopy, Vol. 32, Academic Press, New York, NY 1996, 51–142.
76   P.L. Rinaldi and P. Keifer: J. Magn. Reson. *108*, 259 (1994).
77   A.S. Altieri, K.E. Miller and R.A. Byrd: Magn. Reson. Rev. *17*, 27 (1996).
78   R. Warrass, J.-M. Wieruszeski and G. Lippens: J. Am. Chem. Soc. *121*, 3787 (1999).
79   M.J. Shapiro, J. Chin, A. Chen, J.R. Wareing, Q. Tang, R.A. Tommasi and H.R. Marepalli: Tetrahedron Lett. *40*, 6141 (1999).
80   A.L. Davis, J. Keeler, E.D. Laue and D. Moskau: J. Magn. Reson. *98*, 207 (1992).
81   J. Ruiz-Cabello, G.W. Vuister, C.T.W. Moonen and P.C.M. Van Zijl: J. Magn. Reson. *100*, 282 (1992).
82   J.R. Tolman, J. Chung and J.H. Prestegard: J. Magn. Reson. *98*, 462 (1992).
83   S. Sheng and H. Van Halbeek: J. Magn. Reson. *130*, 296 (1998).

84   R. Wagner and S. Berger: Magn. Reson. Chem. *36*, S44 (1998).

85   G.E. Martin, C.E. Hadden, R.C. Crouch and V.V. Krishnamurthy: Magn. Reson. Chem. *37*, 517 (1999).

86   V.V. Krishnamurthy: J. Magn. Reson. *121*, 33 (1996).

87   R. Marek, L. Kralik and V. Sklenar: Tetrahedron Lett. *38*, 665 (1997).

88   K. Furihata and H. Seto: Tetrahedron Lett. *39*, 7337 (1998).

89   C.E. Hadden, G.E. Martin and V.V. Krishnamurthy: J. Magn. Reson. *140*, 274 (1999).

90   B. Reif, M. Koeck, R. Kerssebaum, J. Schleucher and C. Griesinger: J. Magn. Reson. *112*, 295 (1996).

91   B. Reif, M. Kock, R. Kerssebaum, H. Kang, W. Fenical and C. Griesinger: J. Magn. Reson. *118*, 282 (1996).

92   L. Kay, P. Keifer and T. Saarinen: J. Am. Chem. Soc. *114*, 10663 (1992).

93   M. Von Kienlin, C.T.W. Moonen, A. Van der Toorn and P.C.M. Van Zijl: J. Magn. Reson. *93*, 423 (1991).

94   A.A. Shaw, C. Salaun, J.-F. Dauphin and B. Ancian: J. Magn. Reson. A *120*, 110 (1996).

95   S.L. MacKinnon, P. Keifer and W.A. Ayer: Phytochemistry *51*, 215 (1999).

96   D. Uhrin and P.N. Barlow: J. Magn. Reson. *126*, 248 (1997).

97   E.O. Stejskal and J.E. Tanner: J. Chem. Phys. *42*, 288 (1965).

98   M. Lin and M.J. Shapiro: J. Org. Chem. *61*, 7617 (1996).

99   M. Lin, M.J. Shapiro and J.R. Wareing: J. Am. Chem. Soc. *119*, 5249 (1997).

100   M. Lin, M.J. Shapiro and J.R. Wareing: J. Org. Chem. *62*, 8930 (1997).

101   P.C.M. Van Zijl and C.T.W. Moonen: J. Magn. Reson. *87*, 18 (1990).

102   M. Piotto, V. Saudek and V. Sklenar: J. Biomol. NMR *2*, 661 (1992).

103   R.M. Holt, M.J. Newman, F.S. Pullen, D.S. Richards and A.G. Swanson: J. Mass. Spectrom. *32*, 64 (1997).

104   W.J. Ehlhardt, J.M. Woodland, T.M. Baughman, M. Vandenbranden, S.A. Wrighton, J.S. Kroin, B.H. Norman and S.R. Maple: Drug Metab. Dispos. *26*, 42 (1998).

105   H. Barjat, P.B. Chilvers, B.K. Fetler, T.J. Horne and G.A. Morris: J. Magn. Reson. *125*, 197 (1997).

106   S. Sukumar, M.O-N. Johnson, R.E. Hurd and P.C.M. Van Zijl: J. Magn. Reson. *125*, 159 (1997).

107   J.E. Meier and A.G. Marshall: In: L.J. Berliner and J. Reuben (eds.):Biological magnetic resonance, Vol 9, Plenum Press, New York, NY 1990, 199–240.

108   M. Gueron, P. Plateau and M. Decorps: Prog. Nucl. Magn. Reson. Spectrosc. *23*, 135 (1991).

109   M. Gueron and P. Plateau: In: D.M. Grant and R.K. Harris (eds.):Encyclopedia of nuclear magnetic resonance, John Wiley & Sons, Ltd., West Sussex, England 1996, 4931–4942.

110   G.M. Clore and A.M. Gronenborn: NMR of proteins, CRC Press, Ann Arbor, MI 1993.

111   G. Wagner: Prog. Nucl. Magn. Reson. Spectrosc. *22*, 101 (1990).

112   K. Wuthrich: NMR of proteins and nucleic acids, John Wiley and Sons, New York, NY 1986.

113   L.E. Kay, M. Ikura, R. Tschudin and A. Bax: J. Magn. Reson. *89*, 496 (1990).

114   M. Ikura, L.E. Kay and A. Bax: Biochemistry 29, *4659* (1990).

115   A.M. Gronenborn and G.M. Clore: Anal. Chem. *62*, 2 (1990).

116   G. Wider: Prog. Nucl. Magn. Reson. Spectrosc. *32*, 193 (1998).

117   C. Biamonti, C.B. Rios, B.A. Lyons and G.T. Montelione: Adv. Biophys. Chem. *4*, 51 (1994).

118   G.T. Montelione and G. Wagner: J. Am. Chem. Soc. *111*, 5474 (1989).
119   T.J. Norwood, J. Boyd, J.E. Heritage, N. Soffe and I.D. Campbell: J. Magn. Reson. *87*, 488 (1990).
120   S. Grzesiek, J. Anglister, H. Ren and A. Bax: J. Am. Chem. Soc. *115*, 4369 (1993).
121   R.A. Venters, W.J. Metzler, L.D. Spicer, L. Mueller and B.T. Farmer, II: J. Am. Chem. Soc. *117*, 9592 (1995).
122   M. Sattler and S.W. Fesik: Structure (London) *4*, 1245 (1996).
123   D. Nietlispach, R.T. Clowes, R.W. Broadhurst, Y. Ito, J. Keeler, M. Kelly, J. Ashurst, H. Oschkinat, P.J. Domaille and E.D. Laue: J. Am. Chem. Soc. *118*, 407 (1996).
124   M. Salzmann, K. Pervushin, G. Wider, H. Senn and K. Wuthrich: Proc. Natl. Acad. Sci. USA *95*, 13585 (1998).
125   D. Yang and L.E. Kay: J. Biomol. NMR *13*, 3 (1999).
126   K. Pervushin, R. Riek, G. Wider and K. Wuthrich: J. Am. Chem. Soc. *120*, 6394 (1998).
127   J. Weigelt: J. Am. Chem. Soc. *120*, 10778 (1998).
128   M. Ikura and A. Bax: J. Am. Chem. Soc. *114*, 2433 (1992).
129   C. Zwahlen, P. Legault, S.J.F. Vincent, J. Greenblatt, R. Konrat and L.E. Kay: J. Am. Chem. Soc. *119*, 6711 (1997).
130   K. Pervushin, A. Ono, C. Fernandez, T. Szyperski, M. Lainosho and K. Wuthrich: Proc. Natl. Acad. Sci. USA *95*, 14147 (1998).
131   A.J. Dingley and S. Grzesiek: J. Am. Chem. Soc. *120*, 8293 (1998).
132   F. Cordier and S. Grzesiek: J. Am. Chem. Soc. *121*, 1601 (1999).
133   G. Cornilescu, J.-S. Hu and A. Bax: J. Am. Chem. Soc. *121*, 2949 (1999).
134   A.J. Dingley, J.E. Masse, R.D. Peterson, M. Barfield, J. Feigon and S. Grzesiek: J. Am. Chem. Soc. *121*, 6019 (1999).
135   N. Tjandra, J.G. Omichinski, A.M. Gronenborn, G.M. Clore and A. Bax: Nat. Struct. Biol. *4*, 732 (1997).
136   N. Tjandra and A. Bax: Science (Washington, DC) *278*, 1111 (1997).
137   N. Tjandra, S. Grzesiek and A. Bax: J. Am. Chem. Soc. *118*, 6264 (1996).
138   A. Bax, K.A. Farley and G.S. Walker: J. Magn. Reson. *119*, 134 (1996).
139   K. Furihata and H. Seto: Tetrahedron Lett. *37*, 8901 (1996).
140   R. Wagner and S. Berger: J. Magn. Reson. *120*, 258 (1996).
141   K. Stott and J. Keeler: Magn. Reson. Chem. *34*, 554 (1996).
142   C. Emetarom, T-L. Hwang, G. Mackin and A.J. Shaka: J. Magn. Reson. *115*, 137 (1995).
143   Q.N. Van and A.J. Shaka: J. Magn. Reson. *132*, 154 (1998).
144   V.V. Krishnamurthy: Magn. Reson. Chem. *35*, 9 (1997).
145   A. Kaerner and D.L. Rabenstein: Magn. Reson. Chem. *36*, 601 (1998).
146   D. Klein, J.C. Braekman, D. Daloze, L. Hoffman, G. Castillo and V. Demoulin: Tetrahedron Lett. *40*, 695 (1999).
147   R.C. Crouch, A.O. Davis, T.D. Spitzer, G.E. Martin, M.H.M. Sharaf, P.L. Schiff, Jr., C.H. Phoebe, Jr. and A.N. Tackie: J. Heterocycl. Chem. *32*, 1077 (1995).
148   R.C. Crouch and G.E. Martin: J. Nat. Prod. *55*, 1343 (1992).
149   J.N. Shoolery: Top Carbon-13 NMR Spectrosc. *3*, 28 (1979).
150   J.N. Shoolery and R.E. Majors: Am. Lab. (Fairfield, Conn) *9*, 51 (1977).
151   G.E. Martin, C.E. Hadden, A.N. Tackie, M.H.M. Sharaf and P.L. Schiff, Jr.: Magn. Reson. Chem. *37*, 529 (1999).
152   C.E. Hadden and G.E. Martin: J. Nat. Prod. *61*, 969 (1998).
153   P.A. Keifer: Drug Discovery Today *2*, 468 (1997).

154   P.A. Keifer: Drugs Future *23*, 301 (1998).
155   P.A. Keifer, L. Baltusis, D.M. Rice, A.A. Tymiak and J.N. Shoolery: J. Magn. Reson. A *119*, 65 (1996).
156   C.S. Springer, Jr.: In: R.J. Gillies (ed.): NMR in physiology and biomedicine, Academic Press, San Diego 1994, 75–99.
157   T.M. Barbara: J. Magn. Reson. A *109*, 265 (1994).
158   A. Manzi, P.V. Salimath, R.C. Spiro, P.A. Keifer and H.H. Freeze: J. Biol. Chem. *270*, 9154 (1995).
159   A.E. Manzi and P.A. Keifer: In: R.R. Townsend and A.T. Hotchkiss, Jr. (eds.): Techniques in glycobiology, Marcel Dekker, Inc., New York 1997, 1–16.
160   D. Klein, J.C. Braekman, D. Daloze, L. Hoffman and V. Demoulin: Tetrahedron Lett. *37*, 7519 (1996).
161   D.C. Chauret, T. Durst, J.T. Arnason, P. Sanchez-Vindas, L.S. Roman, L. Poveda and P.A. Keifer: Tetrahedron Lett. *37*, 7875 (1996).
162   J.K. Harper, R. Dunkel, S.G. Wood, N.L. Owen, D. Li, R.G. Cates and D.M. Grant: J. Chem. Soc., Perkin Trans. *21*, 91 (1996).
163   M. Delepierre, A. Prochnicka-Chalufour and L.D. Possani: Biochemistry *36*, 2649 (1997).
164   P. Roux, M. Delepierre, M.E. Goldberg and A.F. Chaffotte: J. Biol. Chem. *272*, 24843 (1997).
165   M. Delepierre, P. Roux, A.F. Chaffotte and M.E. Goldberg: Magn. Reson. Chem. *36*, 645 (1998).
166   M. Delepierre, A. Porchnicka-Chalufour, J. Boisbouvier and L.D. Possani: Biochemistry *38*, 16756 (1999).
167   Gilbert,M., J.-R. Brisson, M.-F. Karwaski, J. Michniewicz, A.-M. Cunningham, Y. Wu, N.M. Young and W.W. Wakarchuk: J. Biol. Chem. *275*, 3896 (2000).
168   P.A. Keifer: Curr. Opin. Biotechnol. *10(1)*, 34 (1999).
169   E.R. Andrew, A. Bradbury and R.G. Eades: Nature *182*, 1659 (1958).
170   D. Doskocilová and B. Schneider: Chem. Phys. Lett. *6*, 381 (1970).
171   D. Doskocilová, D.T. Dang and B. Schneider: Czech J. Phys. B *25*, 202 (1975).
172   L.F. Fuks, F.S.C. Huang, C.M. Carter, W..A. Edelstein and P.B. Roemer: J. Magn. Reson. *100*, 229 (1992).
173   F.O. Zelaya, S. Crozier, S. Dodd, R. McKenna and D.M. Doddrell: J. Magn. Reson. *115*, 131 (1995).
174   F.D. Doty, G. Entzminger and Y.A. Yang: Concepts Magn. Reson. *10(4)*, 239 (1998).
175   R.B. Merrifield: J. Am. Chem. Soc. *85*, 2149 (1963).
176   P.A. Keifer: J. Org. Chem. *61*, 1558 (1996).
177   P.A. Keifer and B. Sehrt: A catalog of ^{1}H NMR spectra of different SPS resins with varying solvents and experimental techniques – an exploration of nano-nmr probe technology, Varian NMR Instruments, Palo Alto, CA 1996.
178   E. Giralt, J. Rizo and E. Pedroso: Tetrahedron *40*, 4141 (1984).
179   R. Epton, P. Goddard and K.J. Ivin: Polymer *21*, 1367 (1980).
180   A. Paio, A. Zaramella, R. Ferritto, N. Conti, C. Marchioro and P. Seneci: J. Comb. Chem. *1*, 317 (1999).
181   J.E. Hochlowski, D.N. Whittern and T.J. Sowin: J. Comb. Chem. *1*, 291 (1999).
182   T. Wehler and J. Westman: Tetrahedron Lett. *37*, 4771 (1996).
183   W.L. Fitch, G. Detre, C.P. Holmes, J.N. Shoolery and P.A. Keifer: J. Org. Chem. *59*, 7955 (1994).

184   S.K. Sarkar, R.S. Garigipati, J.L. Adams and P.A. Keifer: J. Am. Chem. Soc. *118*, 2305 (1996).
185   L.L. Cheng, C.L. Lean, A. Bogdanova, S.C. Wright,Jr., J.L. Ackerman, T.J. Brady and L. Garrido: Magn. Reson. Med. *36*, 653 (1996).
186   L.L. Cheng, M.J. Ma, L. Becerra, T. Ptak, I. Tracey, A. Lackner and R.G. Gonzalez: Proc. Natl. Acad. Sci. USA *94*, 6408 (1997).
187   D.A. Middleton, D.P. Bradley, S.C. Connor, P.G. Mullins and D.G. Reid: Magn. Reson. Med. *40*, 166 (1998).
188   A.M. Tomlins, P.J.D. Foxall, J.C. Lindon, J.K. Nicholson, M.J. Lynch, M. Spraul and J.R. Everett: Anal. Commun. *35*, 113 (1998).
189   K.K. Millis, W.E. Maas, D.G. Cory and S. Singer: Magn. Reson. Med. *38*, 399 (1997).
190   W.C. Hutton, J.R. Garbow and T.R. Hayes: Lipids *34*, 1339 (1999).
191   W.E. Maas, F.H. Laukien and D.G. Cory: J. Am. Chem. Soc. *118*, 13085 (1996).
192   H.C. Dorn: In: D.M. Grant and R.K. Harris (eds.): Encyclopedia of nuclear magnetic resonance, John Wiley & Sons, Ltd., West Sussex, England 1996, 2026–2036.
193   P.A. Keifer: Magn. Reson. Chem. (2000); in press
194   G. Schlotterbeck, L-H. Tseng, H. Haendel, U. Braumann and K. Albert: Anal. Chem. *69*, 1421 (1997).
195   N. Watanabe and E. Niki: Proc. Jpn. Acad. Ser. B *54*, 194 (1978).
196   H.C. Dorn: Anal. Chem. *56*, 747A (1984).
197   K. Albert and E. Bayer: Trends Anal. Chem. *7*, 288 (1988).
198   K. Albert: J. Chromatogr. *703*, 123 (1995).
199   J.C. Lindon, J.K. Nicholson and I.D. Wilson: Adv. Chromatogr. (NY) *36*, 315 (1996).
200   J.C. Lindon, J.K. Nicholson, U.G. Sidelmann and I.D. Wilson: Drug Metab. Rev. *29*, 705 (1997).
201   N. Mistry, I.M. Ismail, M.S. Smith, J.K. Nicholson and J.C. Lindon: J. Pharm. Biomed. Anal. *16*, 697 (1997).
202   J.K. Roberts and R.J. Smith: J. Chromatogr. *677*, 385 (1994).
203   J. Chin, J.B. Fell, M. Jarosinski, M.J. Shapiro and J.R. Wareing: J. Org. Chem. *63*, 386 (1998).
204   K. Hostettmann and J-L. Wolfender: Pestic. Sci. *51*, 471 (1997).
205   B. Vogler, I. Klaiber, G. Roos, C.U. Walter, W. Hiller, P. Sandor and W. Kraus: J. Nat. Prod. *61*, 175 (1998).
206   E. Garo, J.L. Wolfender, K. Hostettmann, W. Hiller, S. Antus and S. Mavi: Helv. Chim. Acta *81*, 754 (1998).
207   K. Albert, G. Schlotterbeck, U. Braumann, H. Haendel, M. Spraul and G. Krack: Angew. Chem. *34*, 1014 (1995).
208   L. Griffiths and R. Horton: Magn. Reson. Chem. *36*, 104 (1998).
209   F.S. Pullen, A.G. Swanson, M.J. Newman and D.S. Richards: Rapid Commun. Mass Spectrom. *9*, 1003 (1995).
210   K.I. Burton, J.R. Everett, M.J. Newman, F.S. Pullen, D.S. Richards and A.G. Swanson: J. Pharm. Biomed. Anal. *15*, 1903 (1997).
211   B.C. Hamper, D.M. Synderman, T.J. Owen, A.M. Scates, D.C. Owsley, A.S. Kesselring and R.C. Chott: J. Comb. Chem. *1*, 140 (1999).
212   D.S. Freedman, J.D. Otvos, E.J. Jeyarajah, J.J. Barboriak, A.J. Anderson and J.A. Walker: Arterioscler. *18*, 1046 (1998).

213   W.H. Gmeiner, W. Cui, D.E. Konerding, P.A. Keifer, S.K. Sharma, A.M. Soto, L.A. Marky and J.W. Lown: J. Biomol. Struct. Dyn. *17*, 507 (1999).

214   A. Williams, S. Bakulin, and S. Golotvin: Poster #2 (NMR prediction software and tube-less NMR – an analytical tool for screening of combinatorial libraries) 1st Annual SMASH Small Molecule NMR Conference, Argonne, IL, Aug 15–18, 1999.

215   P. Styles, N.F. Soffe, C.A. Scott, D.A. Cragg, F. Row, D.J. White and P.C.J. White: J. Magn. Reson. *60*, 397 (1984).

216   H.D.W. Hill: Trans Appl. Supercond. *7*, 3750 (1997).

217   W.A. Anderson, W.W. Brey, A.L. Brooke, B. Cole, K.A. Delin, L.F. Fuks, H.D.W. Hill, M.E. Johanson, V.Y. Kotsubo, R. Nast et al: Bull. Magn. Reson. *17*, 98 (1995).

218   T.A. Logan, N. Murali, G. Wang and C. Jolivet: Magn. Reson. Chem. *37*, 512 (1999).

219   S.D. Hoeltzli and C. Frieden: Biochemistry *37*, 387 (1998).

220   P.J. Hajduk, T. Gerfin, J.-M. Boehlen, M. Haberli, D. Marek and S.W. Fesik: J. Med. Chem. *42*, 2315 (1999).

221   N. Wu, T.L. Peck, A.G. Webb, R.L. Magin and J.V. Sweedler: Anal. Chem. *66*, 3849 (1994).

222   D.L. Olson, M.E. Lacey and J.V. Sweedler: Anal. Chem. *70*, 645 (1998).

223   A.G. Webb: Prog. Nucl. Magn. Reson. Spectrosc. *31*, 1 (1997).

224   D.L. Olson, M.E. Lacey and J.V. Sweedler: Anal. Chem. *70*, 257A (1998).

225   D.L. Olson, M.E. Lacey, A.G. Webb and J.V. Sweedler: Anal. Chem. *71*, 3070 (1999).

226   R. Subramanian, J.V. Sweedler and A.G. Webb: J. Am. Chem. Soc. *121*, 2333 (1999).

227   P. Gfroerer, J. Schewitz, K. Pusecker and E. Bayer: Anal. Chem. *71*, 315A (1999).

228   M.E. Rosen: J. Magn. Reson. A *107*, 119 (1994).

229   D. Marion, M. Ikura and A. Bax: J. Magn. Reson. *84*, 425 (1989).

230   W.F. Reynolds, M. Yu, R.G. Enriquez and I. Leon: Magn. Reson. Chem. *35*, 505 (1997).

231   J.J. Kotyk, N.G. Hoffman, W.C. Hutton, G.L. Bretthorst and J.J.H. Ackerman: J. Magn. Reson. *98*, 483 (1992).

232   J.J. Kotyk, N.G. Hoffman, W.C. Hutton, G.L. Bretthorst and J.J.H. Ackerman: J. Magn. Reson. *116*, 1 (1995).

233   M.P. Foster, C.L. Mayne, R. Dunkel, R.J. Pugmire, D.M. Grant, J.M. Kornprobst, J.F. Verbist, J.F. Biard and C.M. Ireland: J. Am. Chem. Soc. *114*, 1110 (1992).

234   ACD Labs, 133 Richmond St. West, Suite 605, Toronto, Ontario, M5H 2L3, Canada, www.acdlabs.com.

235   V.A. Mandelshtam, H.S. Taylor and A.J. Shaka: J. Magn. Reson. *133*, 304 (1998).

236   V.A. Mandelshtam, H. Hu and A.J. Shaka: Magn. Reson. Chem. *36*, S17 (1998).

237   B.J. Stockman: Prog. Nucl. Magn. Reson. Spectrosc. *33*, 109 (1998).

238   S.B. Shuker, P.J. Hajduk, R.P. Meadows and S.W. Fesik: Science *274*, 1531 (1996).

239   P.J. Hajduk, R.P. Meadows and S.W. Fesik: Science *278*, 497 (1997).

240   H. Kessler: Angew. Chem. *36*, 829 (1997).

241   K.F. Morris and C.S. Johnson, Jr.: J. Am. Chem. Soc. *114*, 3139 (1992).

242   C.S. Johnson,Jr.: Prog. Nucl. Magn. Reson. Spectrosc. *34*, 203 (1999).

243   G.A. Morris and H. Barjat: In: K. Koever, G. Batta and C. Szantay, Jr. (eds.): Methods for structure elucidation by high resolution NMR, Elsevier, Amsterdam 1997, 209–226.

244   N. Birlirakis and E. Guittet: J. Am. Chem. Soc. *118*, 13083 (1996).

245   M.D. Pelta, H. Barjat, G.A. Morris, A.L. Davis and S.J. Hammond: Magn. Reson. Chem. *36*, 706 (1998).

246   H. Barjat, G.A. Morris, S. Smart, A.G. Swanson and S.C.R. Williams: J. Magn. Reson. B *108*, 170 (1995).

247   D. Wu, A. Chen and C.S. Johnson, Jr.: J. Magn. Reson. A *121*, 88 (1996).
248   A. Jerschow and N. Muller: J. Magn. Reson. A *123*, 222 (1996).
249   E.K. Gozansky and D.G. Gorenstein: J. Magn. Reson. B *111*, 94 (1996).
250   D. Wu, A. Chen and C.S. Johnson, Jr.: J. Magn. Reson. A *123*, 215 (1996).
251   H. Barjat, G.A. Morris and A.G. Swanson: J. Magn. Reson. *131*, 131 (1998).
252   S.J. Gibbs and C.S. Johnson, Jr.: J. Magn. Reson. *93*, 395 (1991).
253   A. Chen and M.J. Shapiro: Anal. Chem. *71*, 669A (1999).
254   H. Ponstingl and G. Otting: J. Biomol. NMR *9*, 441 (1997).
255   N. Gonnella, M. Lin, M.J. Shapiro, J.R. Wareing and X. Zhang: J. Magn. Reson. *131*, 336 (1998).
256   D.L. Rabenstein, T. Nakashima and G. Bigam: J. Magn. Reson. *34*, 669 (1979).
257   D.L. Rabenstein, K.K. Millis and E.J. Strauss: Anal. Chem. *60*, 1380A (1988).
258   M. Liu, J.K. Nicholson and J.C. Lindon: Anal. Chem. *68*, 3370 (1996).
259   P.J. Hajduk, E.T. Olejniczak and S.W. Fesik: J. Am. Chem. Soc. *119*, 12257 (1997).
260   J. Klein, R. Meinecke, M. Mayer and B. Meyer: J. Am. Chem. Soc. *121*, 5336 (1999).
261   A.W. Czarnik and S.H. Dewitt: A practical guide to combinatorial chemistry, American Chemical Society, Washington, D.C. 1997.
262   D.L. Rabenstein and D.A. Keire: Pract. Spectrosc. *11*, 323 (1991).
263   U. Holzgrabe, B.W. Diehl and I. Wawer: J. Pharm. Biomed. Anal. *17*, 557 (1998).
264   D.D. Traficante: Concepts Magn. Reson. *4*, 153 (1992).
265   C.K. Larive, D. Jayawickrama and L. Orfi: Appl. Spectrosc. *51*, 1531 (1997).
266   S.W. Gerritz and A.M. Sefler: J. Comb. Chem. *2*, 39 (2000).
267   M. Drew, E. Orton, P. Krolikowski, J.M. Salvino and N.V. Kumar: J. Comb. Chem. *2*, 8 (2000).

Progress in Drug Research, Vol. 55 (E. Jucker, Ed.)
© 2000 Birkhäuser Verlag, Basel (Switzerland)

Prostate cancer and the androgen receptor: Strategies for the development of novel therapeutics

By Laurane G. Mendelsohn

Cancer Research Division
Eli Lilly and Co.
Indianapolis, IN 46285, USA
Email: lgmendelsohn@lilly.com

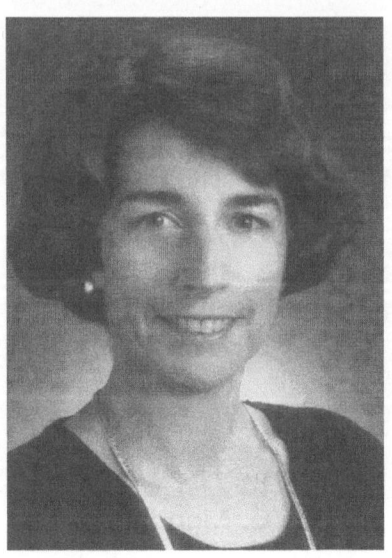

Laurane G. Mendelsohn

obtained a B.S. degree in Chemistry from Syracuse University, Syracuse, N.Y. At the University of Illinois, Champaign Urbana, Ill., she completed a M.S. in Biochemistry in 1971 and a Ph.D. in Biology with a specialization in the Neurosciences in 1974. After postdoctoral studies in enzymology and a fellowship to study Huntington's Disease at the City of Hope in Duarte, Calif., she joined Eli Lilly and Co. in 1979. In the Cancer Research division, her research has focused on developing novel inhibitors of folate-dependent enzymes. More recently, Dr. Mendelsohn has concentrated on developing drugs for the treatment of hormone-refractory prostate cancer. She has published over 50 peer-reviewed papers and seven book chapters. Dr. Mendelsohn is currently a Research Advisor in the Cancer Research Drug Discovery Program at Eli Lilly and Co.

Summary

The early demonstrations that prostate cancer was hormone-sensitive initiated a therapeutic strategy of hormone ablation that is still in use today. Although chemical or surgical castration reduces androgen stimulation of the androgen receptor (AR) and produces tumor regression, little survival benefit is achieved. Patients with metastatic cancer eventually relapse as their tumors progress to hormone independence.

The AR is a member of the steroid receptor family; however, it manifests many unique features including: N-terminal, C-terminal interactions and antiparallel dimerization, unique N-terminal domains for co-factor recruitment, AR-specific co-activators and upstream promoter/enhancer response elements that amplify AR-mediated responses. The AR is regulated by phosphorylation and cross-talk with several signaling pathways, including MAP kinases, PKA and PKC. Non-genomic effects of AR to regulate transcription factors elk-1 and -2 have also been demonstrated. These unique features suggest mechanisms by which novel therapeutics might target and influence AR-mediated actions. Progress in this direction has been realized with the recent synthesis of non-steroidal androgen agonists that may have tissue-selective effects.

Contents

Keywords

Androgen receptor, androgen response element, dihydrotestosterone, hormone-independent prostate cancer, prostate cancer, signal transduction.

Glossary of abbreviations

AF-1, activation function-1 in the N-terminal domain of AR; AF-2, activation function-2 in the C-terminal domain of AR; AI-PCa, androgen-independent prostate cancer; AR, androgen receptor; ARA70, androgen receptor activator; ARIP3, testis-specific interacting protein; ARE, androgen response element; CAB, combined androgen blockade; CAG, codon for glutamine; CBP/pCAF, cyclic-AMP response-element binding protein; DHT, dihydrotestosterone; DU-145, human prostate cancer cell line lacking AR; EGF, epidermal growth factor; GGC, codon for glycine; Her-2/neu, an oncogene with a receptor tyrosine kinase domain related to the EGF receptor; IGF-I, insulin-like growth factor-I; IL-6, interleukin-6; KGF, keratinocyte growth factor; LNCaP, human prostate cancer cell line derived from a lymph node metastasis; LHRH, luteinizing hormone releasing hormone; MMTV-LTR, mouse mammary tumor virus-long terminal repeat; PC3, human prostate cancer cell line lacking AR; PCa, prostate cancer; PIN, prostate intraepithelial neoplasia; PKC, protein kinase C; PKA, protein kinase A, cAMP-activated protein kinase which can be inhibited by PKI; PKI, an inhibitor of protein kinase A; PSA, prostate-specific antigen; PSC 833, [3'-keto-Bmt]-[Val2]-cyclosporine; SBMA, spinal and bulbar muscular atrophy; SMRT, N-CoR, nuclear receptor co-repressor proteins; SRC-1, steroid receptor co-activator-1; TIF2/GRIP1, transcription intermediary factor 2, glucocorticoid receptor interacting protein; TPA, 12-O-tetradecanoylphorbol 13-acetate.

1   Overview

The last fifty years have witnessed considerable progress in the early diagnosis and treatment of prostate cancer (PCa). The use of pre-symptomatic diagnostic screening for elevated serum prostate-specific antigen (PSA), transrectal ultrasonography combined with sextant biopsy procedures and neuron-sparing radical prostatectomy has significantly enhanced the prognosis and long-term survival of patients with organ-confined disease who are detected early [1–2]. For patients with metastatic PCa, however, hormone ablation therapy, either mono-therapy or combined androgen blockade (CAB), provides an initial response rate of approximately 80%, with relapse and progression within 12–24 months [2]. Relapse has been attributed to the emergence of androgen-independent (AI) tumor cells that are refractory to anti-androgen therapy, or to the emergence of phenotypes exhibiting antagonist-dependent growth.

Three factors now make it possible to revisit the androgen receptor (AR) as a therapeutic target for the treatment of metastatic and hormone-refractory PCa: (1) advances in understanding of the molecular regulation of AR action in normal and PCa cells, (2) the development of better models of human PCa, including xenograft models that mimic molecular changes found in metastatic human tumors [3–7], (3) the advent of laser capture microdissection, combined with techniques of molecular biology and immunohistochemistry. Laser capture microdissection facilitates biochemical characterization of tumor biopsy specimens with respect to many markers, e.g., AR status, HER-2/neu, nuclear receptor co-factors and tumor suppressors (p53, pRb) [8, 9]. Thus a patient's tumor can be uniquely characterized at the molecular level. This review will summarize recent advances in understanding the molecular action of the ARs in normal cells, in primary hormone-sensitive PCa and in androgen-independent prostate cancer (AI-PCa). Strategies for the development of novel AR-based therapeutics for advanced metastatic and AI-PCa will be proposed.

2   Biology of the prostate and prostate cancer

2.1   Introduction

The prostate gland is a secretory organ comprising several tissue types: secretory epithelia, which surround the prostatic lumen and ducts, basal epithelia, which serve as a stem cell population for secretory epithelia, supporting stromal cells and small populations of cells of neuroendocrine origin [10]. In the healthy male, the prostate epithelium secretes seminal fluid containing many proteins, including the serine proteinases human kallikrine 2 and PSA, that mediate semen liquefaction. Androgens regulate proliferation and survival of secretory epithelia and expression of these proteinases as well as other tissue-specific genes in the prostate [11]. Basal epithelia are hormone-sensitive; however, their survival is not dependent on the presence of androgen.

In PCa, small foci known as prostatic intra-epithelial neoplasias (PINs) develop as a result of genetic instability in epithelial cell nuclei and concomitant proliferation. These PINs are less well differentiated than normal epithelia and are slow-growing in the early stages. With progression, clonal outgrowth of primary adenocarcinomas occurs. Metastasis to remote sites such as lymph nodes, bone, brain and lungs may develop if the primary tumor is not detected and treated [12].

Prostate tumors are slow-growing and immortal phenotypes emerge as inhibitors of apoptosis, such as bcl-2 become up-regulated following androgen ablation therapy [13–15]. Normal secretory epithelia do not express bcl-2, whereas basal epithelia do. The increase in bcl-2 expression in primary prostate tumors following androgen ablation may reflect proliferation and progression of the stem cell population, or may result from aberrant gene expression in a few residual cells in the primary adenocarcinoma [12]. Classical cytotoxic therapies have poor efficacy in treating PCa, in part because these agents depend on rapid cell cycling to induce apoptosis [2, 16]. Thus, PCa is more a failure of cells to apoptose rather than a hyper-proliferative disorder.

2.2   Incidence and prevalence

It is estimated that 75% of men 80 years and older have histologic PCa, while about 30–40% of men over 50 have PCa. Only about eight percent are clinically diagnosed [17]. In the United States, over 300,000 cases were diagnosed in 1996; over 41,000 men died from the disease [18, 19].

2.3   Treatment of prostate cancer

PCa is androgen-dependent [20]. The earliest therapies included orchiectomy to reduce testosterone, or diethylstilbestrol, 3–5 mg/day, to suppress luteinizing hormone (LHRH) release at the level of the hypothalamus. Diethylstilbestrol was associated with significant rates of cardiovascular disease, e.g., thrombosis [21]. More recently, synthetic analogues of LHRH have been used to achieve chemical castration [22]. This therapy achieves serum castrate levels of testosterone within approximately one month; a concomitant decrease in AR occurs. Response rates for these mono-therapies are approximately 80% with a mean duration of response of 20 months. Although these therapies provide symptomatic relief, there is little effect on survival [23]. Side-effects include: loss of libido, impotence and vasomotor hot flushes [24].

Adrenal androgens are a significant alternative source of residual hormone in patients with PCa [25]. These may have direct, albeit weak agonist activity on the AR, or they may be converted to testosterone or dihydrotestosterone (DHT) [26] in the prostate since essential enzymes are present at significant levels [27–30]. These peripheral sources may contribute as much as 20% of the glandular DHT. In fact, Labrie et al. [31] demonstrated that approximately 50% of intra-prostatic DHT remains after surgical or medical castration. Under these conditions, serum testosterone levels fall to about five to ten percent of presurgical concentrations.

More recently, the availability of antiandrogens, both steroidal, e.g., nilutamide (Anandron™) and non-steroidal, e.g., flutamide (Eulexin™) and bicalutamide (Casodex™), has made possible an approach of combined androgen blockade (CAB) [32]. Although definitive conclusions have not been drawn, patients receiving CAB had increased time to progression [33], shorter periods of terminal disease progression [34] and may have experienced a survival benefit [23, 35]. Other evaluations have been less favorable, however [36, 37], citing fatigue, vasomotor instability and deterioration in muscle strength as significant toxicities [38, 39].

Disease progression after androgen ablation therapy may be treated by secondary hormonal therapies, including ketoconazole or aminogluethimide, to inhibit adrenal steroid production: dexamethasone, or prednisone and mitoxantrone [40, 41].

The most recent clinical initiatives exploit improved understanding of the mechanisms of action of cytotoxic therapies and drug synergy. For example, estramustine, a conjugate of a nitrogen mustard and estradiol, binds to microtubule-associated proteins. A small objective response rate of 19% or less was reported in androgen-independent (AI) PCa. The antimitotic agents, paclitaxel and vinblastine, also induce bcl-2 phosphorylation, which leads to its inactivation and induction of apoptotic cell death [42]. Combination studies of these agents with estramustine in AI PCa produced response rates of greater than 50% [43, 44] with significant palliative benefit. In cell culture studies using human LNCaP cells, Wang et al. [45] showed that estramustine alone, and in combination with the non-immunosuppressive cyclosporine PSC 833, down-regulated expression of the AR by 70 %. The most significant effect, a 90% decrease in phosphorylated AR, was obtained with synergistic concentrations of these agents.

2.4 Androgen independence (AI)

In spite of the advances in the management of primary metastatic PCa, relapse and progression to hormone-refractory or AI cancer is inevitable. Although widely used, the terms hormone-refractory or androgen-independent are not very accurate. Androgen dependence reflects the requirement of androgen for survival; in the absence of androgen, normal prostate epithelial cells apoptose. Androgen stimulates a survival signal and anti-androgens block that signal. AI tumors are refractory to anti-androgen therapy; they survive and proliferate in the absence of androgen; however, they may still be hormone-sensitive. These properties are characteristic of the basal epithelial stem cell population, which has led to speculation that basal cells are the source of metastatic tumors.

The expression of AR in clinical specimens of prostate tumors from relapsed patients has been studied. In contrast to low amounts of AR in the prostate of patients recently treated with anti-hormonal therapy, AI prostate tumors express high levels of AR, similar to pretreatment levels [46, 47]. The re-expressed AR may function as a ligand-independent transactivation factor, i.e., constitutively [48–50]. In addition, the AR may be hyper-sensitive to the presence of low but significant concentrations of residual prostatic andro-gens [31]. Finally, cross-talk between growth factor signaling pathways, including IGF-I receptors, EGF receptors and receptors coupled to protein kinase A (PKA), may influence AR-mediated transactivation [51–53].

Genomic and histologic studies of the AR gene, located on the X chro-mosome, have demonstrated amplification of the Xq11–q13 region in 30% of recurrent prostate cancer cells, but not in specimens from the same patients prior to androgen ablation therapy [54, 55]. Genomic instability may also facilitate the emergence of AR mutations rendering cells responsive in an agonist mode to anti-androgens or other circulating steroids [56]. Clini-cal observations in PCa patients who progress while on anti-androgen ther-apy have documented both flutamide [57, 58] and bicalutamide withdrawal responses [59]. These data indicate a change in phenotype of the AR-medi-ated response to one of antagonist dependence. Recognition of this pheno-type, which occurs in about one-third of all patients, and withdrawal of endocrine therapy may result in 4–6 months clinical benefit for the patients [60]. At the present time, the frequency of such mutations is an area of con-troversy (see website http://www.mcgill.ca/androgendb). However, other explanations for the emergence of "antagonist-dependent" phenotypes are possible (see discussion of non-genomic signaling below).

3 The role of the androgen receptor (AR) in prostate cancer

3.1 The androgen receptor (AR)

The AR is a member of the nuclear receptor superfamily, which includes steroid receptors (Class I receptors), receptors for thyroid hormones, retinoids and vitamin D (Class II receptors) and orphan receptors [61–63]. The amino terminal contains the AF-1 transactivation domain. The DNA binding domain contains two zinc fingers followed by a hinge domain containing the nuclear targeting signal. The carboxy terminal contains the hormone bind-ing domain and, in the absence of ligand, represses AF-1-mediated activation [11, 62]. Several proline-directed serine phosphorylation sites are present, Ser 81, Ser 94 and Ser 650 [64]. The binding of ligand enhances phosphorylation of AR; however, the effect of phosphorylation on AR-mediated transactivation is not clear. Phosphorylation may alter receptor turnover, modulate interaction with nuclear receptor co-factors, or facilitate cross-talk with other signal transduction pathways [11].

The human AR is polymorphic. It has a molecular weight of approximately 98,999 Daltons [65] and consists of approximately 919 amino acids. These polymorphisms include three glutamine-rich domains and two glycine-rich domains that have been associated with increased disease risk. For example, Kennedy's disease (SBMA, spinal and bulbar muscular atrophy) is a sex-linked neurodegenerative disorder in which 40–66 CAG repeats may occur [66]. In contrast, short glutamine-repeat motifs in the second CAG domain (less than 20) [67], or glycine-domains (GGC) of less than 16 repeats, are risk factors for PCa [68, 69]. African-American males have a statistically shorter CAG repeat distribution than Caucasian males (means of 19 and 22 respectively) [70]. This variation may partially explain the higher incidence and more advanced stage of PCa in the U.S. among African-Americans compared to Caucasian males at the time of diagnosis [71]. Greater transactivation efficiency of ARs with fewer glutamine-repeats has been proposed to explain this phenomenon [72]. However, other investigators have not observed this effect. Wilson and colleagues [73] reported an inverse relationship between CAG repeat length and AR mRNA levels. Reduced mRNA for AR resulted in less AR protein as determined in ligand binding assays; however, the affinities of these polymorphic ARs for the androgen ligand, ^{3}H-R1881, were similar [74]. The effect of CAG polymorphisms on the transactivation activity of AR was investigated in transient transfection assays [66]. Longer glutamine repeats did not alter transcriptional activation when assessed using the mouse mammary tumor virus long-terminal repeat (MMTV-LTR) promoter. A recent report suggests that the excessive polyglutamine expansion of AR in SBMA influences induction of apoptosis [75]. Cleavage of AR by caspase-3 resulted in proteolytic fragments that accumulated in peri-nuclear protein aggregates that were pro-apoptotic. This mechanism may be significant in neurodegenerative diseases, but it is less clear that the shortened glutamine or glycine polymorphisms identified in PCa contribute to a decreased apoptotic rate in these cells.

Like other nuclear receptors, AR dimerizes, most likely in an anti-parallel mode, facilitating interaction between the N-terminal and C-terminal (N-C) domains during transactivation of androgen-responsive genes [76–79]. The presence of a second transactivation domain, AF-2, in the ligand binding region has been demonstrated *in vitro* [80, 81]. The N-C interaction of the antiparallel homodimer stabilizes helix 12 and prevents ligand dissociation [82].

3.2 The androgen response element (ARE) and androgen-regulated genes

Hormone response elements for androgen receptors have been reported for a number of genes. The response element is a dyad comprising two non-identical hexamer base-pair elements separated by a three base-pair bridge [83]. The sequence difference between the two dyads is consistent with the cooperative binding of an antiparallel AR homodimer.

In reporter-based assays of AR transactivation, the MMTV-LTR promoter has been used to measure of the efficacy of AR transactivation [84–86]. However, this promoter responds to other steroid receptors, including glucocorticoid, progesterone and mineralocorticoid receptors. This promiscuity is inconsistent with the selectivity of hormone action *in vivo*, suggesting that other regulatory co-factors or additional promoter/enhancer elements influence tissue-specific responsiveness to receptors in this subfamily. Other consensus sequences, which influence the binding affinity of AR to the ARE [87], have been identified. Some androgen responsive genes: prostatic binding protein C3 [88], mouse sex-limited protein [89] and PSA [90–92], are regulated by enhancer/promoters. The PSA gene promoter element has been examined in detail. The proximal promoter has two AREs: ARE I and ARE II, and a core TATA box [93]. A promoter/enhancer located approximately –4.2 kb upstream contains at least 4 tandem non-consensus AREs that interact synergistically to provide tissue specificity and response amplification [94]. These promoter/enhancer elements have a weak affinity for AR; they are only activated in the presence of high receptor concentrations.

3.3 Nuclear receptor co-regulatory proteins

The nuclear receptor co-factor family of proteins includes the p160 proteins (SRC-1, TIF-2/GRIP-1), CBP (cyclic-AMP response-element binding protein) and its homolog p300, and p/CAF(p300/CBP-associated factor) [95, 96]. All three families are histone acetyltransferases that modulate nuclear transcription through covalent modification of chromatin. Members of these families bind to most nuclear receptors through LXXLL motifs [97] and auxiliary domains [98]. Binding of co-factors to receptors stabilizes the receptor-DNA complex and enhances transcriptional activation [99]. In contrast to this mechanism, ARs recruit co-activators through interaction with the N-terminal domain [81, 82]. Several AR-selective proteins have also been identified, including ARA70 [100], ARA54 [101], ARA55 [102] and a testis-specific co-activator (ARIP3) which interacts with the zinc-finger domain [103]. ARA70, also identified in thyroid cancer cells as ELE1 [81], can interact with basal transcription factors and may interact more broadly with other steroid receptors. A recent report demonstrated that ARA70 significantly enhanced estradiol activation of AR [104] and conferred agonist activity on the antagonists bicalutamide or hydroxyflutamide [105]. However, other investigators [106] find that ARA70 displays only weak co-activator function. Differences in assay methodology may well account for diverse observations of laboratories exploring the role of this protein. ARA54 enhanced DHT-stimulated transactivation of AR (wild type) and, notably, also enhanced estradiol and hydroxyflutamide-stimulated transactivation of the LNCaP mutant AR. Characterization of the binding domains for co-activator recruitment is currently an active area of investigation.

In addition to co-activator proteins, co-repressor proteins regulate nuclear receptor transactivation activity. Notably, co-repressors, such as SMRT or N-CoR [107], have not demonstrated interaction with AR; however, this is an active area of investigation. The interaction of antagonist drugs with some nuclear receptors has been shown to alter the composition and ratio of co-activators/co-repressors recruited to the hormone response element, e.g., tamoxifen and the estrogen receptor, RU486 and the progesterone receptor [108].

Thus the AR and its ARE transactivation pathway exhibit unique biochemical features that distinguish it from the other steroid receptors. These include N-C terminal interaction, anti-parallel receptor dimerization, AR-specific N-terminal motifs for co-activator recruitment, AR-specific and tissue-specific co-activators and transactivation through promoter/enhancer response elements that amplify AR-mediated responses in the presence of high levels of AR.

3.4 Androgen-independent activation of the AR: Cross-talk between signaling pathways and the AR

The AR can be activated by alternative signaling pathways in the absence of ligand. For example, forskolin-induced activation of PKA resulted in hormone-independent activation of the AR [52]. Both flutamide and bicalutamide blocked this effect, indicating an AR-mediated response. Using human prostatic tissue explants, Nakhla et al. [109] showed that estradiol in combination with sex-hormone binding globulin could activate AR, resulting in PSA production. These effects were not blocked by anti-estrogens, but were inhibited by anti-androgens or the PKA inhibitor, PKI. In cell-based assays, Culig et al. [110] demonstrated synergistic enhancement of low concentrations of androgen by LHRH, which stimulates cAMP production. Secretion of PSA was measured and androgen antagonists blocked this effect. Marelli and colleagues [111] evaluated the effects of LHRH agonist on the IGF-I and IGF-I receptor-mediated responses. In the AI DU-145 cell line or using AR-transfected cells, they observed LHRH agonist-induced inhibition of proliferation and reduction of receptor phosphorylation. These effects were mediated through different signaling pathways, depending on the AR-status of the cells. In other studies employing co-transfection of cells with artificial ARE-driven promoters and AR expression vectors, the growth factors IGF-I, KGF and EGF activated AR-mediated transactivation [110]. Bicalutamide inhibited these effects, confirming that the responses were mediated through the AR. Clearly, important cross-talk occurs between the AR and growth factor signaling pathways.

Activation of the protein kinase C (PKC) pathway has been reported to have both stimulatory and inhibitory effects on the AR. PKC, activated by phorbol myristate acetate (TPA) may phosphorylate a co-factor that enhances AR-mediated transactivation [112]. Alternatively, TPA, through activation of the AP-1 transcription factor (c-jun/c-fos heterodimer) and binding to the TPA response element, may diminish AR transactivation of ARE [113]. Direct binding of c-jun to the AR protein has also been reported [114]. The effects of PKC activation and the role of AP-1 in modulating AR activity may be significantly influenced by the cellular and promoter context of the experimental paradigm; thus, extrapolating these results to the normal cellular context is not possible at this time.

Recently several investigators have demonstrated effects of IL-6 to synergistically activate AR in the presence of low androgen, or in the absence of androgen. Ligand-independent activation resulted in a stimulation of either reporter-based responses or PSA secretion and a decrease in proliferation of cultured cells [115]. Inhibitors of the PKA, PKC and MAP kinase pathways decreased reporter-based responses, indicating the importance of these intracellular signaling pathways in mediating IL-6 effects. Other investigators have demonstrated IL-6 effects to enhance proliferation [116] or act as an autocrine growth factor [117]. In view of the clinical significance of high IL-6 levels in serum of metastatic PCa patients, understanding the mechanism by which IL-6 induces AR activation may have significant clinical impact [118].

Activation of the HER-2/neu-AR signaling pathway has been reported in PCa. Using LAPC-4 cells which have a wild type AR or LNCaP cells which have a mutated AR, Sawyers and colleagues [5] studied ligand-independent activation of AR in parental and hormone-independent sublines. Co-transfection of HER-2/neu tyrosine kinase activity and PSA promoter/enhancer ARE-reporter constructs resulted in increased expression of either PSA or reporter proteins. The addition of an androgen agonist resulted in synergy of induction. Importantly, the activation of AR by HER-2/neu was blocked by bicalutamide in the parental LNCaP line, but not in the hormone-independent cells. These studies underscore the importance of promoter and cellular contexts for studies of ligand-independent transactivation by AR.

3.5 The phosphorylated AR

As mentioned earlier, the AR contains several phosphorylation sites. Phosphorylation of AR significantly influences ligand binding and transactivation [45, 119–122]. The presence of agonists enhances AR phosphorylation, while antagonists such as bicalutamide and the functional antagonist estramustine reduce levels of phospho AR in treated cells. Interestingly, in LNCaP cells, forskolin treatment to activate PKA results in activation of phosphatases, leading to de-phosphorylation of AR. The consequences of these effects on specific AR phosphorylation sites and the influence on co-factor interaction and AR transactivation need further exploration.

3.6 Non-genomic mechanisms of AR signaling

Mitogen-activated protein (MAP) kinase pathways are known to regulate rapid and slow effects of several steroid receptors. In AR-positive cells, activation of MAP kinase kinase1 phosphorylates AR, stimulates AR-mediated transcription, and leads to apoptosis [53]. In AR-transfected PC3 cells, activation of AR stimulated the MAP kinases Erk-1 and -2. These effects had two time components, a rapid phase which occurred over seconds, and a slower phase; the rapid phase was consistent with a non-genomic mechanism of action. These activities were enhanced by androgen agonists. Provocatively, both androgen antagonists, hydroxyflutamide and bicalutamide, were partial agonists in this system [123]. In these studies, activation of AR by DHT also increased activation of the transcription factors Elk-1 and -2, and the classical androgen antagonists displayed partial agonist activity in these assays. These observations provide a rationale for understanding the clinical phenomenon of withdrawal responses observed in PCa patients who become refractory to these antagonists and yet have no evidence of mutated AR [57].

3.7 The AR in prostate cancer

Androgens are growth and survival factors for normal and for PCa cells. Castration in the normal male leads to down-regulation of AR and involution of the prostate. Since the AR protein is very labile in the absence of ligand, it is rapidly degraded. In animal models of PCa, androgen ablation enhances rates of apoptosis [124]. In contrast, activation of genes regulated by the AR stimulates prostate cell proliferation and inhibits apoptosis [125]. Re-expression of AR in tumors from patients who progress following androgen ablation therapy may represent clonal selection of tumor cells capable of surviving despite lower serum androgen concentrations. Furthermore, estimates of residual prostatic DHT concentrations as high as 50–60% of pre-treatment values [27, 31] suggest that the ablative strategy has been only partially successful. Thus, PCa patients treated with androgen ablation therapy may relapse as tumor cells evolve mechanisms of survival in a low androgen environment.

Mutations in the AR have been documented in some primary tumor specimens, but are found with greater frequency in specimens from relapsing patients. Some of these mutations result in changes in specificity. The AR mutation identified in LNCaP cells, threonine 877 to alanine, enables the AR to respond broadly to other steroid agonists, including estrogen and progesterone. It has been identified frequently in hormone-refractory prostate tumors [126]. Many other mutations have been identified [56, 127]; however, the frequency and phenotypic consequences of these mutations are poorly understood [128].

4 Strategies for the development of novel therapeutics

Elucidation of the biochemical mechanisms of AR-mediated effects has proven to be more challenging than for other nuclear receptors. The silver lining to this cloud is that the unique biochemistry of AR-mediated responses provides a number of more selective mechanisms that may be targeted for the development of PCa therapeutics. These are outlined below.

4.1 Disruption of AR transactivation

As identified in the discussion above, the N-C domains of AR interact in an AR-unique fashion that is required for stabilization of ligand binding and recruitment of co-activators. Inhibitors of the N-C interaction or co-activator binding to the AF-1 domain would be highly AR-specific. Initially, peptide antagonists fashioned after the consensus binding motifs could be used to confirm inhibition of AR-mediated responses *in vitro* using techniques such as yeast-2 hybrid or immunoprecipitation. Similar assays could then be used to screen compound libraries for novel agents that mimic these activities. An important feature of this approach would be the response used to assess transactivation efficiency in whole cell assays. Based on the recent literature demonstrating that responses are often promoter-specific and cell context-specific, it would be important to use native promoter/enhancer response elements [94] instead of the MMTV-LTR, and to utilize a prostate cell line wherever possible.

It may be possible to search for novel AR antagonists that could recruit co-repressors to the receptor complex, or to use existing antagonists to identify tissue-specific co-repressors that may interact with AR. This approach was utilized by Horwitz and colleagues [108] who demonstrated that partial agonists, tamoxifen or RU486, influenced the composition and ratio of co-activator/co-repressor proteins associated with the nuclear receptors.

4.2 Phosphorylation pathways

As reported above, the phosphorylation of AR has an important influence on transactivation efficiency. By exploring the effects of inhibitors of the signaling pathways, including MAP kinase, PKC and PKA, on AR phosphorylation, it may be possible to determine the most important signaling cascade to target, particularly in AI-PCa. These studies would be best carried out using cell lines mimicking the refractory patient, where the AR gene is upregulated and the effect on promoter/enhancer activation can be evaluated. In addition, the acute effect of liganded AR to induce phosphorylation of erk-1 and -2 is an exciting observation [123]. This observation may provide a simple model for screening for novel AR antagonists that inhibit this activity.

4.3 Tissue-selective modulators of androgen action

The possibility of developing tissue-selective androgen receptor modulators or "SARMs" has been proposed [129]. Indeed progress has already been made with the synthesis of non-steroidal androgen agonists that repress LHRH secretion [130]. Full exploration of the effects of these agents on AR phosphorylation, co-factor recruitment, promoter/enhancer activation, cross-talk between AR and signal transduction pathways and also the non-genomic effects of AR, promises greater insight into the complexity of AR function. Although much remains to be elucidated regarding the role of AR in AI-PCa, sufficient detail exists to begin harvesting this information through the development of novel therapeutics.

References

1   P.C. Walsh, A.W. Partin and J.I. Epstein: J. Urol. *152*, 1831 (1994).
2   R.J. Long, K.P. Roberts, M.J. Wilson, C.J. Ercole and J.L. Pryor: Andrology *18*, 15 (1997).
3   M. Nagabhushan, C.M. Miller, T.P. Pretlow, J.M. Giaconia , N.L. Edgehouse, S. Schwartz, H.J. Kiung, R.W. White DeVere, P.H. Gumerlock, M.I. Resnick et al.: Cancer Res. *56*, 3042 (1996).
4   C.W. Gregory, K.G. Hamil, D. Kim, S.H. Hall, T.G. Pretlow, J.L. Mohler and F.S. French: Cancer Res. *58*, 5718 (1998).
5   N. Craft, Y. Shostak, M. Carey and C.L. Sawyers: Nat. Medicine *3*, 280 (1999).
6   Z. Culig, J. Hoffmann, M. Erdel, I.E. Eder, A. Hobisch, A. Hittmair, G. Bartsch, G. Utermann, M.R. Schneider, K. Parcyzk et al.: Br. J. Cancer *81*, 242 (1999).
7   D.B. Agus, C. Cordon-Cardo, W. Fox, M. Drobnjak, A. Koff, D.W. Golde and H.I. Scher: J. Natl. Cancer Inst. *91*, 1869 (1999).
8   N.L. Simone, R.F Bonner, J.W. Gillespie, M.R. Emmert-Buck and L.A. Liotta: Trends Genet. *14*, 272 (1998).
9   N.L. Simone, A.T. Remaley, L. Charboneau, E.F. Petricoin, J.W. Glickman, M.R. Emmert-Buck, T.A. Fleisher and L.A. Liotta: Amer. J. Path. *156*, 445 (2000).
10 R.S. Kirby, T.J. Christmas and M.J. Brawer: Prostate cancer, an imprint of Times Mirror International, Mosby, London 1996.
11 J.M. Kokontis and S. Liao: Vitamins and Hormones *55*, 219 (1999).
12 J.T. Isaacs: Urol. Clin. North Am. *26*, 263 (1999).
13 R.J. Raffo, H. Perlman, M.W. Chen, M.L. Day, J.S. Streitman and R. Buttyan: Cancer Res. *55*, 443 (1995).
14 T.J. McDonnell, P. Troncoco, S. M. Brisbay, C. Logothetis, L.W. Chung, J.T. Hsieh and S.M. Tu: Cancer Res. *52*, 6940 (1992).
15 K.S. Chaudhary, P.D. Abel and E.N. Lalani: Environmental Health Perspectives *107* (Suppl. 1), 49 (1999).
16 P.N. Lara and F.J. Myers: Cancer Investigation *17*, 137 (1999).
17 H.B. Carter and D.S. Coffey: Prostate *16*, 39 (1990).
18 S.L. Parker, T. Tong, S. Bolden and P.A. Wingo: CA Cancer J. Clin. *65*, 5 (1996).
19 E. Ruijter, C. van de Kaa G. Miller, D. Ruiter, F. Debruyne and J. Schalken: Endocrine Reviews *20*, 22 (1999).
20 C. Huggins and C.V. Hodges: Cancer Res. *1*, 293 (1941).
21 P. Henriksson and O. Edhag: Br. Med. J. *293*, 413 (1986).
22 R. Sharifi and M. Soloway: J. Urol. *143*, 68 (1990).
23 D.J. McLeod, E.D. Crawford and E.P. DeAntoni: Eur Urol. *32* (Suppl. 3), 70 (1997).
24 A. Radmeijer, K. Bormacher and F. Neumann: In: F.H. Schroder (ed): Treatment of prostate cancer, facts and controversies, Wiley-Liss, New York 1990, 131.
25 M.E. Harper, A. Pike, W.B. Peeling and K.G. Griffiths: J. Endocrinol. *60*, 117 (1974).
26 J.E. Foote and E.D. Crawford: Semin. Urol. *4*, 291 (1988).
27 J. Gellar: Semin. Oncol. *12*, 28 (1985).
28 R. A. Hiipakka and S. Liao: In: L.J. Degroot (ed): Endocrinology, ed. 3, WB Saunders, Philadelphia 1995.
29 J. Imperato-McGinley and T. Gautier: Trends Genet. *2*, 130 (1986).
30 J.D. McConnell: Urol. Clin. North Am. *18*, 1 (1991).

31   F. Labrie, I. Luthy, R. Veilleux, J. Simard, A. Belanger and A. Dupont: Prog. Clin. Biol. Res. *43A*, 145 (1987).

32   D.W.W. Newling, Brit. J. Urol. *77*, 776 (1996).

33   M. Hussain, M. Wolf, E. Marshall et al.: Clin. Oncol. 12, 1868 (1994).

34   L. Denis: Prostate *27*, 233 (1995).

35   L.J. Denis and K. Griffiths: Seminars in Surgical Oncology *18*, 52 (2000).

36   M.A. Eisenberger, B.A. Blumenstein, E.D. Crawford, G. Miller, D.G, McCleod, P.J. Loehrer, G. Wilding, K Sears, D.J. Calkin, I.M. Thompson Jr.: N. Engl. J. Med. *339*, 1036 (1998).

37   A.J. Dowling and I.F. Tannock: Cancer Treatment Reviews *24*, 283 (1998).

38   Z. Wajsman: Eur. Urol. *34* (Suppl. 3), 25 (1998).

39   U.E. Studer and R.D. Mills: Eur. Urol. *34* (Suppl. 3), 29 (1998).

40   M.J.P. Pilat, J.M. Kamradt and K.J. Pienta: Cancer Metastasis Reviews *17*, 373 (1999).

41   D.M. Reese and E.J. Small: Urol. Clin. North Am. *26*, 311 (1999).

42   S. Haldar, A. Basu and C.M. Croce: Cancer Res. *57*, 229 (1997).

43   B.J. Roth: Seminars in Oncology *23*, 49 (1996).

44   W.K. Oh and P.W. Kantoff: J. Urol. *160*, 1220 (1998).

45   L.G. Wang, X.M. Liu, D.R. Budman and W. Kreis: Biochem. Pharm. *58*, 1115 (1999).

46   A. Hobisch, Z. Culig, C. Radmayr, G. Bartsch, H. Klocker and A. Hittmair: Cancer Res. *55*, 3068 (1995).

47   R.W. de Vere White, F. Meyers, S.G. Chi, S. Chamberlain, D. Siders, F. Lee, S. Stewart and P.H. Gumerlock: Eur. Urol. *31*, 1 (1997).

48   J.A. Simental, M.Sar, M.V. Lane, F.S. French and E.M. Wilson: J. Biol. Chem. *266*, 510 (1991).

49   G. Jenster, H.A.G.M. van der Korput, J. Trapman and A.O. Brinkman: J. Biol. Chem. *270*, 7341 (1995).

50   N.L. Weigel and Y. Zhang: J. Mol. Med. *76*, 469 (1999).

51   Z. Culig, A. Hobisch, M.V. Cronauer, C. Radmayr, J. Trapman, A. Hittmair, G. Bartsch and H. Klocker: Cancer Res. *54*, 5474 (1994).

52   L.V. Nazareth and N.L. Weigel: J. Biol. Chem. *271*, 19900 (1996).

53   M.T. Abreau-Martin, A. Chari, A.A. Palladino, N.A. Craft and C.L. Sawyers: Mol. and Cell Biol. *19*, 5143 (1999).

54   T. Visakorpi, E. Hyytinen, P. Koivisto, M. Tanner, R. Keinanen, C. Palmberg, A. Palotie, T. Tammela, J. Isola and O.P. Kallioniemi: Nat. Genet. *9*, 401 (1995).

55   P. Koivisto, J. Kononen, C. Palmberg, T. Tammela, E. Hyytinen, J. Isola, J. Trapman, K. Cleutjens, A. Noordzij, T. Viasakorpi et al.: Cancer Res. *57*, 314 (1997).

56   W.D. Tilley, G. Buchana, T.T. Hickey and J.M. Bentel: Clin. Cancer Res. *2*, 277 (1996).

57   H.I. Scher and W.K. Kelly: J. Clin. Onc. *11*, 1566 (1993).

58   W.D. Figg, A.O. Sartor, M.R. Cooper, A, Thibault, R.C. Bergan, N. Dawson, E. Reed, C. E. Myers: Am. J. Med. *98*: 412 (1995).

59   E.J. Small, P.R. Carroll: Urology *43*, 408 (1994).

60   W.K. Kelly: Eur. Urol. *34* (Suppl.), 18 (1999).

61   M.J. Tsai and B.W. O'Malley: Ann. Rev. Biochem. *63*, 451 (1994).

62   Z.X Zhou, M. Sar, C.H. Wong and E.M. Wilson: Recent Progress in Hormone Research *49*, 249 (1994).

63   D.J. Mangelsdorf, C. Thummel, M. Beato, P. Herrlich, G. Schutz, K. Umesono, B. Blumberg, P. Kastner, M. Mark, P. Chambon et al.: Cell *83*, 835 (1995).

64   Z.X. Zhou, M.V. Lane, J.A. Kemppainnen and E.M Wilson: Mol. Endocrinol. *9*, 600 (1995).
65   C.S. Choong and E. M. Wilson: J. Mol. Endo. *21*, 235 (1998).
66   A.R. La Spada, E.M. Wilson, D.B. Lubahn, A.E. Harding, K.H. Fishbeck, Nature *352*, 77 (1991).
67   E. Giovannucci, M.J. Stampfer, K. Krithivas, M. Brown, A. Brufsky, J. Talcott, C.H. Hennkens and P.W. Kantoff: Proc. Natl. Acad. Sci. *94*, 3320 (1997).
68   J.M. Hakimi, M.P. Schoenberg, R.H. Rondinelli, S. Piantadosi and E.R. Barrack: Clin. Cancer Res. *3*, 1599 (1997).
69   J.L. Stanford, J.J. Just, M. Gibbs, K.G. Wicklund, C.L. Neal, B.A. Blumenstein and E.A. Ostrander: Cancer Res. *57*, 1194 (1997).
70   R.A. Irvine, M.C. Yu, R.K. Ross and G.A. Coetzee: Cancer Res. *55*, 1937 (1995).
71   V.V. Boring, T.S. Suites and C.W. Heath: Cancer Journal Clinics *43*, 7 (1992).
72   N.L. Chamberlain, E.D. Driver and R.L. Miesfeld: Nucl. Acids Res. *22*, 3181 (1994).
73   C.S. Choong, J.A. Kemppainen, Z.X. Zhou and E.M. Wilson: Mol. Endo. *10*, 1527 (1996).
74   Z.X Zhou, M.V. Lane, J.A. Kemppainen, F.S. French and E.M. Wilson: Mol. Endo. *9*, 208 (1995).
75   L.M. Ellerby, A.S. Hackman, S.S. Propp, H.M. Ellerby, S. Rabizadeh, N.R. Cashman, M.A. Trifiro, L. Pinsky, C.L. Wellington, G.S. Salvesen et al.: J. Neurochem. *72*, 185 (1999).
76   E. Langley, Z.X. Zhou and E.M. Wilson: J. Biol. Chem. *270*, 29983 (1995).
77   P. Doesburg, C.W. Kuil, C.A. Berrevoets, K. Steketee, P.W. Faber, E. Mulder, A.O. Brinkman and J. Trapman: Biochemistry *35*, 1052 (1997).
78   T. Ikonen, J.J. Palvimo and O.A. Janne: J. Biol. Chem. *272*, 29821 (1997).
79   E. Langley, J.A. Kemppanainen and E.M. Wilson: J. Biol. Chem. *273*, 92 (1998).
80   R. Snoek, P.S. Rennie, S. Kasper, R.J. Matusik and N. Bruchovsky: J. Steroid Biochem. & Mol. Biology *59*, 243 (1996).
81   F. Alen, F. Claessens, E. Schoenmakers, J.V. Swinnen, G. Verhoeven, W. Rombauts and B. Peeters: Mol. Endocrinol. *13*, 117 (1999).
82   B. He, J.A. Kemppainen, J.J. Voegel, H. Groenemeyer and E.M. Wilson: J. Biol. Chem. *274*, 37219 (1999).
83   M.C. Luke and D.S. Coffey: J. Androl. *15*, 41 (1994).
84   P. Dabre, M. Page and R.J.B. King: Mol. Cell Biol. *6*, 2847 (1986).
85   A. Cato, D. Hendeson and H. Ponta: EMBO J. *6*, 363 (1987).
86   J. Ham, A. Thompson, M. Needham, P. Webb and M. Parker: Nucleic Acids Res. *16*, 5263 (1988).
87   P.J. Roche, S.A. Hoare and M.G. Parker: Mol. Endo. *6*, 2229 (1992).
88   J. Tan, K.B. Marschke, K.C. Ho, S.T. Perry, E.M. Wilson and F.S. French: J. Biol. Chem. *267*, 4456 (1992).
89   Y.M. Ning and D.M. Robins: J. Biol. Chem. *274*, 30624 (1999)
90   P.H.J. Reigman, R.J. Vlietstra, H.A.G.M. van der Korput, A.O. Brinkman and J. Trapman: Mol. Endo. *5*, 1921 (1991).
91   P. Murtha, D.J. Tindall and C.Y.F. Young: Biochem. *32*, 6459 (1993).
92   E.R. Schuur, G.A. Henderson, L.A. Kmetec, J.D. Miller, H.G. Lamparski and D.R. Henderson: J. Biol. Chem. *271*, 7043 (1996).
93   K.B. Cleutjens, C.C. van Eekelen, H.A. van der Korput, A.O. Brinkman and J.J. Trapman: J. Biol. Chem. *271*, 6379 (1996).
94   W. Huang, Y. Shostak, P. Tarr, C. Sawyers and M. Carey: J. Biol. Chem. *274*, 26756 (1999).

95   H. Shibata, T.E. Spencer, S.A. Onate, G. Jenster, S.Y. Tsai, M.J. Tsai and B.W.O. O'Malley: Recent Progress in Hormone Research *52*, 141 (1997).

96   J. Torschia, C.K. Glass and M.G. Rosenfeld: Curr. Opin. Cell Biol. *10*, 373 (1998).

97   E.M. McInerney, D.W. Rose, S.E. Flynn, S. Westin, T.M. Mullern, A. Krones, J. Inostroza, J. Torchia, R.T. Nolte, N. Assa-Munt et al.: Genes and Development *12*, 3357 (1998).

98   H. Hong, B.D. Darimont, H. Ma, L. Yang, K.R. Yamamoto and M.R. Stallcup: J. Biol. Chem. *274*, 3496 (1999).

99   D.P. Edwards: Vitamins and Hormones *55*, 165 (1999).

100   S. Yeh and C. Chang: Proc. Natl. Acad. Sci.: *93*, 5517 (1996).

101   H.Y. Kang, S. Yeh, N. Fujimoto and C. Chang: J. Biol. Chem. *274*, 8570 (1999).

102   N. Fujimoto, S. Yeh, H.Y. Kang, S. Inui, H.C. Chang, A. Mixokami and C. Chang: J. Biol. Chem. *274*, 8316 (1999).

103   A.M. Miolanen, U. Karvonen, H. Poukka, W. Yan, J. Toppari, O.A. Janne and J.J.Palvimo: J. Biol. Chem. *274*, 3700 (1999).

104   S. Yeh, H. Miyamoto, H. Shima and C. Chang: Proc. Natl. Acad. Sci. *95*, 5527 (1998).

105   H. Miyamoto, S. Yeh, G. Wildong and C. Chang: Proc. Natl. Acad. Sci. *95*, 7379 (1998).

106   T. Gao, K. Brantley and M.J. McPhaul: Mol. Endo. *13*, 1645 (1999).

107   L. Xu, C.K. Glass and M.G. Rosenfeld: Curr. Opin. Genetics & Development *9*, 140 (1999).

108   G.S. Takimoto, J.D. Grahma, T.A. Jackson, L. Tung, R.L. Powell, L.D. Horwitz and K. Horwitz: J. Steroid Biochem. & Mol. Bio. *69*, 45 (1999).

109   A.M. Nakhla, N.A. Romas and W. Rosner: J. Biol. Chem. *272*, 6838 (1997).

110   Z. Culig, A. Hobisch, A. Hittmair, M.V. Cronauer, C. Radmayr, J. Zhang, G. Bartsch and H. Klocker: The Prostate *32*, 106 (1997).

111   M.M. Marelli, R.M. Moretti, D. Dondi, M. Motta and P. Limonta: Cancer Res. *52*, 6940 (1992).

112   P.E. De Ruiter, R. Teuwen, J. Trapman, R. Dijkema and A.O. Brinkman: Mol. Cell Endo. *110*, 41 (1995).

113   K. Tillman, J.L. Oberfield, X.W. Shen, A. Bubulya and L. Shemshedini: Endocrine *9*, 193 (1998).

114   N. Sato, M.D. Sadar, N. Bruchovsky, F. Saatcioglu, P.S. Rennie, S. Sato, P.H. Lange and M.E. Gleave: J. Biol. Chem. *272*, 17485 (1997).

115   A. Hobisch, I.E. Eder, T. Putz, W. Horniger, G. Bartsch, H. Klocker and Z. Culig: Cancer Res. *58*, 4640 (1998).

116   M. Okamoto, C. Lee and R. Oyasu: Cancer Res. *57*, 141 (1997).

117   T.D.K. Chung, J.J. Yu, M.T. Spiotto, M. Bartkowski and J. W. Simons: The Prostate *38*, 199 (1999).

118   D.E. Drachenberg, A.A. Elgamel, R. Rowbotham, M. Peterson and G.P. Murphy: The Prostate *41*, 127 (1999).

119   T. Ikonen, J.J. Palvimo, P.J. Kallio, P. Reinikainen and O.A. Janne: Endocrinol. *135*, 1359 (1994).

120   G. Jenster, P.E. de Ruiter, H.A.G.M. van der Korput, G.G.J.M. Kuiper, J. Trapman and A.O. Brinkman: Biochem. *33*, 14064 (1994).

121   A.O. Brinkmann, L.J. Blok, P.E. De Ruiter, P. Doesburg, K. Steketee, C.A. Berrevoets and J. Trapman: J. Steroid Biochem. & Molec. Biol. *69*, 307 (1999).

122   L.G. Wang, X.M. Liu, W. Kreis and D.R. Budman: Biochem. Biophys. Res. Comm. *259*, 21 (1999).

123   H. Peterziel, S. Minl, A. Schonert, M. Becker, H. Klocker and A.C.B. Cato: Oncogene *18*, 6322 (1999).
124   H.F. English, N. Kyprianou and J.T. Isaacs: The Prostate *15*, 233 (1989).
125   J.T. Isaacs: Vitam. Horm. *49*, 433 (1994).
126   J. Veldscholte, C. Ris-Stalpers, G.G.J.M. Kuiper, G. Jenster, C. Berrovoets, E. Classen, H.C.K. van Rooij, J. Trapman, A.O. Brinkman and E.A. Mulder: Biochem. Biophys. Res. Comm. *173*, 534 (1990).
127   Z. Culig, A. Hobisch, M.V. Cronauer, A.C. Cato, A. Hittmair, C. Radmayr, J. Eberle, G. Bartsch and H. Klocker: Mol. Endo. *7*, 1541 (1993).
128   G. Jenster, J. Trapman and A.O. Brinkmann: In: T.P. Burris and E.R.B. McCabe (eds.): Nuclear receptors and genetic disease, Academic Press, London, UK 2000 (in press)
129   A. Negro-Vilar: J. Clin. Endo. & Metabol. *84*, 3459 (1999).
130   L.G. Hamann, N.S. Mani, R.L. Davis, X.N. Wang, K.B. Marschke and T.K. Jones: J. Med. Chem. 42, 210 (1999).

Progress in Drug Research, Vol. 55 (E. Jucker, Ed.)

Quantitative structure-activity relationships of cardiotonic agents

By Satya P. Gupta

Department of Chemistry, Birla Institute of Technology and Science, Pilani 333031, India

Satya P. Gupta

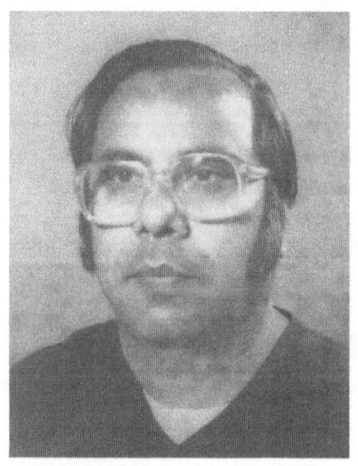

Satya P. Gupta is at present a professor of chemistry at Birla Institute of Technology and Science (BITS), Pilani. He obtained his D.Phil. degree in quantum chemistry in 1971 from the University of Allahabad, Allahabad, India. Before joining BITS in 1973, Dr. Gupta spent a couple of years at Tata Institute of Fundamental Research (TIFR), Bombay, where he worked with Prof. G.Govil on the structure and function of biomembrane. For the past several years, Dr. Gupta has been deeply involved in the theoretical aspects of drug design and for the excellence of his work in this area the Ranbaxy Research Foundation Award, a coveted national award, has been bestowed upon him, and he was made a Fellow of the National Academy of Sciences, India.

Summary

Quantitative structure-activity relationships (QSARs) of different cardiotonic agents are presented. A critical analysis of all QSARs provides a very vivid picture of the mechanisms of varying cardiotonic agents. The cardiotonics can be broadly put into 2 categories: cardiac glycosides and nonglycoside cardiotonics, which include phosphodiesterase of type III (PDE III) inhibitors, sympathomimetic (adrenergic) stimulants, A1-selective adenosine antagonists, Ca2+ channel activators and vasopressin antagonists. For cardiac glycosides, QSARs reveal that the position of carbonyl oxygen in their lactone moiety and shifting of the lactone ring from its original position or its replacement by another group would be crucial for their activity. The carbonyl group or its isostere like CN is indicated to be the sole binding entity and the hydrogen bonding through this group is considered to be the most likely binding force. For nonglycoside cardiotonics that include PDE III inhibitors and A1-selective antagonists, a five-point model has been established for their activity, the salient features of which are: (1) the presence of a strong dipole, (2) an adjacent acidic proton, (3) a methyl-sized lipophilic space, (4) a relatively flat overall topography and (5) a basic or hydrogen-bond acceptor site opposite to the dipole. For Ca2+ channel activators, the importance of steric, electrostatic, lipophilic and hydrogen-bonding properties of molecules is indicated, while for vasopressin antagonists the lipophilic and electronic properties are suggested to be the most important.

Contents

Keywords

Cardiotonic agents, cardiac glycosides, nonglycoside cardiotonics, phosphodiesterase of type III inhibitors, A_1-selective adenosine antagonists, Ca^{2+} channel activators, vasopressin antagonists, quantitative structure-activity relationship (QSAR).

Glossary of abbreviations

AM1, Austin model 1 (a quantum mechanical method); cAMP, cyclic adenosine monophosphate; ATP, adenosine triphosphate; ATPase, adenosine triphosphatase; AV, antrioventricular; AVP, arginine vasopressin; CNDO/2, complete neglect of differential overlap/second version; D_2, molar concentration of drugs leading to 50% of the maximum inotropic effect; E, steric parameter representing ratio of volumes of two moieties; E_s, Taft's steric parameter; EC_{50}, concentration of drugs required to increase developed tension to 50% of isoprenaline maximum; cGMP, cyclic guanine monophosphate; IC_{50}, molar concentration of drugs leading to 50% inhibition of the enzyme; MR, molar refractivity index; PA, proton affinity parameter; PDE III, phosphodiesterase of type III; pK_a, $-\log K_a$ (K_a: dissociation constant of acid); pK_i, $-\log K_i$ (K_i: binding affinity constant); QSAR, quantitative structure-activity relationship; 3D-QSAR, three-dimensional QSAR; S, selectivity factor = $K_i(A_1$-receptor$)/K_i(A_2$-receptor$)$; SA, sinoatrial; V_w, van der Waals volume; π, hydrophobic constant, σ, Hammett's electonic constant; n, number of data points; r, correlation coefficient; s, standard deviation; $F_{x,y}$, F-ratio between the variances of calculated and observed activities (x: number of independent variables; y = n–x–1).

1   Introduction

In technologically advanced countries, more people die from diseases of the heart and blood vessels than from any other single cause. The diseases related to the heart (cardiac diseases) arise from the irregularity in the functioning of the heart and the blood vessels. The heart is a kind of muscular pump, which by rhythmic contraction functions to convert the chemical energy of nutrient materials, such as glucose and fatty acids, supplied to it by its own blood vessels (the coronary arteries) into the mechanical energy necessary to force the viscous blood through the systemic blood vessels. The function of the blood and the circulatory system as a whole is to maintain an optimal environment for cellular functions by supplying appropriate concentrations of nutritive materials, oxygen, hormones and antibiotics, and by removing waste materials and foreign matter such as invading microorganisms.

Part of the energy imparted to the blood during the contraction of the heart muscle is transiently stored as potential energy in the elastic walls of the large arteries. This stored energy enables the pulsating pumping action of the heart to provide a peripheral tissue blood flow that is almost constant throughout each period of contraction (systole) and relaxation (diastole) of the heart.

The contraction and relaxation of the heart are associated with the electro-physiological phenomena of the cell membranes and most of the cardiac diseases are the consequence of the abnormalities in these electrophysiological phenomena [1–3].

The contraction of most mammalian hearts is initiated by and is proportional to the influx of Ca^{2+} ions that occurs during the transmembrane action potential. This in turn causes the release of additional Ca^{2+} ions from the sarcoplasmic reticulum of cardiac fibres. The Ca^{2+} ions that enter the cell play an important role in excitation-contraction coupling of the heart since they serve to replenish intracellular stores from which the ions are released to activate the contractile mechanisms. Drugs (such as verapamil and nifedipine) or ions (such as Mn^{2+}, Co^{2+}, Ln^{3+}) that can block the entry of Ca^{2+} ions into the cell produce a considerable depression of contractility when given in large doses, resulting in cardiac failure.

Of all the heart diseases, cardiac failure is the most fatal and the most predominant. It is a state in which the heart fails to maintain an adequate circulation for the needs of the body, despite an adequate venous filling pressure. The acute occlusion of a major branch of a coronary artery may precipitate cardiac failure. There occurs a complete loss of contractile power in the region of a myocardial infarct and impaired contractility in the adjacent hypoxic regions. The situation is further complicated by the occurrence of arrhythmias originating from the ischemic region.

In the failing heart, the capacity to develop force during systole is reduced and thus a greater end-diastolic volume is needed to perform any given level of external work. In congestive heart failure, therefore, one can assume the following sequence of events: (1) the mismatch of work capacity and load results in decreased systolic ejection and an increased end-systolic volume in the ventricles; (2) since the blood initially continues to enter the ventricles during diastole at almost the normal rate, the end-diastolic volume and pressure increase; (3) if this sequence progresses, the ventricular volume increases and, therefore, in cardiac failure the heart is abnormally enlarged.

2   Cardiotonic agents

Cardiotonic agents or cardiotonics are the drugs that act on the myocardium and increase the force of myocardial contraction (positive inotropic effect) and thus are of great value in the treatment of heart failure. The increase in the force of myocardial contraction leads to increased cardiac output, decreased heart size, venous pressure and blood volume, diuresis and relief of edema in patients with heart failure. Apart from the positive inotropic effect, cardiotonics also slow down the ventricular rate in atrial fibrillation and flutter.

Cardiotonic agents can be broadly put into two categories: cardiac glycosides and nonglycoside cardiotonics.

2.1 Cardiac glycosides

Cardiac glycosides are the combination of an aglycone or genin and one to four sugars. The aglycone is chemically similar to bile acids and to steroids, such as adrenocortical and sex hormones, and constitutes the pharmacologically active portion of the glycosides. The sugars modify the water and lipid solubility of the glycoside molecules and thus affect their potency and duration of action. Glycosides are obtained from dried leaves of foxglove, *Digitalis purpurea* (digitoxin) or *Digitalis lanata* (digitoxin, digoxin), and from the seeds of *Strophanthus gratus* (ouabain). The term digitalis genin or simply digitalis is frequently used to refer to the entire group of cardiac glycosides.

The cardiac glycosides can be divided into two major classes: cardenolides and bufadienolides. The normal perhydrocyclopentanophenanthrene nucleus is characteristic of the genin portion of all the members of both classes. Attached to the 17-position of this steroid nucleus is an unsaturated lactone ring: a 5-membered in the cardenolide series and a 6-membered (α-pyrone) in the bufadienolide series. A prototype of cardenolides is digitoxigenin (1) and that of bufadienolides, bufogenin (2).

The most probable mechanism underlying the positive inotropic effect of digitalis or glycosides appears to be their ability to inhibit the sodium pump by inhibiting the enzyme Na^+, K^+-activated ATPase. The inhibition of this enzyme leads to an increase in intracellular accumulation of Na^+ ions and a depletion of intracellular K^+ ions, resulting in an enhancement in the amount of free Ca^{2+} ions inside the cell [4–9]. However, in spite of the evidence that the positive inotropy results from the inhibition of the pump and a resultant elevation of intracellular free Ca^{2+} ions, some other possible mechanisms of digitalis action have also been suggested. A number of studies have shown that a very low concentration of digitalis causes stimulation of the pump and a concomitant positive inotropic effect [10]. Other studies attribute the effect of digitalis to an alteration in Ca^{2+} binding by sarcolemal phospholipids [11]. The question of alternative modes of action has been discussed [12, 13], but a prominent inotropic effect is not expected until there is some inhibition of active transport of Na^+ and K^+ ions [14].

2.2 Nonglycoside cardiotonics

Among the nonglycoside cardiotonics, the most important are the inhibitors of cardiac phosphodiesterase (PDE) of type III [15]. Of the different molecular forms of PDE present in cardiac muscle, it is PDE III, a low K_m, cyclic adenosine monophosphate (cAMP) specific form of the enzyme, whose inhibition leads to the cardiotonic effect [16, 17]. That the cardiotonic effect originates through the inhibition of this form of the enzyme is supported by the observation that cardiotonic agents produce selective concentration of cAMP but not of cGMP (cyclic guanine monophosphate), potentiate the positive inotropic response to isoproterenol and restore contractility to isolated potassium-depolarized cardiac muscle [18–22].

The other class of nonglycoside cardiotonics can be sympathomimetic (adrenergic) stimulants. Direct β-stimulants cause an increase in force (inotropic) and rate (chronotropic) of contraction of cardiac muscle, leading to an increase in cardiac output, work and myocardial oxygen consumption. This is accomplished by an increase in intracellular concentration of cAMP in target tissues [23, 24]. β-Sympathomimetics bind to membrane receptors and activate adenylate cyclase via guanine nucleotide binding [25]. Adenylate cyclase catalyzes the conversion of ATP to cAMP.

Cardiotonic activity has also been found to be associated with the antagonists of endogeneous adenosine at A1 inhibitory receptors in the heart [26]. Adenosine is released in high concentrations during congestive heart failure [27], which can slow down the conduction in the sinoatrial (SA) and antrioventricular (AV) nodes and reduce atrial contractility [28–30] and thus may further damage the heart. The negative effects of adenosine on the heart appear to be related to a reduction in the duration of the action potential in response to a direct inhibition of Ca^{2+} channels [31–34] and/or to a reduction in Ca^{2+} flux into the cell due to an increased K^+ conductance and hyperpolarization of the cell membrane [32, 35, 36]. Thus, the endogeneous adenosine antagonists may indirectly increase intracellular Ca^{2+} concentration and activate the contractile system without increase in cAMP levels and without the related risk of dangerous arrhythmias [37]. In fact, all the PDE III inhibitors, by increasing cAMP content, exert favourable hemodynamic effects in patients with cardiac failure, but most of them may exacerbate ventricular arrhythmias, provoke myocardial ischemia, accelerate the progression of the underlying disease and increase the mortality rate [38, 39]. Therefore, studies of adenosine antagonists acting at A_1 receptors offer a creative possibility in the treatment of cardiac failure.

Drugs acting directly on the Ca^{2+} channel, producing agonistic effects, serve to induce Ca^{2+} currents by stabilizing the open channel state to initiate positive inotropic responses [39]. Therefore, Ca^{2+} channel activators can also be utilized for the treatment of heart failure.

Another possibility for the treatment of cardiac failure may lie in the investigation of vasopressin antagonists. The arginine vasopressin (AVP) is well known for its pressor response and antidiuretic activity in mammals. It is a neurophysical nonpeptide hormone which interacts with vascular V_{1a} and renal V_2 receptors, leading to vasoconstriction and antidiuresis, respectively [40–42]. Because vasopressin is elevated in some patients with congestive heart failure, where peripheral resistance is also increased, V_{1a} antagonists may decrease systematic vascular resistance, increase cardiac output and prevent vasopressin-induced coronary vasoconstriction, and thus may be useful as cardiotonic agents [43].

For the design and development of any kind of cardiotonics, it is however essential that we clearly know the mechanism of their action. In this respect, the quantitative structure-activity relationship (QSAR) study has acquired a very important place. It tries to explain the variations in biological activities of a given series of compounds in terms of the variations in physicochemical, structural and conformational properties of the molecules [44]. A detailed analysis of QSARs on any kind of drugs, therefore, provides an excellent picture of the mechanism of drug action and a rationale for the development of the drugs. Our several reviews written in the recent past on the QSARs of various drugs [45–53] have been of value in gaining in-depth understanding of the nature of drug-receptor interactions and in formulating ways for the development of therapeutically useful drugs. The QSARs on cardiotonics are presented with the same objectives.

3   QSAR results and discussion

3.1   Cardiac glycosides

As already mentioned, the inotropic effects of the cardiac glycosides are thought to occur through the inhibition of the enzyme Na^+, K^+-ATPase. For

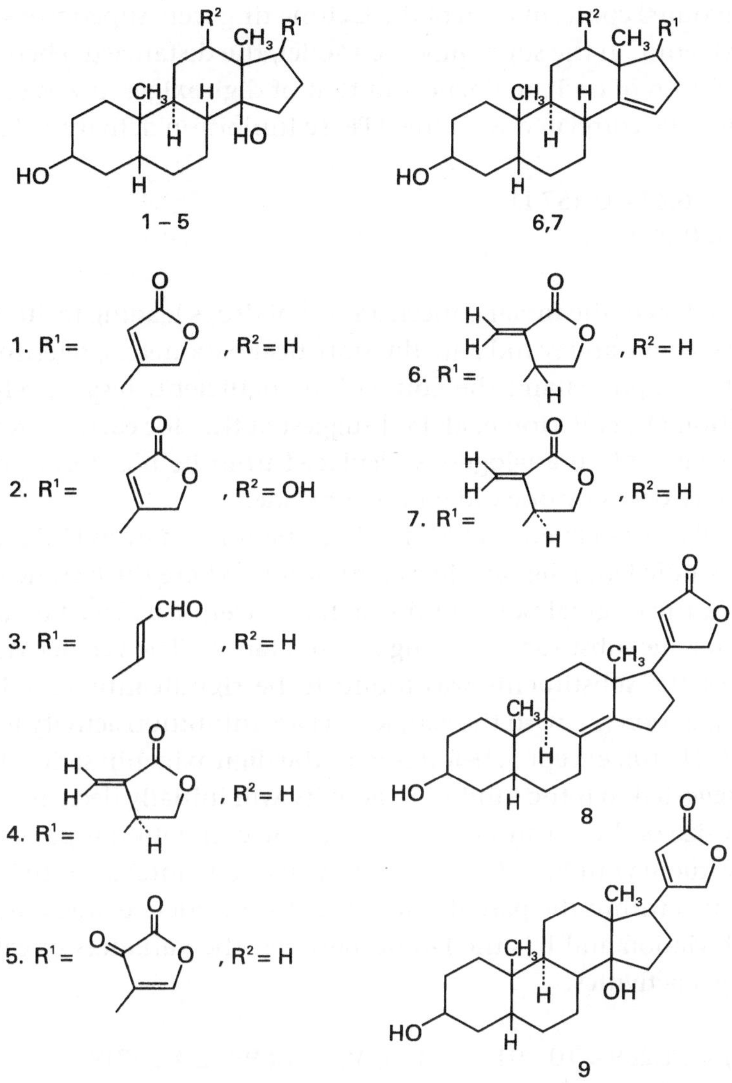

Fig. 1
Cardenolides studied by Fullerton et al. [54].

a set of 9 cardenolides as shown in Figure 1, it was shown [54, 55] that the ATPase inhibition activity of these compounds was a function of the position of the carbonyl (C=O) oxygen of the lactone moiety relative to that in digitoxigenin (1), when structurally similar parts of a compound with energetically favoured conformation of the lactone ring were superimposed upon the digitoxigenin. In the superimposed model, the distance (D) between the carbonyl oxygen of each analogue and that of digitoxigenin was calculated and shown to be correlated with the ATPase inhibition activity as [54]

$$\log(1/IC_{50}) = 6.47 - 0.457\,D \tag{1}$$
$$n = 9,\ r = 0.997$$

where IC_{50} refers to the molar concentration of drugs leading to 50% inhibition of the enzyme and n and r are the statistical parameters, referring to the number of data points and the correlation coefficient, respectively. Thus, from Equation (1), Fullerton et al. [54] suggested that for each 2.2 Å that the carbonyl oxygen of an analogue is displaced from its position in digitoxigenin, activity drops by one order of magnitude.

A molecular size-related analysis has been performed by us [56] on a series of recently studied [57] digitalis-like compounds, where the lactone ring was shifted from the original position through a spacer or replaced by different guanylhydrazone substituent-bearing chains (Tab. 1). The van der Waals volume (V_w) of the substituents was found to be significantly correlated, as shown by Equation (2), with the Na^+, K^+-ATPase inhibition activity for all the compounds (1–10), except 5, belonging to the digitoxigenin series. This correlation suggested that the inhibition activity will initially decrease with the increase in size of the substituent, but since the correlation is parabolic, the larger substituent with $V_w > 1.113 \times 10^2$ Å^3 will be advantageous. In Equation (2), the figures within the parentheses are 95% confidence intervals, s is the standard deviation and F is the F-ratio between the variances of calculated and observed activities.

$$\log(1/IC_{50}) = 11.269 - 10.901\,(\pm 8.416)\,V_w + 4.899\,(\pm 4.267)V_w{}^2 \tag{2}$$
$$n = 9,\ r = 0.921,\ s = 0.14,\ F_{2,6} = 16.86$$

However, in the derivation of Equation (2), compound 5 has not been included, as it behaves as an outlier. Its observed activity (6.80) is much higher than predicted by Equation (2) (5.63). In the whole series, compound 5 has the highest activity. Cerri et al. [57] have suggested that in the case of this compound, the association of a basic guanidine group and a polarized system, which closely resembles the α,β-unsaturated lactone system present

Table 1.
Digitalis-like compounds and their biological activities [57].

Compd	R	$\log(1/IC_{50}{}^a)$	$\log E_{max}{}^b$	$\log(1/IC_{50}{}^c)$	$V_w{}^d$ (10^2 Å^3)
1	(E)-CH=N-N=C(NH2)	5.80	2.42	5.40	0.737
2	(E)-CH=N-NH(2-imidazolinyl)	5.20	2.11	4.77	1.073
3	(E)-CH=N-NH[2-(1,4,5,6-tetrahydro-pyrimidinyl)]	5.30	1.79	5.30	1.158
4	CH2-NH-N=C(NH2)2	5.70	2.22	5.10	0.775
5	(E,E)-CH=CH-CH=N-N=C(NH2)	6.80	2.15	6.40	1.003
6	(E,Z)-CH=CH-CH=N-NH(2-imidazolinyl)	5.20	–	–	1.261
7	(E,E)-CH=CH-CH=N-NH(2-imidazolinyl)	5.60	2.13	5.05	1.261
8	(E,E,E)-(CH=CH2)2-CH=N-N=C(NH2)2	5.10	1.99	4.82	1.269
9	(E)-CH=CH(2,5-dihydro-5-oxo-3-furyl)	5.40	2.04	4.85	0.969
10	2,5-dihydro-5-oxo-3-furyl(digitoxigenin)	6.30	2.30	6.22	0.663
11	digoxin[e]	6.30	2.26	6.40	

[a]Concentration required to inhibit 50% of Na+, K+-ATPase activity.
[b]Maximal % increase in force of contraction.
[c]Concentration producing 50% of the maximal increase in force of contraction.
[d]Calculated according to I. Moriguchi, Y. Kanada and K. Komatsu: Chem. Pharm. Bull. (Tokyo) 24, 1799 (1976).
[e]Not the substituent but the molecule (structure 4a). Since it does not belong to the series, it was not included in our correlation study.

in digitoxigenin, permits a very strong interaction with the receptor, resulting in a very high inhibition of the enzyme. For a series of cardiotonic steroids, Bohl et al. [58] observed that a linear relationship existed between the Na+, K+-ATPase inhibitory activity of the compounds and their calculated energy of interaction with the digitalis receptor.

Cerri et al. [58] showed that a highly significant correlation existed between Na+, K+-ATPase inhibitory potency and the inotropic potency in isolated atria ($r^2 = 0.73$, $n = 10$ including digoxin). However, for a set of 6 compounds in the series, for which the arrhythmogenic concentrations were also evaluated, a strong correlation was found to exist between the arrhythmogenic activity and the Na+, K+-ATPase inhibitory potency ($r^2 = 0.99$) [58]. This is a highly disappointing point for the development of therapeutically useful cardiotonics.

Though for a set of cardenolides, the Na+, K+-ATPase inhibition activity was found to be correlated with dipole moment (r = 0.95) [59], various qualitative structure-activity relationships (SARs) have presented some pictorial models of the actions of glycosides [60–64]. Basic studies had shown that the steroid ring system, the 17β-lactone and a 3β-sugar moiety were essential features for the activity of glycosides and it was therefore assumed that these features were involved in the drug-receptor interactions. Repke [65] suggested that the lactone ring, containing a carbonyl group conjugated with a double bond, was the functional group of the glycoside for interaction with the receptor. The carbonyl group was assumed to form a hydrogen bond with the receptor [66] and the binding energy was calculated to be about 20 kJ/mol [67], roughly equivalent to the binding energy of an average hydrogen bond. In naturally occurring cardiac glycosides, the lactone ring is always in β-orientation with respect to the steroid nucleus. Inversion of this ring to an α-configuration does not, for steric reasons, permit the steroid ring to approach the enzyme surface. This results in instability of the initial complex – the hydrogen bond breaks and the compound becomes inactive [68, 69].

Thomas et al. [62, 70] found that the lactone ring could be replaced by an open-chain α,β-unsaturated moiety (Fig. 2a). They postulated that the lactone or its open-chain analogues could be bonded to the receptor by a "two-point" attachment, involving a hydrogen bond and an ion-dipole interaction, in which the fractional positive charge on C20 was supposed to be involved (Fig. 2b). But this "two-point" attachment concept was very empirical. A more rigorous approach was adopted by Fullerton et al. [71]. For a group of compounds, these authors obtained an excellent correlation between the biological activity and the position of the carbonyl group or its equivalent (e.g., CN) and therefore concluded that any further speculation about other binding centers was superfluous. These authors insist that the carbonyl group or its isostere (CN) is the sole binding entity and that the rest of the side chain performs a purely passive role of positioning the carbonyl group. The hydrogen bonding through this group was considered to be the most likely binding force.

The enzyme Na+, K+-ATPase has been shown to consist of two or possibly three subunits of polypeptides designated as α, β, and γ. Of these three subunits, α is thought to contain the main locus of the receptor for glycosides

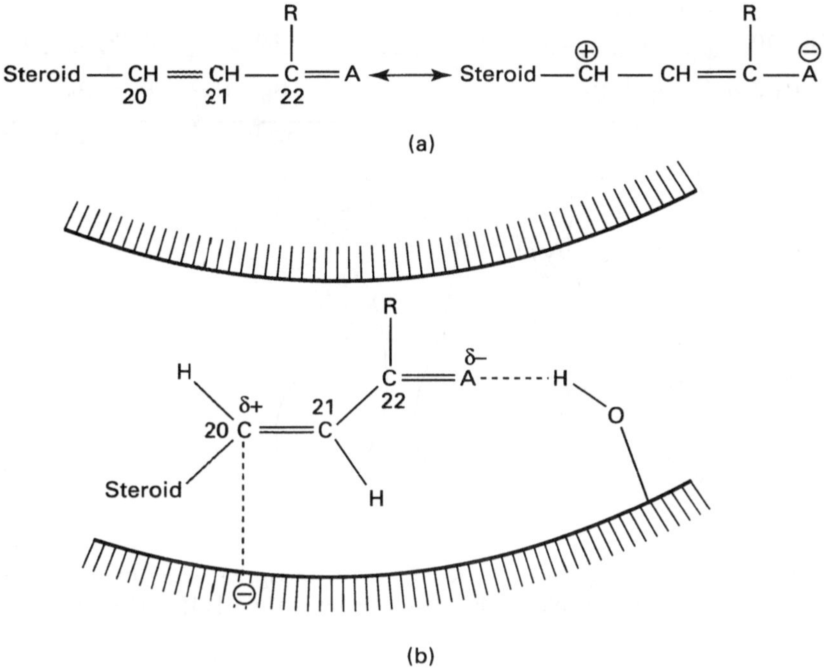

Fig. 2
(a) An open chain α,β-unsaturated moiety (A = a hetero atom),which can replace lactone ring at 17-position of digitalis. R is usually an oxygen- or nitrogen-containing group. (b) Interaction of the open chain with the digitalis receptor – a "two-point" attachment model of Thomas et al. [62, 70], involving a hydrogen bond and an ion-dipole interaction. The chain is shown as lying within a cleft on the enzyme surface. The charge distribution on atoms is due to the resonance phenomenon as shown in (a). Reprinted with permission from [62]. © 1974 American Chemical Society.

[64, 72–76]. Eight major hydrophobic sequences were identified, and it was suggested that these sequences represent the eight transmembrane domains of the unit [77]. A model showing the above features was published by Wallick et al. [78] (Fig. 3). The hydrophobic sequences are labelled H_1 to H_8; the extracellular domains are specified by H regions on either side. For example, the first extracellular domain is designated as H_1-H_2. This model of Wallick et al. was based on the work of Shull et al. [79].

The first two extracellular domains of the α-subunit, i.e., H_1-H_2 and H_3-H_4, are the putative binding sites. Since these domains contain several free carboxylic groups, providing several binding possibilities for ligands with dif-

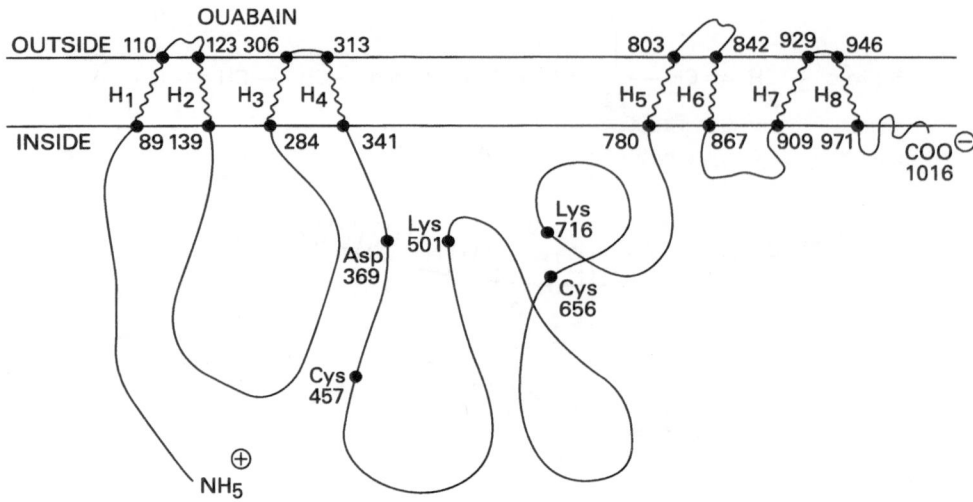

Fig. 3
Wallick et al.'s model of α-subunit of Na+, K+-ATPase. H_1 to H_{8h} represent the transmembrane hydrophobic sequences of the subunit. Reprinted with permission from [64]. © 1990 Academic Press.

ferent degrees of ionization, Quadri et al. [80] studied the effect of the basicity of the substituents at the 17β-position of the digitalis skeleton on binding to the enzyme. They measured the Na+, K+-ATPase binding affinity of a series of 13 hydrazone derivatives of digitoxigenin (Tab. 2) and tried to correlate it with the pK_a of the compounds. A significant correlation was obtained between the two (Eq. 3), suggesting that a great portion of the variance in the activity (about 75%, $r^2 = 0.749$) can be accounted for by changes in the basicity of the compounds. The positive coefficient associated with pK_a indicates that the higher the pK_a value (the greater the tendency to protonate), the higher the binding affinity.

$$\log (1/IC_{50}) = 4.195 + 0.238 \,(\pm\, 0.042)\, pK_a \qquad (3)$$
$$n = 13, \ r = 0.865, \ s = 0.47, \ F_{1,11} = 32.81$$

However, the statistically most significant models were achieved when an additional parameter V_w (van der Waals volume) or MR (molar refractivity index) was also added (Eqs. 4 and 5).

248

Table 2.
Hydrazone derivatives of digitoxigenin and their biological and physicochemical properties [80].

Compd	R^a	$\log(1/IC_{50}{}^b)$	pK_a	V_w (Å³)	MR	PA (kcal/mol)
1	a	7.0	9.35	82.8	27.588	226.23
2	b	5.1	1.78	78.8	27.189	217.46
3	c	5.7	6.34	116.5	40.139	221.99
4	d	4.6	3.44	112.2	38.561	217.16
5	e	6.7	8.42	104.8	35.168	227.47
6	f	6.6	10.36	120.2	39.923	232.98
7	g	6.0	8.05	116.0	40.463	229.24
8	h	5.7	5.76	107.3	36.856	224.58
9	i	5.2	8.62	148.0	53.921	229.89
10	j	6.7	9.49	98.2	32.096	227.87
11	k	4.7	0.86	90.4	35.180	219.93
12	l	4.5	2.37	123.9	39.742	215.67
13	m	4.7	3.58	101.9	35.397	216.48

[a]For substituents see Figure 4.
[b]Concentration required to inhibit 50% of [³H] ouabain binding to Na⁺, K⁺–ATPase.

$$\log (1/IC_{50}) = 6.422 + 0.275\ (\pm 0.021)\ pK_a - 0.023\ (\pm 0.004)\ V_w \qquad (4)$$
$$n = 13,\ r = 0.973,\ s = 0.23,\ F_{2,10} = 89.81$$

$$\log (1/IC_{50}) = 6.310 + 0.263\ (\pm 0.020)\ pK_a - 0.061\ (\pm 0.010)\ MR \qquad (5)$$
$$n = 13,\ r = 0.974,\ s = 0.23,\ F_{2,10} = 91.86$$

From these models it appears that an increase in the molecular size of the compound would have an adverse effect, which may be due to some steric role. The increase in binding affinity with the increase in basicity confirms the Thomas hypothesis [64] that an ion-pair interaction takes place between a carboxylate residue of the enzyme and the hydrazone group at 17β-position when the latter is in the cationic form. The decrease in activity with the increase in molecular size (accounted for by both V_w and MR) may be due to the limited bulk tolerance of the receptor site.

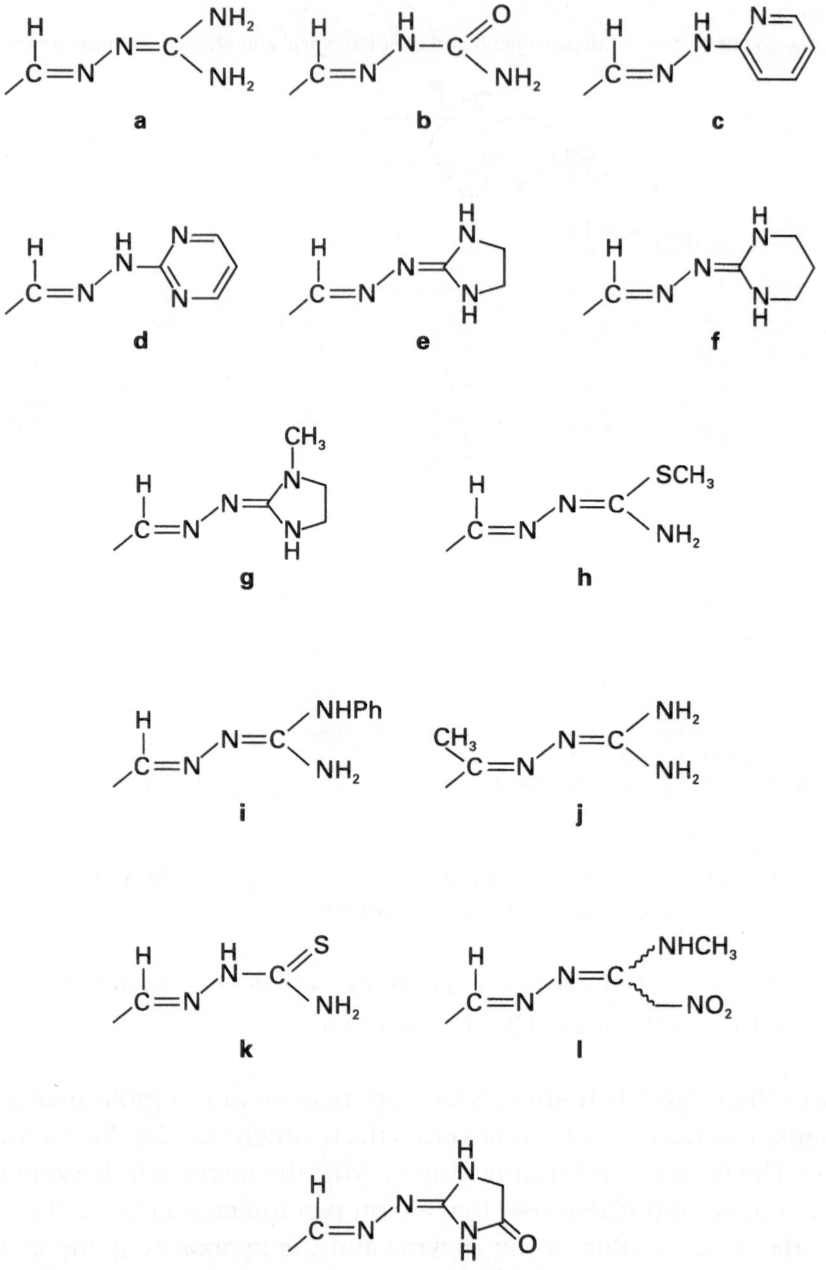

Fig. 4
The R-substituents of Table 2.

A good linear correlation (r = 0.91) was found [74] between the experimental variable pK_a and the proton affinity parameter PA, calculated by semi-empirical quantum mechanical method AM1 [81]. Hence the use of PA in place of pK_a had also resulted in good correlations (Eqs. 6 and 7) [80].

$$\log (1/IC_{50}) = -24.171 + 0.144 \ (\pm 0.022) \ PA - 0.023 \ (0.007) \ V_w \tag{6}$$
$$n = 13, \ r = 0.903, \ s = 0.43, \ F_{2,10} = 21.97$$

$$\log (1/IC_{50}) = -24.475 + 0.147 \ (\pm 0.017) \ PA - 0.074 \ (0.015) \ MR \tag{7}$$
$$n = 13, \ r = 0.944, \ s = 0.33, \ F_{2,10} = 40.87$$

A calculation was made on the differences in the interaction energy of cardiotonic steroids with the digitalis receptor by Bohl et at. [81] using empirical molecular electrostatic potentials. A linear relationship was observed between the interaction energies and the Na^+, K^+-ATPase inhibitory activity of the compounds.

The mechanism by which the sugar component of cardiac glycosides confers its effect is not well known. It was only proposed that the sugars protect the 3-hydroxyl group from epimerization and/or conjugation [82]; either of these biotransformations leads to a relatively inactive compound. Yoda et al. [83–86] were the first to carry out systematic studies on the role of the sugar in the action of glycosides. They found that glycosides with 6-deoxy sugars (i.e., those with 5'-methyl groups) were the most potent of all glycosides and concluded that this group was a key factor in the interaction of the glycoside moiety with the receptor. These authors proposed that binding of cardiac glycosides occurs in two steps: first, binding of the steroid, and then a slower interaction of the sugar residues [85, 86]. They established that it was the first sugar of multiple sugar glycosides that makes the major contribution to the binding.

Although the classical SAR studies indicated the importance of the 3β- and 14β-hydroxyl groups of the steroid ring in binding, subsequent studies showed that activity was not abolished if these groups were removed. The 3β-hydroxyl group does not contribute to binding but provides an essential point of attachment for the sugar residues. Although the removal of the 14β-hydroxyl group does not abolish activity, its presence significantly increases the activity, and it probably has a direct binding role. Naaido et al. [87] suggested that this group may be involved in hydrogen bonding with the recep-

3

Table 3.
Grayanotoxins (**3**) and their inotropic activity [88].

Compd	R	V_w (10^2 Å^3)
1	H	0.013
2	OH	0.081
3	OCOCH$_3$	0.423
4	OCOC$_2$H$_5$	0.577
5	OCO-n-C$_3$H$_7$	0.731
6	OCO-n-C$_4$H$_9$	0.885
7	OCO-n-C$_5$H$_{11}$	1.039
8	OCO-n-C$_6$H$_{13}$	1.193
9	OCOCH$_2$CH$_2$Cl	0.712
10	OCOC$_6$H$_{11}$	1.039
11	OCOC$_6$H$_5$	0.963
12	OCO-t-C$_4$H$_9$	0.785
13	OCOCH(OH)CH$_3$	0.595

tor surface. However, in a series of grayanotoxins (3), Shirai et al. [88] found that acylation of an equivalent 14β-hydroxyl group increased inotropic potency. They synthesized a series of 14β-acylated grayanotoxins (Tab. 3) and measured their positive inotropic potency (in terms of the molar concentration, D_2, for 50% of the maximum inotropic effect) in guinea pigs, which was found to be significantly correlated with the van der Waals volume of the 14-substituents as [88].

$$\log (1/D_2) = 3.751 \ (\pm 1.592) \ V_w - 3.371 \ (\pm 1.296) \ V_w^2 + 5.653 \qquad (8)$$
$$n = 12, \ r = 0.894, \ s = 0.252, \ F_{2,9} = 17.84$$

Since Equation (8) represents a parabolic correlation, an optimum value of $V_w = 0.556 \times 10^2$ Å^3 is obtained. This suggests that although the bulkiness of the 14-substituent may favour the activity, only a moderate size will be tolerated. Shiral et al., however, suggested that some electronic characteristics of 14-substituents and an overall hydrophilic-lipophilic balance of the molecule would also be related to the development of the inotropic effect.

In the derivation of Equation (8), compound 12 was not included because of its aberrant behaviour. Equation (8) predicts very high activity for this compound as compared to its observed activity. Its low observed activity may be due to the steric effect of the t-butyl group present in its R-substituent.

Hydroxy groups at positions other than 3 and 14 of the steroid ring generally decrease the activity [89,90]. This means that the portion of the receptor that binds the steroid has hydrophobic characteristics, or else that the additional hydroxyl groups interfere with the tight fit of the molecule in the receptor cleft.

Extensive studies on glycosides established the clinical applicability of two compounds: digoxin (**4a**) and digitoxin (**4b**) [64].

4a: R=OH ; 4b: R=H

3.2 Nonglycoside cardiotonics

3.2.1 PDE III inhibitors

Amrinone (**5**) and milrinone (**6**) are the forerunners of nonglycoside cardiotonic agents. They are bipyridine derivatives with well established inotropic activity and vasodilatory properties [91–93]. Both these compounds

5   **6**

and their analogues have been reported to be the selective inhibitors of PDE III [94, 95]. Recent molecular modelling studies on milrinone and certain heterocyclic phenyl imidazoles have supported a possible correlation between positive inotropic response and selective PDE inhibition, coming out from the finding that these substances mimic the structural and electronic features of cAMP at the enzyme active binding site [96–100]. It was assumed that agonists and antagonists compete for a common receptor site.

For a fairly large series of amrinone, milrinone and milrinone analogues, Boggia et al. [101] performed a partial least square analysis on their positive inotropic activity to find that the most important factor to account for the variation in the activity was the volume. These authors concluded that the activity was due in part to the close fitting of some substituents to the receptor sites and that with the increasing volume of the substituents perhaps some other parts of the receptor might also participate in the interaction with the molecule. Results on subfamilies indicated that the charge on the carbonyl oxygen (6-O) and possibly on neighbouring atoms could be important, together with the volume.

The local effect of volume on the cardiotonic activity of milrinone analogues was also described by Fornia et al. [102], using Zupan's descriptors.

In another series of milrinone analogues, Cody et al. [103] observed that analogues lacking a 2-substituent, or with the N1 position blocked by a methyl group, did not show cardiac activity (stimulation of myocardial membrane Ca^{2+}-ATPase). A 2-methyl (or a 2'-methyl) substituent was found to give a twist conformation to the molecule, which was observed to possess better activity than the planar conformation. Thus, Cody et al. proposed that for maximal stimulation of Ca^{2+}-ATPase, a 2-CH_3, an N1-H, an electronegative 5-substituent (such as CN, NH2, or Br) and a twist angle greater than 40° between rings are essential. From this, it appears that the N1-H moiety is involved in the hydrogen bonding with the receptor and that the elec-

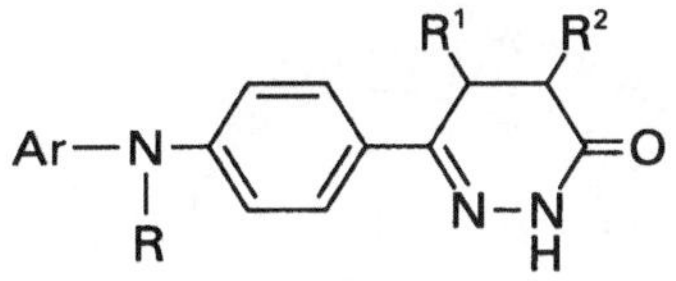

7

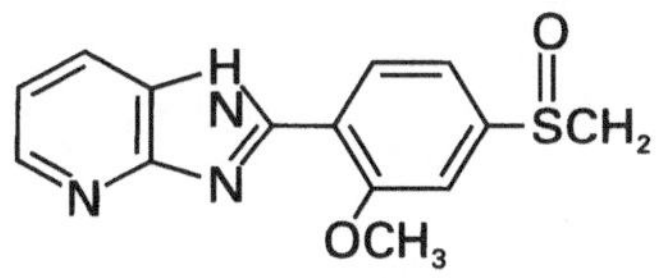

8

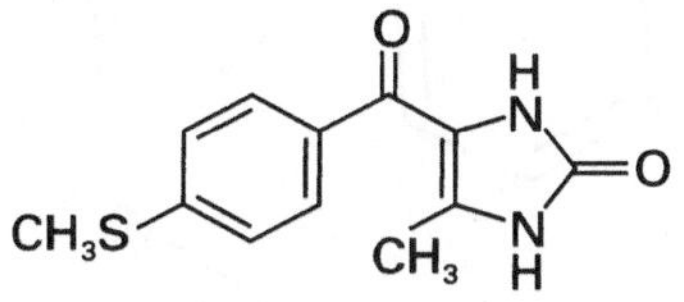

9

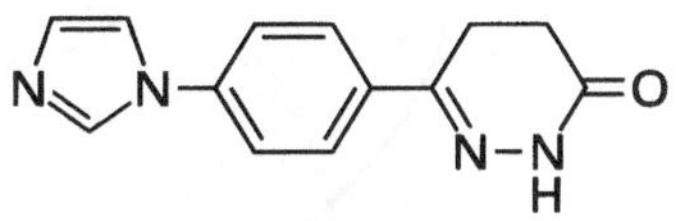

10

tronegative substituent at the 5-position either leads to the formation of a charge-transfer complex with the receptor or binds electrostatically with it. The 2-methyl group, in addition to providing a twist conformation to the molecule, may also be involved in the hydrophobic interaction with the receptor.

Okushima et al. [104] found a marked cardiotonic activity in some phenylpyridazinone derivatives (7) and observed that the most active compound in the series was the one that had Ar = 4-pyridyl, R = H, R_1 = CH_3 and R_2 = H [105]. On the basis of this observation, Okushima et al. suggested that these substituents were optimal for the cardiotonic activity of pyridazinones and proposed a model for their interaction with the receptor as shown in Figure 5 [105].

The discovery of amrinone and milrinone had stimulated the development of several other compounds, e.g., sulmazole (8) [106], fenoximone (9) [107], CI-914 (10) [108] and CI-930 (11) [108], which could replace the glycosides in the treatment of heart failure. Sulmazole (8) had been tested clinically as an orally active replacement for digoxin (4a), but because of its undesirable toxicological effects and substantial metabolism, its further development for chronic oral use was suspended [109, 110]. Attempts to obtain an inotropic agent with a better profile of pharmacological effects led to the development of an isomer of sulmazole, isomazole (12) [111–113], which was

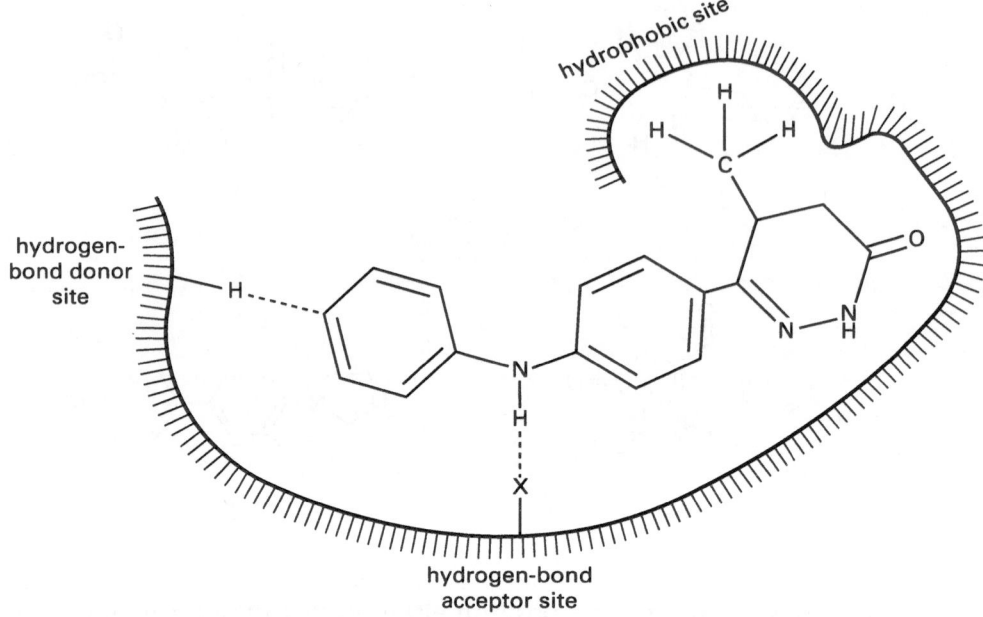

Fig. 5
Okushima et al.'s hypothetical model for the interaction of a cardiotonic phenylpyridazinone with the receptor [105]. Reprinted with permission from [105]. © 1987 American Chemical Society.

11

12

found to be more potent than sulmazole [114]. On the basis of this encouraging result, Barraclough et al. [115] prepared a series of sulmazole analogues (Tab. 4) and studied their structure-activity relationships. They failed in their attempt to find any correlation between *in vitro* inotropic activity and pK_a, protonation site, or logP value. However, they, reported a reasonably good linear correlation (r = 0.81) between the activity and the charge density at the imidazo nitrogen atom calculated by the CNDO/2 method. This report

Table 4.
Sulmazole analogues and their *in vitro* inotropic activity [115].

1 - 10   11 - 16

Compd	X	Y	$\log(1/C_{50}{}^a)$	$Q_N{}^b$
1	H	S(O)	4.70	−0.266
2	5-OCH$_3$	S(O)	3.00	−0.255
3	6-OCH$_3$	S(O)	3.63	−0.246
4	7-OCH$_3$	S(O)	4.10	−0.281
5	6-NH$_2$	O	4.64	−0.256
6	6-NH$_2$	S(O)	3.91	−0.279
7	6-Cl	S(O)	3.76	−0.258
8	6-CH$_3$	S(O)	3.00	−0.226
9	6-OH	S(O)	4.80	−0.276
10	H	O	4.01	−0.263
11	H	S(O)	3.61	−0.258
12	4-OCH$_3$	S(O)	3.73	−0.243
13	6-OCH$_3$	S(O)	3.75	−0.249
14	7-OCH$_3$	S(O)	5.08	−0.282
15	7-NH$_2$	S(O)	3.72	−0.238
16	H	O	4.01	−0.259

[a]Concentration required to give 50% increase in basal contractile force.
[b]Charge at imidazo nitrogen calculated by CNDO/2 method.

was found to be consistent with an earlier finding of these authors regarding sulmazole analogues with varying heterocyclic ring systems [112].

Calculations of the electrostatic potential field in the plane of the imidazopyridine ring and in a series of planes parallel to the system revealed the trend that active molecules had an electrostatic potential minimum adjacent to the formally sp^2 imidazo nitrogen [115]. Molecular mechanics calculations predict that the most stable conformers of sulmazole analogues are essentially planar with little (< 5°) or no deviation of the aryl ring from the plane of the heterocyclic ring [115].

In their study, Barraclough et al. [115] also observed that inotropic activity of sulmazole analogues is sensitive to both the nature and the position of pyridine ring substituents. The 6-position of sulmazole appeared to be the

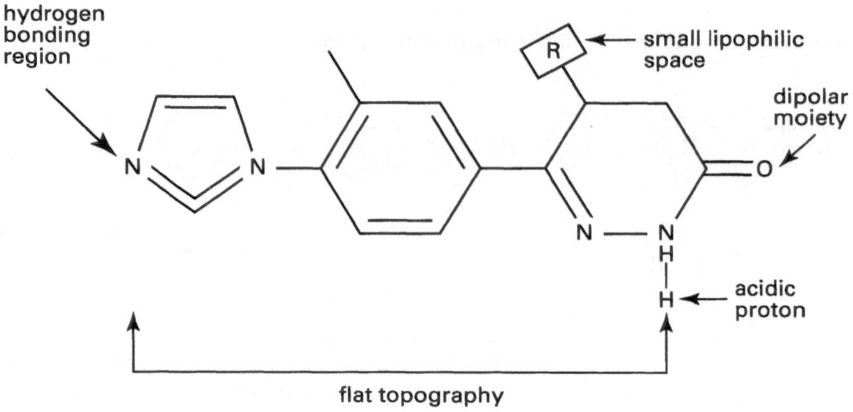

Fig. 6
A hypothetical five-point model for positive inotropic activity of PDE III inhibitors, illustrated with CI-930 (**11**). Reprinted (with slight modification for clarity) with permission from [98]. © 1987 American Chemical Society.

most tolerant toward substituents and a methoxy substituent was best tolerated at the 4-position of isomazole. Overall, electron-releasing substituents, such as methoxy and amino, were better tolerated than lipophilic or electron-withdrawing groups by any analogue.

Initial studies with amrinone [116] had suggested that inhibition of cAMP PDE III was not a component of the mechanism of its cardiotonic action, but Bristol et al. [108] found the *in vivo* inotropic potency of all important non-glycoside cardiotonics (**5, 6, 8–11**) to be significantly correlated (r = 0.89) with their PDE III inhibition potency.

The molecular modelling studies on these structurally different cardiotonics suggested several spatial and electronic similarities among them and led Moos et al. (unpublished results) to suggest a hypothetical five-point model for positive inotropic activity, the salient features of which were as follows: (1) the presence of a strong dipole (carbonyl) at one end of the molecule; (2) an adjacent acidic proton; (3) a methyl-sized lipophilic space; (4) a relatively flat overall topography; (5) a basic or hydrogen-bond acceptor site opposite to the dipole. This model got firm support from the subsequent studies on several pyridazinone-like PDE-inhibiting cardiotonics [94, 98, 117–121]. A refined form of it is represented by Figure 6 [98].

258

13, Papaverine: n = 1, R = 3,4–(OCH$_3$)$_2$

Table 5.
Some papaverine analogues (**13**) and their cAMP specific PDE inhibition activity [122].

Compd	n	4-R	log(1/C$_{50}$[a])	V$_w$[b] (10^2 Å^3)
1	0	NH$_2$	5.13	0.884
2	0	NHCH$_2$CH$_2$Cl	5.46	1.335
3	0	NHCOCH$_2$Cl	5.30	1.363
4	0	N(CH$_2$CH$_2$Cl)$_2$	5.28	1.786
5	0	NHCOCH=CHCOOCH$_3$ (cis)	5.28	1.743
6	0	NHCOCH=CHCOOCH$_3$ (trans)	4.85	1.743
7	0	NHCOCH=CH$_2$	4.92	1.333
8	1	NH$_2$	5.13	1.038
9	1	NHCH$_2$CH$_2$Cl	5.39	1.489
10	1	NHCOCH$_2$Cl	5.41	1.522
11	1	N(CH$_2$CH$_2$Cl)$_2$	5.28	1.940
12	1	NHCOCH=CHCOOCH$_3$ (cis)	5.40	1.897
13	1	NHCOCH=CHCOOCH$_3$ (trans)	5.10	1.897
14	1	NHCOCH=CH$_2$	5.00	1.487
15	1	3,4-(OCH$_3$)$_2$	5.06	1.419

[a]Against bovine heart cAMP specific phosphodiesterase.
[b]Calculated for the whole –(CH$_2$)$_n$–C$_6$H$_4$–R group.

Cyclic AMP specific phospodiesterase inhibition activity of some other classes of compounds has also been analyzed. Some papaverine analogues (**13**) were studied for their inhibition potency against bovine heart enzyme by Walker et al. [122]. Gupta et al. [123] correlated their activity data, as given in Table 5, with van der Waals volume (V$_w$) of the substituent as shown by Equation (9).

$$\log (1/IC_{50}) = 5.245 - 0.157\ V_w + 0.355\ I \tag{9}$$
$$n = 13,\ r = 0.920,\ s = 0.08,\ F_{2,10} = 27.38$$

Table 6.
Mesoionic 1,3,4-thiadiazopyrimidines and their cAMP specific PDE inhibition activity [125].

$R_6 = Et$

Compd	R_2	R_6	$\log(1/IC_{50}{}^a)$	$V_w (R_6)$ (10^2 Å^3)	$\pi (R_6)$
1	H	H	3.11	0.056	0.00
2	H	Me	2.94	0.245	0.56
3	H	Et	3.26	0.399	1.02
4	H	n-Pr	3.60	0.553	1.55
5	H	i-Pr	3.60	0.503	1.53
6	H	s-Bu	3.63	0.657	1.70
7	H	t-Bu	3.81	0.657	1.98
8	H	Amyl	3.81	0.861	2.65
9	H	Bz	4.28	0.939	2.01
10	H	p-Cl-Bz	5.02	1.104	2.66
11	H	Ph	4.62	0.785	1.96
12	Me	Me	2.61	0.245	0.56
13	Me	Et	2.77	0.399	1.02
14	Et	Me	2.62	0.245	0.56
15	Et	Et	2.70	0.399	1.02

^{a}Against bovine heart cAMP specific phophodiesterase.

The indicator variable I = 1 stands for the presence of chlorine atom(s) in the R-substituent. Thus, while a negative coefficient of V_w suggested a detrimental effect of molecular size of R-substituent, a positive coefficient of I indicated an advantageous role of chlorine atom(s), if any, present in it. In deriving Equation (9), however, the cis isomers of compounds 6 and 13 were not included, as to account for the configurational effect another variable was needed, but the remaining compounds in the series were not the subject of configuration.

Prabhakar et al. [124] found the bovine heart cAMP PDE inhibition activity of a series of mesoionic 1,3,4-thiadiazolopyrimidines (Tab. 6) [125] to be significantly correlated with V_w of R_6-substituents (Eq. 10).

$$\log(1/IC_{50}) = 2.677 + 1.810 \ (\pm 0.583) \ V_w \ (R_6) - 0.585 \ (\pm 0.377) \ I(R_2) \qquad (10)$$
$$n = 15, \ r = 0.944, \ s = 0.26, \ F_{2,12} = 48.97$$

The indicator parameter $I(R_2)$ has been used with a value of unity for any R_2-substituent. The negative coefficient of this parameter suggested that an R_2-substituent may produce some steric effects, while R_6-substituent might be involved in a dispersion interaction with the receptor and increase the activity with an increase in its size.

We, however, found $\pi(R_6)$ as a good replacement of $V_w(R_6)$ (Eqs. 11a,b) and thus hydrophobic interaction also seems to be a possibility.

$$\log(1/IC_{50}) = 0.607 \ (\pm 0.293) \ \pi \ (R_6) - 0.621 \ (\pm 0.507) \ I \ (R_2) + 2.817 \qquad (11a)$$
$$n = 15, \ r = 0.898, \ s = 0.35, \ F_{2,12} = 24.87$$
$$\log \ (1/IC_{50}) = 0.381 \ (\pm 0.146) \ \pi \ (R_6) - 0.573 \ (\pm 0.224) \ I \ (R_2)$$
$$+ \ 0.851 \ (\pm 0.259) \ D + 2.946 \qquad (11b)$$
$$n = 15, \ r = 0.983, \ s = 0.15, \ F_{3,11} = 104.64$$

This appears to be more plausible as it is one of the points of the five-point model of PDE-inhibiting cardiotonics (Fig. 6). Thus, mesoionic thiadiazolopyrimidines of Table 6 are very close to the model, i.e., they have a strong dipole (carbonyl), an adjacent acidic proton (if R_8 = H), a lipophilic R_6 moiety, a basic or hydrogen-bond acceptor site (N3) opposite to the dipole and almost a flat topography. In Equation (11b), the use of additional indicator variable D, with a value of 1 for an aromatic R_6-substituent (as in compounds 9–11), leading to a significant improvement in the correlation and exhibiting more positive effects of an aromatic substituent than an aliphatic substituent, supports the assumption of flat topography, since aromatic substituents are usually flat and may lie in the molecular plane.

3.2.2 Sympathomimetic (adrenergic) stimulants

Several adrenergic stimulants have been studied for their cardiotonic effects and their SARs published [126, 127]. Direct β-stimulants have been more important; on the basis of several SAR studies, Carlstrom et al. [128] proposed the following requirements for the cardiotonic effect of a β-stimulant: (1) an aromatic six-membered ring system, (2) an extended ethylamine side chain, approximately perpendicular to the ring system, (3) a positively charged tetracovalent nitrogen atom, (4) a hydrophilic and a hydrophobic group (cis to phenolic OH) at the β-carbon, (5) an R-configuration at the β-carbon. All these points can be represented by a model as **14**.

Pratesi et al. [130–132], however, observed that the selectivity of sympatholytics towards α- or β-adrenergic receptors is dependent upon the cationic head, i.e., the inductive and steric effects of the alkyl group and hydrogen bonding or the basicity of the nitrogen. In a study on a series of **15**, Pratesi et al. [133] found the tracheal and atrial bindings of the compounds to be well correlated with a steric parameter E (Eqs.12 and 13), which is the ratio of van der Waals volumes of α and β moieties in R where the $N-C_\alpha-C_\beta$ sequence is located.

$$pD_2 \text{ (tracheal)} = 5.99 + 1.87\ E - 0.45\ E^2 \tag{12}$$
$$n = 9, r = 0.99$$

$$pD_2 \text{ (atrial)} = 6.64 + 3.24\ E - 1.09\ E^2 \tag{13}$$
$$n = 9, r = 0.98$$

$$Y = 35.42 + 30.59\ E_s \tag{14}$$
$$n = 9, r = 0.843$$

Similarly, Tessel et al. [134] examined the effects of a series of **16** on the maximal chronotropism of isolated guinea pig atria and found the maximal change (Y) in atrial rate from control to be correlated with Taft's steric parameter as shown by Equation (14). Though Equation (14), as well as those obtained by Pratesi et al. (Eqs. 12 and 13), are based on small numbers of data points, they do indicate some steric effects in the binding of the compounds with the receptor.

16

3.2.3 A$_1$-selective adenosine antagonists

Although bipyridine derivatives, such as amrinone (**5**) and milrinone (**6**), have been classified as PDE III inhibitors, they have also been found at elevated concentrations to displace endogeneous adenosine from its cardiac receptors [135–139]. Therefore, in order to obtain pure adenosine antagonists, devoid of inhibitory effect on PDE, Mosti et al. [140–142] synthesized a number of milrinone analogues (**17a–c**) in which the 1,6-dihydro-6-oxopyridine moiety of the parent drug was variously functionalized. Some of these compounds were found to possess better inotropic activity than milrinone and an inhibition of the negative influence exerted by endogeneous adenosine appeared to be involved in their contractile activity [143–145]. From crystallographic and quantum chemical studies, their different inotropic (positive or negative) activities were suggested to be the function of the steric and electronic properties of the substituent at their 2-position [144, 146, 147].

17a   **17b**   **17c**

18a   **18b**   **18c**

19   **20**

Since the purine nucleoside adenosine contains the pyrimidine moiety as an integral part of the molecule, Dorigo et al. [148] synthesized a series of compounds (**18a–c**), characterized by the pyrimidine nucleus bearing an electron donor dimethyl-amino group at position 2 and a variety of functional groups at positions 5 and 6, and investigated their cardiotonic activity by determining their effects on the contractile force and the frequency rate of spontaneously beating atria isolated from guinea pigs. These authors also performed crystallographic studies on two of these compounds (**19** and **20**) and molecular modelling studies on them and some selected analogues and observed that the structural requirements for the inotropic activity of these compounds were: (a) the presence of a dipole area (carbonyl group), (b) a nearby acidic proton donor (OH attached to carbonyl carbon), (c) a hydrogen-bond acceptor site (pyrimidine or aminic nitrogen), (d) an overall planar topography of the molecular area containing the preceding points (encircled in **20**). These requirements seem to be short of only one point, the presence of a small lipophilic area, to exactly match the five-point model of PDE III inhibitors (Fig. 6). The highest inotropic activity associated with **20** in the series, however, led Dorigo et al. [148] to suggest the importance of a prop-

21 (SF40)

erly sized lipophilic group, like a phenyl moiety in 6-substituent, to fit the lipophilic pocket with bulk tolerance in the receptor. In the series of **17** also, the high potency associated with **21** was attributed to the presence of, additionally, the substituted cyclohexane moiety. Orsini et al. [147] had also observed that the presence of a small lipophilic area, near the dipole, at position 4 in the series of **18** and at position 4 or 5 in the series of **17**, would be advantageous. Thus, there can be two beneficial lipophilic areas located on the opposite side of the pyrimidine ring in 18 or of the pyridone ring in **17**. The presence of even a small lipophilic area in pyrimidine analogues (**18**) complements for them the five-point model as described for PDE inhibitors.

The *in vitro* A_1-adenosine receptor binding affinity of some 8-arylxanthine analogues (Tab. 7) studied by Jacobson et al. [149] was found [150] to be significantly correlated with van der Waals volume and hydrophobic constant of phenyl ring B substituents as shown in Equation (15).

$$pK_i = 2.508 \, (\pm 0.412) \, V_w \, (3',5') + 0.280 \, (\pm 0.041) \, \pi \, (4')$$
$$+ \, 0.220 \, (\pm 0.092) \, \pi_X + 7.518 \tag{15}$$
$$n = 17, \, r = 0.929, \, s = 0.22, \, F_{3,13} = 27.43$$

Equation (15) suggests that substituents of the meta positions might be involved in some dispersion interactions while that of the para position might be involved in hydrophobic interaction with the receptor. The bridge moiety X also appears to have some hydrophobic interaction with the receptor, but when only compounds 1–10 were taken, where X = CSNH was constant, a more significant correlation (Eq. 16) was obtained [150], suggesting that changes only in ring substituents can largely account for the variance in the activity; their interactions with the receptor are quite effective.

Table 7.
1,3-Dipropyl-8-phenylxanthines and their A_1-adenosine receptor binding affinity [149].

Compd	X	R	pK_i	V_w (3'5') (10^2 Å^3)	π (4')	π_X
1	CSNH	4'-NCS	8.18	0.112	1.15	−0.17
2	CSNH	3'-NCS	8.62	0.494	0.00	−0.17
3	CSNH	4'-Me	7.80	0.112	0.56	−0.17
4	CSNH	4'-OMe	7.48	0.112	−0.02	−0.17
5	CSNH	4'-F	7.81	0.112	0.14	−0.17
6	CSNH	2',3',4',5',6'-F$_5$	8.04	0.230	0.14	−0.17
7	CSNH	4'-CN	7.78	0.112	−0.57	−0.17
8	CSNH	4'-Br	8.14	0.112	0.86	−0.17
9	CSNH	4'-NO$_2$	7.80	0.112	−0.28	−0.17
10	CSNH	4'-SO$_3^-$	6.44	0.112	−4.76	−0.17
11	SO$_2$	3'-SO$_2$Cl	8.60	0.554	0.00	−1.86
12	SO$_2$	4'-Me	7.14	0.112	0.56	−1.86
13	COCH$_2$	4'-NHCOOCMe$_3$	7.28	0.112	−1.27	−0.55
14	COCH$_2$	4'-NH$_2$	7.40	0.112	−1.23	−0.55
15	XX[a]	4'-NCS	7.60	0.112	1.15	−1.09
16	YY[b]	4'-NCS	8.16	0.112	1.15	−1.69
17	CO	4'-CH$_2$Br	7.94	0.112	0.79	−1.08

[a]XX = COCH$_2$ArNHCSNH.
[b]YY = COCH$_2$NHCSNH

$$pK_i = 2.175 \ (\pm 0.416) \ V_w \ (3',5') + 0.281 \ (\pm 0.031) \ \pi \ (4') + 7.535 \qquad (16)$$
$$n = 10, \ r = 0.972, \ s = 0.15, \ F_{2,7} = 59.95$$

Similarly, for another series of xanthine analogues (Tab. 8) studied by Jacob-son et al. [151], the A_1-receptor binding data were found to be correlated with the molecular size of the substituents (Eq. 17) [150]. In Equation (17), the indicator variable I_Y is equal to 1 for Y = O and zero for Y = S, and I_R is equal to 1 for R = Pr and zero for R = Me or Et.

Table 8.
8-Substituted xanthine analogues and their A_1-adenosine receptor binding affinity [151].

Compd	X	Y	R	R^1	pK$_i$	V$_w$ (R^1) (10^2 Å^3)
1	O	O	Me	H	5.07	0.056
2	O	O	Pr	H	6.35	0.056
3	O	O	Me	c-pentyl	7.96	0.757
4	O	O	Pr	c-pentyl	9.05	0.757
5	S	O	Me	c-pentyl	7.99	0.757
6	S	O	Pr	c-pentyl	9.18	0.757
7	O	O	Me	2-furyl	6.46	0.608
8	O	O	Pr	2-furyl	7.43	0.608
9	S	O	Me	2-furyl	6.74	0.608
10	S	O	Pr	2-furyl	7.49	0.608
11	O	O	Me	3-furyl	7.14	0.608
12	O	O	Me	2-thienyl	6.63	0.717
13	O	O	Me	3-thienyl	6.82	0.717
14	O	O	Pr	2-thienyl	7.79	0.717
15	O	O	Pr	3-thienyl	8.00	0.717
16	S	O	Me	2-thienyl	6.66	0.717
17	S	O	Pr	2-thienyl	7.45	0.717
18	O	O	Me	phenyl	7.07	0.785
19	O	O	Et	phenyl	7.35	0.785
20	O	O	Pr	phenyl	7.99	0.785
21	S	O	Me	phenyl	7.42	0.785
22	S	O	Pr	phenyl	7.79	0.785
23	S	S	Me	c-pentyl	7.39	0.757
24	S	S	Pr	c-pentyl	8.31	0.757
25	O	S	Me	c-pentyl	6.69	0.757
26	O	S	Pr	c-pentyl	7.81	0.757
27	O	S	Me	phenyl	5.86	0.785
28	O	S	Et	phenyl	6.00	0.785

$$pK_i = 2.950 \ (\pm 0.575) \ V_w \ (R^1) + 0.545 \ (\pm 0.257) \ I_Y$$
$$+ 1.066 \ (\pm 0.207) \ I_R + 4.394 \tag{17}$$
$$n = 28, \ r = 0.831, \ s = 0.54, \ F_{3,24} = 17.85$$

The positive coefficients of both I_Y and I_R suggested that at 4-position the oxygen was more beneficial than sulfur and that at N1 and N3 the propyl group was optimal. At 2-position, the change between O and S was not shown to be very effective. In a Free-Wilson analysis, Sharma et al. [150] had found the activity contributions of X, Y, and R substituents as: X (O = –0.057, S = 0.102), Y (O = 0.232, S = –0.857), R (Me = –0.437, Pr = 0.545, Et = –0.211).

From Equation (17), the size of R^1-substituent at the 8-position was suggested to have the dominant effect. However, from the Free-Wilson analysis, Sharma et al. [150] had shown that the activity contribution of only c-pentyl (~ 1.0) was significant and all other substituents, except 3-furyl, had negative contributions. For furyl, though positive, it was only 0.122. Thus, at position 8, a c-pentyl group seems to be most appropriate, probably due to steric fitting. Thus, the xanthine analogues, too, particularly of the type in Table 8, fulfil almost all the requirements of the five-point model. They have a dipole area (4-O), a nearby acidic proton (N9-H), a hydrogen-bond acceptor site (N7), a properly sized lipophilic area (4-Pr) near the dipole area and an overall flat topography. A properly sized R^1 group opposite to 4-Pr constitutes an additional site of hydrophobic or steric interaction.

A large series of 8-styrylxanthine analogues (22) was studied particularly for A_2-selective adenosine antagonist activity [152] and a selectivity factor S was defined as the ratio of $K_i(A_1)$ to $K_i(A_2)$. Ojha et al. [153] correlated this selectivity factor with molecular and electronic properties of C-ring substituents as shown by Equation (18).

22

$$\log (S) = 1.052 \, (\pm 0.324) \, V_w \, (3',5') + 0.760 \, (\pm 0.230) \, \sigma \, (2',4')$$
$$- 0.655 \, (\pm 0.108) \, I_R + 1.166 \, (\pm 0.104) \, I_{R1} + 0.323 \qquad (18)$$
$$n = 48, \, r = 0.907, \, s = 0.36, \, F_{4,43} = 50.00$$

Thus, like Equation (16) obtained for A_1-receptor affinity, Equation (18), too, suggests that for A_2-receptor binding also the molecular size of meta substituents at the phenyl ring will be advantageous. Also the electron-withdrawing substituents at 2'- and 4'-positions seem to increase the selectivity towards the A_2-receptor. Therefore, to increase the selectivity towards A_1, the electron-releasing substituents at ortho and para positions can be of great value.

Insofar as the substituents at the xanthine ring are concerned, the two indicator variables I_R and I_{R1} have been used, with a value of 1 each, to account for the effect of Pr relative to Me at R and of Me relative to H at R^1. The negative coefficient of I_R indicates that a propyl group at R will reduce the selectivity towards A_2 but a methyl group at R^1 will increase it. Therefore, the selectivity towards A_1 will increase if R = Pr and R^1 = H, which, as already discussed, are among the essential features required for A_1-selective adenosine antagonist activity of xanthine analogues (Tabs. 7 and 8).

3.2.4 Ca^{2+} channel activators

The compounds that were initially studied [154] for Ca^{2+} channel activation, e.g., Bay K 8644 (23), CGP 28 392 (24) and PN 202 791 (25), were from the 1,4-dihydropyridine series, which have been basically exploited for the development of Ca^{2+} channel antagonists [40]. A nondihydropyridine Ca^{2+} chan-

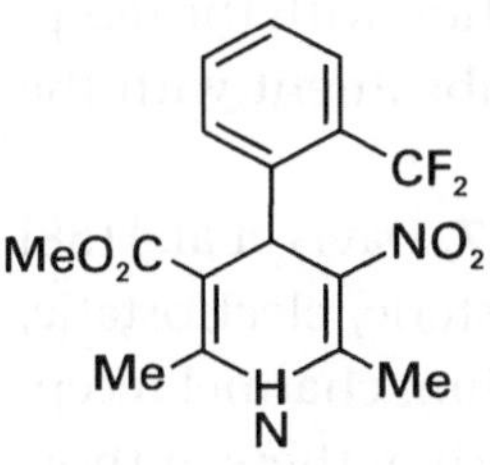

23

Bay K 8644

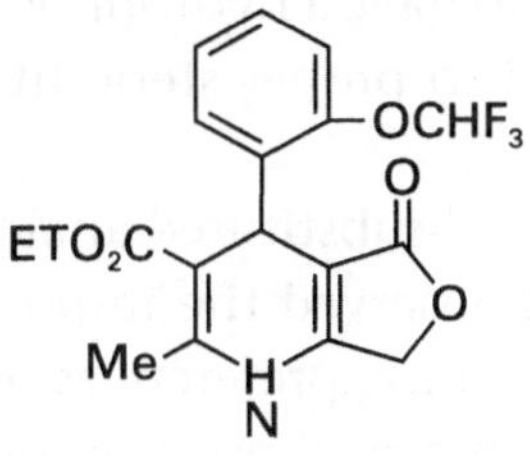

24

CGP 28 392

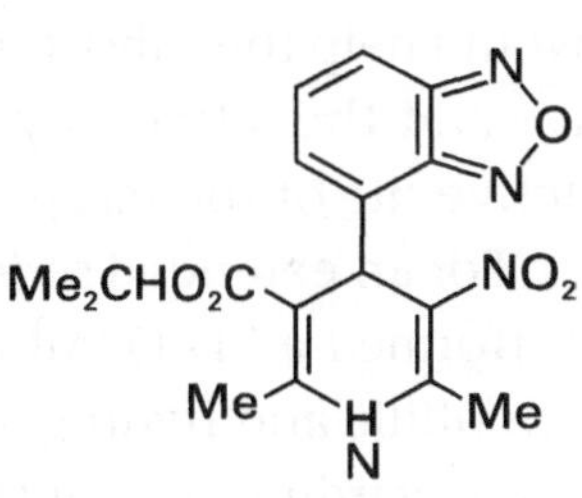

25

PN 202 791

26   **27**

nel activator, FPL 64176 (**26**), that activated the channels in cardiac and vascular tissues with a novel mechanism and site of action, was investigated by McKechnie et al. [155]. Several other compounds (**27**) related to it were then synthesized and studied for their Ca^{2+} channel activation and inotropic activity by Baxter et al. [156]. An attempt was then made to correlate these activities with physicochemical parameters [156]. For a small set of 2'-substituted active congeners, the inotropic activity was shown to be correlated with the hydrophobic constant and Verloop's STERIMOL width parameter B_5 [157] of the substituents as shown by Equation (19).

$$\log (1/EC_{50}) = 0.42\ (\pm 0.15)\ \pi + 0.33\ (\pm 0.19)\ B_5 - 1.97 \tag{19}$$
$$n = 8,\ r = 0.889,\ s = 0.22,\ F_{2,5} = 9.3$$

The EC_{50} refers to the concentration required to increase developed tension to 50% of the isoprenaline maximum. Baxter et al. could not find any good correlation for Ca^{2+} channel activation.

Equation (19) suggested that the hydrophobic property and the width of the substituent would be beneficial to the inotropic activity; the former would help the substituent to have a hydrophobic interaction with the receptor and the latter may lead to proper steric fit of the substituent with the active site of the receptor.

For an extended series of 2'-substituted analogues of **27**, Davis et al. [158] performed a 3D-QSAR and observed the importance of steric, electrostatic, lipophilic and hydrogen-bonding preferences of the calcium channel receptor. Regarding the substituents at 2'-position of the aryl ring, these authors found that lipophilic benzyl substituents lead to the most active compounds and the small hydrophilic substituents to the least active compounds. Of the

270

larger substituents, benzyl substituents and their isosteres are more effective than phenethyl substituents and their isosteres once log P has been accounted for. Also para substituents on benzyl or phenethyl groups have a small unfavourable effect on the activity once their lipophilicity has been accounted for.

For electrostatic and hydrogen-bonding interactions, it can be assumed that the bridge carbonyl group can be involved in electrostatic interaction and N1-H and 3-COOCH$_3$ group can be involved in hydrogen bonding.

Compounds belonging to 1,4-dihydropyridine (DHP) series were usually found to act as Ca^{2+} channel antagonists. Attempts were, therefore, made to find out how a few of them, e.g., 23–25, could act as Ca^{2+} channel activators. Studies of the crystal structures of 1,4-DHP antagonists bearing ortho- or meta- substituents in the phenyl ring have indicated that the activity correlates with the planarity of the 1,4-DHP ring– it increases with increasing ring planarity [159–161], but the conformational analysis of the activator analogues of **23** did not indicate any significant correlation existing between the activator properties and the degree of ring flattening [162]. The differentiating features for activator and antagonist actions of 1,4-DHPs have been attributed to the differences in the hydrogen bonding patterns [163]. From diffraction analyses it has been observed that the hydrogen bond acceptors to 1,4-DHP-amine of activators are not restricted to a single significant interaction [162] which is polarized along the line of sight of the N1-H bond, as was noted for antagonists. The activator analogues of **23** have been found to tend to have multiple DHP-amine contacts which are uniformly distributed ± 60° from the N1-H bond in the vertical N1-C4 plane of the DHP ring [162]. This flexibility of bonding to the amine acceptor group may have consequences with regard to the activator ligands binding to the ion-conducting open channel state.

Based on force field and quantum mechanical calculations, a hypothesis on the molecular mechanism of Ca^{2+} channel activators was proposed by Höltje and Marrer [164]. From the careful investigation of the molecular electrostatic fields of some 1,4-DHP derivatives, these authors discovered a unique area of molecular potentials, where Ca^{2+} agonists and antagonists possess potentials with opposite sign. Höltje and Marrer [164] further demonstrated that calcium channel activators and blockers can exert an opposite effect on the electrostatic potential of the binding site in the receptor. The activators were found to decrease the electrostatic potential, which could probably affect the calcium channel proteins, resulting in an increased influx of Ca^{2+} ions into the cells. On the other hand, the antagonists were found to increase this potential, triggering a structural change of the channel that could result in a reduction of calcium influx.

3.4.5 Vasopressin antagonists

Various peptide analogues of arginine vasopressin (AVP) were studied for their antagonistic activity [40–43] but found to possess poor oral bioavailability, with some having agonistic activity [165, 166]. Therefore, some authors recently tried [167–169] to investigate nonpeptide AVP antagonists that could have oral bioavailability. We performed a QSAR study on V_{1a} antagonistic activity of a series of 1-(1-benzoyl-4-piperidyl)quinolines (28) studied by Ogawa et al. [168]. The use of data of Table 9 revealed Equation (20), which suggests that a lipophilic 4-substituent at the phenyl ring up to an optimum value of $\pi_4 = 1.84$, and any electron-releasing substituent at any position will be quite advantageous to the activity.

28

$$\log (1/IC_{50}) = 0.434 \ (\pm 0.137) \ \pi_4 - 0.118 \ (\pm 0.114) \ (\pi_4)^2$$
$$- 0.369 \ (\pm 0.250) \ \sigma - 0.498 \ (\pm 0.232) \ I_{2,3} + 6.005 \qquad (20)$$
$$n = 29, \ r = 0.892, \ s = 0.23, \ F_{4,24} = 23.30$$

A lipophilic 4-substituent may be involved in a hydrophobic interaction with the receptor; its electron-releasing ability or that of any other substituent present at any other position may increase the electron density at the bridge carbonyl oxygen, enhancing its ability to form a stronger hydrogen bond with

Table 9.
1-(1-Benzoyl-piperidyl)-3,4-dihydro-2-(1H)-quinolines (**28**) and their V_{1a} receptor binding affinity [168].

Compd	R	$\log(1/IC_{50}{}^a)$	π_4	σ
1	2-Cl	5.00	0.00	0.23
2	3-Cl	5.36	0.00	0.37
3	4-Cl	5.92	0.71	0.23
4	2-Me	5.08	0.00	−0.17
5	3-Me	5.89	0.00	−0.07
6	4-Me	6.30	0.56	−0.17
7	2-NO$_2$	5.08	0.00	0.78
8	3-NO$_2$	5.51	0.00	0.71
9	4-NO$_2$	5.70	−0.28	0.78
10	2-OAc	5.85	0.00	0.31
11	3-OAc	5.43	0.00	0.39
12[b]	4-OAc	6.31	−0.64	0.31
13	2-OH	5.82	0.00	−0.37
14	3-OH	5.20	0.00	0.12
15	4-OH	5.89	−0.67	−0.37
16	4-NH$_2$	5.43	−1.23	−0.66
17	4-CO$_2$Me	5.46	−0.01	0.45
18	4-CONH$_2$	4.96	−1.49	0.36
19	4-NHAc	5.55	−0.97	0.00
20	4-CN	5.51	−0.57	0.66
21	4-NMe$_2$	6.33	0.18	−0.83
22	4-F	5.85	0.14	0.06
23	4-Br	6.30	0.86	0.23
24	4-OMe	6.21	−0.02	−0.27
25	4-OEt	6.68	0.38	−0.24
26	4-OPr	6.49	1.05	−0.25
27	4-OBu	6.38	1.55	−0.32
28	4-Et	6.30	1.02	−0.15
29	4-Pr	6.48	1.55	−0.13
30	4-Bu	6.46	2.13	−0.16

[a]Concentration of the compound leading to 50% inhibition of [^{3}H]AVP binding to its specific site at the receptor.
[b]Not included in the derivation of Equations (20) and (21).

the receptor. It can be assumed that a bridge CO group might be involved in the hydrogen bond formation.

In Equation (20), $I_{2,3}$ is an indicator parameter used with a value of unity for a 2- or 3-substituent at the phenyl ring. A negative coefficient of it indi-

Satya P. Gupta

cates that these substituents would be sterically unfavourable to the activity, though their electron-releasing ability will have the beneficial effect. Thus the 4-substituents seem to be the most advantageous. On taking only the 4-substituted analogues, a much better correlation (Eq. 21) was obtained, suggesting that a lipophilic and electron-releasing 4-substituent plays the most dominating role in V_{1a} inhibition.

$$\log (1/IC_{50}) = 0.433 \, (\pm 0.108) \, \pi_4 - 0.119 \, (\pm 0.089) \, (\pi_4)^2$$
$$- 0.405 \, (\pm 0.231) \, \sigma_4 \, + 6.006 \tag{21}$$
$$n = 19, \, r = 0.93, \, s = 0.17, \, F_{3,15} = 31.95$$

In deriving Equations (20) and (21), compound 12 was, however, not included, as it exhibited an aberrant behaviour. Both of these equations predicted very low activity for this compound as compared to its observed activity. No apparent reasons could be found to explain this anomaly.

4   Concluding remarks

The greatest contribution of QSAR studies has been that they have provided a systematic and fairly complete understanding in quantitative terms of the roles of various physicochemical properties in drug design. Combined with molecular modelling or computer graphics, they have provided clear pictures of drug-receptor interaction and the recognition of active sites at the receptors. The present review has discussed QSARs on various classes of cardiotonics and in each class a conclusive picture of drug-receptor interaction has emerged. In cardiac glycosides, the position of carbonyl oxygen of the lactone moiety and shifting of lactone ring from its original position or its replacement by another group are shown to be crucial for their activity. A bulky, basic and polarized system is indicated to be a good replacement of the lactone ring. According to Thomas et al. [62, 70], the lactone ring could be successfully replaced by an open-chain α,β-unsaturated moiety (Fig. 2a). Whatsoever, according to Fullerton et al. [71], be it lactone ring or its open-chain analogues, the carbonyl group or its isostere (e.g. CN) is the sole binding entity. The hydrogen bonding through this group is considered to be the most likely binding force.

274

The findings of Quadri et al. [80] (Eqs. 3–7) for the hydrazone derivatives of digitoxigenin (Tab. 2) supported the role of the basic nature of hydrazone substituents at the 17β-position (the lactone ring replacement) and thus confirmed the Thomas hypothesis [64] that an ion-pair interaction can take place between a carboxylate residue of the enzyme and a hydrazone group at the 17β-position, when the latter is in the cationic form. This hypothesis of Thomas had, however, appeared superfluous to Fullerton et al. [71]. However, whatever the nature of the interaction between a hydrazone substituent and the receptor, Equations (4–7) suggested that the bulk of the substituent would have steric effects.

The binding of cardiac glycosides has been indicated to occur in two steps: first the binding of the steroid and then a slower interaction of the sugar residue [85, 86]. For the former, the 14β-OH group was suggested to be important for the activity due to its ability to form the hydrogen bond with the receptor surface [87], but in a series of grayanotoxins (3), the acylation of the equivalent 14β-hydroxyl group was found to increase the activity with the increase in the size of the acyl group up to the tolerable limit of the active site (Eq. 8) [88].

For nonglycoside cardiotonics – PDE III inhibiting agents – molecular modelling and other SAR studies on pyridazinone-like compounds led to the establishment of a five-point model (Fig. 6) for their inotropic activity. QSAR results (Eqs. 11a,b) on some other kinds of cAMP PDE inhibitors (Tab. 6) also led to support for this model. This five-point model was found to be valid even for the cardiotonic activity of A_1-selective adenosine antagonists like 18a–c. The QSAR results (Eqs. 15–18) for different xanthine series (Tabs. 7 and 8, and 22) and some of the essential features of these molecules, like carbonyl group, acidic proton, basic nitrogen and flat topography, suggest that probably all types of A_1-selective adenosine antagonists would follow the five-point model.

A different five-point model as depicted by 14 has been established for β-stimulating cardiotonics also, but in some cases of β-stimulants, as in 15 and 16, steric factors have also been found to be important (Eqs. 12–14).

For Ca^{2+} channel activators, e.g., 27, 3D-QSAR pointed out the importance of steric, electrostatic, lipophilic and hydrogen-bonding properties of molecules [158]. Equation (19), obtained for a small series of 27, corroborates the role of lipophilic and steric factors. The derivatives of 1,4-dihydropyridine (1,4-DHP) that can act as Ca^{2+} channel activators, e.g., 23–25, differ from those acting as antagonists in respect of the modes of hydrogen bonding with the receptor. Both agonist and antagonist analogues of 1,4-DHP possess a unique area of molecular potentials with opposite sign. The molecular potential of a simple receptor site model is reduced by the interaction of activators and increased by the interaction of antagonists. This is thought to be the basis of the increased and decreased influx of calcium ions into the cells.

The hydrophobic and electronic factors appeared to be important in the action of vasopressin antagonists (28) also (Eqs. 20 and 21) along with the hydrogen bonding.

Thus, in most of the cases, a set of common structural features – a five-point model – is required for the inotropic activity of the compounds. The hydrogen bonding seems to play the most important role in all the cases.

Acknowledgements

The financial assistance provided by University Grants Commission, New Delhi, the other necessary facilities provided by our Institute and the assistance rendered in the preparation of the manuscript by my students and colleagues, Suresh Babu Mekapati and Anita Paleti, are thankfully acknowledged. I also express high appreciation to my wife, Kanak, who always bears with me during my involvement in writing such articles.

References

1   W.C. Bowman and M.J. Rand: Textbook of pharmacology, 2nd ed., Blackwell Scientific Publications, London 1980, Ch. 22 and 23.
2   R.E. Thomas: In: M.E. Wolf (ed.): Burger's medicinal chemistry, 4th ed., John Wiley and Sons, New York 1981, Part III, p. 47.
3   (a) B.F. Hoffman and J.T. Bigger, Jr.: In: A.G. Gilman, L.S. Goodman,T.W. Rall and F. Murad (eds.): Goodman and Gilman's the pharmaceutical basis of therapeutics, 7th ed., Macmillan Publishing Company, New York 1985, p. 716; (b) J.T. Bigger, Jr. and B.F. Hoffman: In: (a), p. 748; (c) P. Rudd and T.F. Blaske: In: (a), p. 784; (d) P. Needleman, P.B. Corr and E.M. Johnson, Jr.: In: (a), p. 806; (e) M.S. Brown and J.L. Goldstein: In: (a), p. 827.
4   D.G. Allen and J.R. Blinks: Nature (London) 273, 509 (1978).
5   J.W. Deitmer and D.J. Ellis: J. Physiol. (London) 284, 241 (1978).
6   D.C. Gadsby and P.F. Cranefield: Proc. Natl. Acad. Sci. USA 76, 1783 (1979).

7   C.O. Lee and M. Dagostino: Biophys. J. *40*, 185 (1982).

8   D.A. Eisner, W.J. Lederer and R.D. Vaughan-Jones: J. Physiol. (London) *335*, 723 (1983).

9   J.R. Blinks, W.G. Wier, J.P. Morgan and P. Hess: In: H. Xoshita, Y. Hagiwara and S. Ebashi (eds.): Advances in pharmacology and therapeutics II, Vol.3: Cardio-renal and cell pharmacology, Pergamon Press, Oxford 1982, p. 205.

10   D. Noble: Cardiovasc. Res. *14*, 495 (1980).

11   A. Gervais, L.K. Lane, B.N. Annes, G.E. Lindermayer and A. Schwartz: Circ. Res. *40*, 8 (1977).

12   R.Weingart: In: Cardiac glycosides, Part 1: Handbook of experimental pharmacology, Springer-Verlag, Berlin 1981, Vol. 56/1, p. 221.

13   E. Marbin and R.W. Tsien: J. Physiol. (London) *329*, 589 (1982).

14   T.J. Hougen and T.W. Smith: Circ. Res. *42*, 856 (1978).

15   R.E. Weishaar, M. Quade, D. Boyd, J. Schenden and H.R. Kaplan: Drug Dev. Res. *3*, 517 (1983).

16   S.F. Campbell, N.J. Cussans, J.C. Danilewicz, A.G. Evans, A.L. Ham, A.A. Jaxa-Chamiec, D.A. Robers and J.K. Stubbs: Roy. Soc. Chem. (Spl. Publ.), No. *54*, 47 (1984).

17   R.E.Weishaar, M.H. Cain and J.A. Bristol: J. Med. Chem. *28*, 537 (1985).

18   A.A. Alousi, L.H. Watton, G.Y. Leshur and A.E. Farah: Roy. Soc. Chem. (Spl. Publ.) No. *50*, 65 (1984).

19   T. Kariya, L.T. Willey and R.C. Dage: J. Cardiovasc. Pharmacol. *4*, 50 (1982).

20   T. Kariya, L.T. Willey and R.C. Dage: J. Cardiovasc. Pharmacol. *6*, 50 (1984).

21   R.E. Weishaar, M. Quade, J.A. Schenden, D.K. Boyd and D.B.Evans: Pharmacologist *25*, 551 (1983).

22   R.E. Weishaar, M. Quade, J.A. Schenden, D.K. Boyd and D.B.Evans: Proc. Fed. Am. Soc. Exp. Biol. *44*, 1792 (1985).

23   G.A. Robinson, R.W. Butcher and E.W. Sutherland: Cyclic AMP, Academic Press, New York 1971.

24   E.W. Sutherland, G.A. Robinson and R.W. Butcher: Circulation *37*, 279 (1968).

25   S. Swillens and J.E. Dumont: Life Sci. *27*, 1013 (1980).

26   G.S. Francis: Am. Heart J. *118*, 642 (1989).

27   W.H. Newman, S.J. Grossman, M.B. Franskis and J.G. Webb: J. Mol. Cell. Cardiol. *16*, 577 (1984).

28   L. Belardinelli, A. West, R. Crampton and R.M. Berne: In: R.M. Berne, T.W. Rall and R. Rubio (eds.): Regulatory function of adenosine, Nihoff, Boston 1983.

29   M. Endoh, M. Maruyama and N. Taira: In: J.W. Daly, Y. Kuroda, J.W. Phillis, and H. Schmizu, VI (eds.): Physiology and pharmacology of adenosine derivatives, Raven Press, New York 1983, p. 127.

30   A. Pelleg, T. Mitsouka and E.L. Michelson: J. Pharmacol. Exp. Ther. *242*, 791 (1987).

31   L. Belardinelli and G. Isenberg: Am. J. Physiol. *244*, H 734 (1983).

32   M. Bohm, R. Bruckner, I. Hackabarth, B. Haubitz, R. Linhart, W. Meyer, B. Schmidt, W. Schmidz and H. Scholz: J. Pharmacol. Exp. Ther. *230*, 483(1984).

33   E. Cerbai, U. Klockner and G. Isenberg: Am. J. Physiol. *255*, H 872 (1988).

34   M. Prostan and V.M. Varagic: Arch. Int. Pharmacodyn. *294*, 137 (1988).

35   G. Jochem and H. Nawrathm: Experientia *39*, 1347 (1983).

36   S. Visentin, S.N. Wu and L. Belardinelli: Am. J. Physiol. *258*, H1070 (1990).

37   W.F. Lubbe, T. Podzuweit and L.H. Opie: J. Am. Cell. Cardiol. *19*, 1622 (1992).

38   (a) M. Packer: Am. Coll. Cardiol. *12*, 1299 (1988); (b) M. Packer, J.R. Carver, R.J.Rode-

Satya P. Gupta

heffer, R.J. Ivanhoe, R. Dibianco, S.M. Zeldis, G.H. Hendrix, W.J. Bommer, D. Elkayam, M.L. Kukin et al.: N. Engl. J. Med. *325*, 1468 (1991).

39   D.J. Triggle: In: J.C. Emmett (ed.): Comprehensive medicinal chemistry, Vol. 3, Pergamon Press, Oxford 1990, p. 1047.
40   M. Manning and W.H. Sawyer: J. Recept. Res. *13*, 195 (1993).
41   L.B. Kinter, W.F. Huffman and F.L. Stassen: Am. J. Physiol. *254*, F165 (1988).
42   F.A. Laszlo, Jr. and D. De Wied: Pharmacol. Rev. *43*, 73 (1991).
43   J.D. Albright and P.S. Chan: Current. Pharm. Des. *3*, 615 (1997).
44   H. Kubinyi: QSAR: Hansch analysis and related approaches, VCH Publishers, Weinheim - New York 1993.
45   S.P. Gupta, P. Singh and M.C. Bindal: Chem. Rev. *83*, 633 (1983).
46   S.P. Gupta: Chem. Rev. *87*, 1183 (1987).
47   S.P. Gupta: Chem. Rev. *89*, 1765 (1989).
48   S.P. Gupta: Chem. Rev. *91*, 1109 (1991).
49   S.P. Gupta: Chem. Rev. *94*, 1507 (1994).
50   S.P. Gupta: Prog. Drug. Res. *45*, 67 (1995).
51   S.P. Gupta: Current Pharm. Des. *4*, 455 (1998).
52   S.P. Gupta: Prog. Drug Res. *53*, 53 (1999).
53   R. Garg, S.P. Gupta, H. Gao, S.B. Mekapati, A.K.Debnath and C. Hansch: Chem. Rev. *99*, 3525 (1999).
54   D.S. Fullerton, K. Yoshioka, D.C. Rohrer, A.H.L. From and K. Ahmed: Science *205*, 917 (1979).
55   D.C. Rohrer, D.S. Fullerton, K. Yoshioka, A.H.L. From and K. Ahmed: ACS Symp. Ser. No.112, 259 (1979).
56   S.P. Gupta and A. Paleti: Personal communication.
57   A. Cerri, F. Serra, P. Ferrari, E. Folpini, G. Padoani and P. Melloni: J. Med. Chem. *40*, 3484 (1997).
58   M. Bohl, K. Ponsold and G. Reck: J. Steroid Biochem. *21*, 373 (1984).
59   K.R.H. Repke, F. Dittrich, P. Berlin and H.H. Portius: Ann. N.Y. Acad. Sci. *242*, 737 (1974).
60   C.S. Davies and R.P. Halliday: In: A. Burger (ed.): Medicinal chemistry, 3rd Ed., Vol. 5, Part 2, John-Wiley, New York 1970, p. 1065.
61   T.W. Guntert and H.H. Linde: Experientia *33*, 697 (1977).
62   R. Thomas, J. Boutagy and A. Gelbart: J. Pharm. Sci. *63*, 1649 (1974).
63   C.K. Chiu and T.R. Watson: J. Med. Chem. *28*, 509 (1985).
64   R. Thomas, P. Gray and J. Andrews: Adv. Drug. Res. *19*, 311 (1990).
65   K. Repke: Internist *7*, 418 (1966).
66   K. Repke and H.J. Portius: Arzneim.-Forsch. *14*, 1073 (1964).
67   W. Schonfeld, J. Weiland, C. Lindig, M. Masnyk, M.M. Kabat, A. Kurek, J. Wicha and K.R.H. Repke: Naunyn Schmiedebergs Arch. Pharmacol. *329*, 414 (1985).
68   K.K. Chen and R.C. Elderfield: J. Pharmacol. Exp. Ther. *70*, 338 (1940).
69   W.A. Jacobs: J. Biol. Chem. *88*, 519 (1930).
70   R. Thomas, J. Boutagy and A. Gelbart: J. Pharmacol. Exp. Ther. *191*, 219 (1974).
71   D.S. Fullerton, K. Ahmed, A.H.L. From, R.H. McParland, D.C. Rohrer and J.F. Griffin: In: A.S.V. Burgen, G.C.K. Roberts and M.S. Tute (eds.): Molecular graphics and drug design, Elsevier, Amsterdam 1986, p. 257.
72   B. Forbush, III.: Curr. Top. Membr. Transp. *19*, 167 (1983).

73   M.P. Goeldner, C.G. Hirth, B. Rossi, G. Ponzio and M. Lazdunski: Biochemistry *22*, 4685 (1983).

74   B. Rossi, G. Ponzio and M. Lazdunski: EMBO J. *1*, 859 (1982).

75   B. Rossi, G. Ponzio, M. Lazdunski, M. Goeldner and C. Hirth: Curr. Top. Membr. Transp. *19*, 271 (1983).

76   C. Hall and A. Ruoho: Proc. Natl. Acad. Sci. USA *77*, 4529 (1980).

77   P.L. Jörgensen, E. Skriver, H. Hebert and A.B. Maunsbach: Ann. N.Y. Acad. Sci. *402*, 207 (1982).

78   E.T. Wallick, T.L. Kirley and A. Schwartz: In: E. Erdman, K. Greeff and J.C. Skou (eds.): Cardiac glycosides 1785–1985, Steinkoff Verlag, Darmstadt 1986, p. 27.

79   G.E. Shull, A. Schwartz and J.B. Lingrel: Nature (London) *316*, 691 (1985).

80   L. Quadri, A. Cerri, P. Ferrari, E. Folpini, M. Mabilia and P. Melloni: J. Med. Chem. *39*, 3385 (1996).

81   M.J.S. Dewar and K.M. Dieter: J. Am. Chem. Soc. *108*, 8075 (1986).

82   K. Repke and L.T. Samuels: Biochemistry *3*, 689 (1964).

83   A. Yoda, S. Yoda and A.M. Sarrif: Mol. Pharmacol. *9*, 766 (1973).

84   A. Yoda: Ann. N.Y. Acad. Sci. *242*, 598 (1974).

85   A. Yoda and S. Yoda: Mol. Pharmacol. *11*, 653 (1975).

86   A. Yoda and S. Yoda: Mol. Pharmacol. *13*, 352 (1977).

87   B.K. Naaido, T.R. Witty, W.A. Remers and H.R. Besch, Jr.: J. Pharm. Sci. *63*, 1391 (1974).

88   N. Shirai, J. Sakakibara, T. Kaiya, S. Kobayashi, Y. Hotta and K. Takeya: J. Med. Chem. *26*, 851 (1983).

89   A. De Pover and T. Godfraind: Naunyn Schmiedebergs Arch. Pharmacol. *321*, 135 (1982).

90   L. Brown, B. Lorenz and R.E. Thomas: Biochem. Pharmacol. *32*, 2767 (1983).

91   A.E. Farah and A.A. Alousi: Life Sci. *22*, 1139 (1978).

92   A.A. Alousi, J.M. Carter, M.J. Montenaro, D.J. Fort and R.J. Ferrari: J. Cardivasc. Pharmacol. *5*, 792 (1983).

93   A. Ward, R.N. Brogdein, R.C. Heel, T.M. Speight and G.S. Avery: Drug *26*, 468 (1983).

94   R.E. Weishaar, S.D. Burrows, D.C. Koybylarz, M.M. Quade and D.B. Evans: Biochem. Pharmacol. *35*, 787 (1986).

95   M. Ito, T. Tanaka, M. Saitoh, H. Msuoka, T. Nahano and H. Hidaka: Biochem. Pharmacol. *37*, 2041 (1988).

96   I. Sirkar, L.D. Bradley, G. Bobowsky, J.A. Bristol and D.B. Evan: J. Med. Chem. *28*, 1405 (1985).

97   A.A. Hagedorn, III, P.W. Erhardt, W.C. Lumma, Jr., R.A. Wohl, R.E. Cantor, Y.L. Chou, W.R. Ingebresten, D. Pang, C.A. Pease and J. Wiggins: J. Med. Chem. *30*, 1342 (1987).

98   H.W. Moos, C.C. Humblet, I. Sircar, C. Rithner, R.E. Weishaar, J.A. Bristol and A.T. McPhail: J. Med. Chem. *30*, 1963 (1987).

99   P.W. Erhardt, A.A. Hagedorn, III and M. Sabio: Mol. Pharmacol. *33*, 1 (1987).

100   P.W. Erhardt and Y. Chou: Life Sci. *49*, 553 (1991).

101   R. Boggia, M. Forina, P. Fossa and L. Mosti: Quant. Struct.-Act. Relat. *16*, 201 (1997).

102   M. Forina, R. Boggia, L. Mosti and P. Fossa: Farmaco *52*, 411 (1997).

103   V. Cody, A. Wojtczak, F.B. Davis and S.D. Blass: J. Med. Chem. *38*, 1990 (1995).

104   (a) H. Okushima, A. Narimatsu and R. Furuya: JP Kokai 8 015, 8 016 (1983); (b) H. Okushima, A. Narimatsu and I. Shimooda: JP Kokai 140 016 (1983).

105   H. Okushima, A. Narimatsu, M. Kobayashi, R. Furuya, K. Tsuda and Y. Kitada: J. Med. Chem. *30*, 1157 (1987).

106   W. Diederen and R. Kadatz: Arzneim.-Forsch. *31*, 141 (1981).

107   R.A. Schnettler, R.C. Dage and J.M. Grisar: J. Med. Chem. *25*, 1477 (1982).

108   J.A. Bristol, I. Sirkar, W.H. Moos, D.B. Evans and R.E. Weishaar: J. Med. Chem. *27*, 1099 (1984).

109   P.W. Erhardt: J. Med. Chem. *30*, 231 (1987).

110   D. El Allaf, V. D'Orio and J. Calier: Arch. Int. Physio. Biochim. *92*, 10 (1985).

111   D. Barraclough, R. Firmin, R. Iyer, W.R. King, J.C. Lindon, M.S. Nobbs, S. Smith, C.J. Wharton and J.M. Williams: J. Chem. Soc. Perkin Trans. *2* ,1839 (1988).

112   D.W. Robertson, E.E. Beedle, J.H. Krushinski, G. Don Pollock, H. Wilson, V. Wyss and J.S. Hayes: J. Med. Chem. *28*, 717 (1985).

113   D.W. Robertson and J.S. Hayes: Drugs Future *10*, 295 (1985).

114   G. Allan, D. Cambridge, M.J. Follenfant, D. Stone and M.V. Whiting: Br. J. Pharmacol. *93*, 387 (1988).

115   P. Barraclough, J.W. Black, D. Cambridge, D. Collard, D. Firmin, V.P. Gerskowitch, R.C. Glen, H. Giles, A.P. Hill, R.A.D. Hull et al.: J. Med. Chem. *33*, 2231 (1990).

116   A.A. Alousi, A.E. Farah, G.Y. Lesher and C.J. Opalka: Circ. Res. *45*, 666 (1979).

117   I. Sirkar, R.E. Weishaar, D. Kobylarz, W.H. Moos and J.A. Bristol: J. Med. Chem. *30*, 1955 (1987).

118   R.E. Weishaar, M.M. Quade, J.A. Schenden and D.B. Evans: J. Cyclic Nucleotide Protein Phosphor. Res. *10*, 551 (1985).

119   R.E. Weishaar, M. Quade, J.A. Schenden, D.K. Boyd and D.B. Evans: Eur. J. Pharmacol. *119*, 205 (1985).

120   D.B. Evans, R.E. Potoczak, R.P. Steffen, W.E. Burmeister, R.W. McNish, J.A. Schenden and H.R. Kaplan: Drug Dev. Res. *9*, 143 (1986).

121   S.A. Harrison, D.H. Reifsnyder, B. Gallis, G.G. Cadd and J.A. Beavo: Mol. Pharmacol. *29*, 506 (1986).

122   K.A. Walker, M.R. Boots, J.F. Stubbins, M.E. Rogers and C.W. Davis: J. Med. Chem. *26*, 174 (1983).

123   S.P. Gupta, C. Garg and J.K. Gupta: Res. Commun. Chem. Pathol. Pharmacol. *61*, 265 (1988).

124   Y.S. Prabhakar, A. Handa and S.P. Gupta: J. Pharmacobio-Dyn. *7*, 366 (1984).

125   R.A. Glenon, M.E. Rogers, J.D. Smith, M.K. El-Said and J.L. Egle: J. Med. Chem. *24*, 658 (1981).

126   A.M. Lands, T.G., Brown, Jr.: In: A. Burger (ed.): Drugs affecting the peripheral nervous system, Vol. 1, Marcel Dekker, New York 1976, p. 399.

127   D.J. Triggle, in ref. 60, p.1235.

128   D. Carlstrom, R. Bergin and G. Falkenberg: Quart. Rev. Biophys. *6*, 257 (1973).

129   P.N. Patil, J.B. Lapidiu and A. Tye: J. Pharm. Sci. *59*, 1205 (1970).

130   P. Pratesi: International symposium on pharmaceutical chemistry, Florence, 1962, Butterworths, London 1963, p. 435.

131   P. Pratesi and E. Grana: Adv. Drug Res. *2*, 127 (1965).

132   P. Pratesi, L. Villa and E. Grana: Farmaco *21*, 409 (1966).

133   P. Pratesi, L. Villa and E. Grana: Farmaco *30*, 315 (1975).

134   R.E. Tessel, J.E. Wooda, R.E. Counsell and G.P. Basmadjian: J. Pharmacol. Exp. Ther. *192*, 319 (1975).

135   P. Dorigo and I. Maragno: Br. J. Pharmacol. *32*, 623 (1986).

136   C.Q. Earl, J. Linden and W.B. Weglicki: J. Cardiovasc. Pharmacol. *8*, 864 (1986).

137 W.J. Parson, V. Ramkumar and G.L. Stiles: Mol. Pharmacol. *33*, 441 (1988).

138 P. Dorigo, R.M. Gaion and I. Maragno: Cardiovasc. Drug Ther. *4/2*, 509 (1990).

139 M. Ungerer, M. Bohm, R.H.G. Schwinger and E. Erdman: Naunyn Schmiedebergs Arch. Pharmacol. *341*, 577 (1990).

140 L. Mosti, G. Menozzi, P. Schenone, P. Dorigo, R.M. Gaion, F. Benetollo and G. Bombieri: Eur. J. Med. Chem. *24*, 517 (1989).

141 L. Mosti, G. Menozzi, P. Schenone, P. Dorigo, R.M. Gaion and P. Belluco: Farmaco *47*, 427 (1992).

142 L. Mosti, P. Schenone, M. Iester, P. Dorigo, R.M. Gaion and D. Fraccarollo: Eur. J. Med. Chem. *28*, 853 (1993).

143 P. Dorigo, R.M. Gaion, P. Belluco, P.A. Borea, L. Guerra, L. Mosti, M. Floreani and F. Carpendo: Gen. Pharmacol. *23*, 535 (1992).

144 P. Dorigo, R.M. Gaion, P. Belluco, D. Fraccarollo, I. Maragno, G. Bombieri, F. Benetollo and F. Orisini: J. Med. Chem. *36*, 2475 (1993).

145 P. Dorigo, D. Fraccarollo, G. Santostasi, R.M. Gaion, I. Maragno, M. Floreani, F. Carpendo, M. Iester, L. Mosti and P. Schenone: Farmaco *49*, 19 (1994).

146 F. Orsini, F. Benetollo, G. Bombieri and L. Mosti: Eur. J. Med. Chem. *25*, 425 (1990).

147 F. Orsini, F. Benetollo, G. Bombieri and L. Mosti: Eur. J. Med. Chem. *28*, 637 (1993).

148 P. Dorigo, D. Fraccarollo, G. Santostasi, I. Maragno, M. Floreani, P.A. Borea, L. Mosti, L. Sansebastino, P. Fossa, F. Orsini et al.: J. Med. Chem. *39*, 3671 (1996).

149 K.A. Jacobson, S. Barone, U. Kammula and G.L. Stiles: J. Med. Chem. *32*, 1043 (1989).

150 R.C. Sharma, P. Singh, T.N. Ojha and S. Tiwari: Drug Des. Discov. *12*, 169 (1994).

151 K.A. Jacobson, L. Kiriasis, S. Barone, B.J. Bradbury, U. Kammula, J.M. Campagne, S. Secunda, J.W. Daly, J.L. Neumeyer and W. Pfeiderer: J. Med. Chem. *32*, 1873 (1989).

152 K.A. Jacobson, C. Gallo-Rodrigsez, N. Melman, B. Fischer, M. Mailard, A. Van Bergen, P.J. Van Galen and K. Yishai: J. Med. Chem. *36*, 1333 (1993).

153 T.N. Ojha, S. Tiwari, R.C. Sharma and P. Singh: Indian J. Chem. *34B*, 452 (1995).

154 R.A. Janis, P. Silver and D.J. Triggle: Adv. Drug Res. *16*, 309 (1987).

155 K. McKechnie, P.G. Killingback, I. Naya, S.E. O'Connor, G.W. Smith, D.W. Wattam, E. Wells, Y.M. Whitehead and G.E. Williams: Br. J. Pharmacol. *98*, 673P (1989).

156 A.J.G. Baxter, J. Dixon, F. Ince, C.N. Manners and S.J. Teague: J. Med. Chem. *36*, 2739 (1993).

157 A. Verloop, W. Hoogenstraaten and J. Tipker: In: E.J. Ariëns (ed.): Drug design, Vol. VII, Academic Press, New York 1976, p. 165.

158 A.M. Davis, N.P. Gensmantel, E. Johansson and D.P. Marriot: J. Med. Chem. *37*, 963 (1994).

159 D.J. Triggle, D.A. Langs and R.A. Janis: Med. Res. Rev. 9, 123 (1989).

160 R. Fossheim, K. Svarteng, A. Mostad, C. Romming, E. Shefter and D.J. Triggle: J. Med. Chem. *25*, 126 (1982).

161 R. Fossheim, A. Joslyn, A.J. Solo, E. Luchowski, A. Rutledge and D.J. Triggle: J. Med. Chem. *31*, 300 (1988).

162 D.A. Langs, Y.W. Kwon, P.D. Strong and D.J. Triggle: J. Comput-Aided Mol. Des. *5*, 95 (1991).

163 R. Fossheim: Acta Chem. Scand. *B41*, 581 (1987).

164 H.-D. Holtje and S. Marrer: J. Comput-Aided Mol. Des. *1*, 23 (1987).

165 S.C. Mah and K.G. Hofbauer: J. Pharmacol. Exp. Ther. *245*, 1028 (1988).

166 W.F. Huffman, C. Albrightson-Winslow, B. Brickson, H.G. Bryan, N. Caldwell, G. Dytko,

D.S. Eggleston, L.B. Kinter, M.L. Moore, K.A. Newlander et al.: J. Med. Chem. *32*, 880 (1989).

167   C. Serradeil-Le Gal., J. Wagnon, C. Garcia, C. Lacour, P. Guiraudou, B. Christople, G. Villanova, D. Nistato, J.P. Maffrand, G. Le Furr et al: J. Clin. Invest. *92*, 224 (1993).

168   H. Ogawa, Y. Yamamura, H. Miyamato, K. Kondo, H. Yamishita, K. Nakaya, T. Chihara, T. Mori, M. Tominaga and Y. Yabuuchi: J. Med. Chem. *36*, 2011 (1993).

169   H. Ogawa, H. Yamashita, K. Kondo, Y. Yamamura, H. Miyamoto, K. Kan, K. Kitano, M. Tanaka, K. Nakaya, S. Nakamura et al.: J. Med. Chem. *39*, 3547 (1996).

Index Vol. 55

Index of titles
Vol. 1–55 (1959–2000)

Author and paper index
Vol. 1–55 (1959–2000)

Problems in preparation, testing and use of diphtheria, pertussis and tetanus vaccines *19*, 229 (1975)	D. D. Banker
Phosphodiesterase 4 (PDE4) inhibitors in asthma and chronic obstructive pulmonary disease *53*, 193 (1973)	Mary S. Barnette
Recent advances in electrophysiology of antiarrhythmic drugs *17*, 33 (1973)	A. L. Bassett A. L. Wit
Chirality and future drug design *41*, 191 (1993)	Sanjay Batra Manju Seth A. P. Bhaduri
Drugs for treatment of patients with high cholesterol blood levels and other dyslipidemias *43*, 9 (1994)	Harold E. Bays Carlos A. Dujovne
Stereochemical factors in biological activity *1*, 455 (1959)	A. H. Beckett
Natriuretic hormones II *45*, 245 (1995)	Elaine J. Benaksas E. David Murray, Jr. William J. Wechter
Molecular modelling and quantitative structure-activity analysis of anti-bacterial sulfanilamides and sulfones *36*, 361 (1991)	P. G. De Benedetti
Industrial research in the quest for new medicines *20*, 143 (1976) The experimental biologist and the medical scientist in the pharmaceutical industry *24*, 38 (1980)	B. Berde
Newer diuretics *2*, 9 (1960)	K. H. Beyer, Jr. J. E. Baer
Recent developments in 8-amino-quinoline antimalarials *28*, 197 (1984)	A. P. Bhaduri B. K. Bhat M. Seth
Studies on diphtheria in Bombay *19*, 241 (1975)	M. Bhaindarkar Y. S. Nimbkar
Bitoscanate in children with hookworm disease *19*, 6 (1975)	B. Bhandari L. N. Shrimali
Recent studies on genetic recombination in *Vibriocholerae* *19*, 460 (1975)	K. Bhaskaran

Interbiotype conversion of cholera vibrios by action of mutagens *19*, 466 (1975)	P. Bhattacharya S. Ray
Experience with bitoscanate in hook-worm disease and trichuriasis in Mexico *19*, 23 (1975)	F. Biagi
Analysis of symptoms and signs related with intestinal parasitosis in 5,215 cases *19*, 10 (1975)	F. Biagi R. López J. Viso
Untersuchungen zur Biochemie und Pharmacologie der Thymoleptika *11*, 121 (1968) The role of adipose tissue in the distribution and storage of drugs *28*, 273 (1984)	M. H. Bickel
The β-adrenergic-blocking agents, pharmacology, and structure-activity relationships *10*, 46 (1966)	J. H. Biel B. K. B. Lum
Prostaglandins *17*, 410 (1973)	J. S. Bindra R. Bindra
In vitro models for the study of antibiotic activities *31*, 349 (1987)	J. Blaser S. H. Zinner
The red blood cell membrane as a model for targets of drug action *17*, 59 (1973)	L. Bolis
Epidemiology and public health. Importance of intestinal nematode infections in Latin America *19*, 28 (1975)	D. Botero
Clinical importance of cardiovascular drug interactions *25*, 133 (1981) Serum electrolyte abnormalities caused by drugs *30*, 9 (1986)	D. Craig Brater
Update of cardiovascular drug interactions *29*, 9 (1985)	D. Craig Brater Michael R. Vasko
Some practical problems of the epidemiology of leprosy in the Indian context *18*, 25 (1974)	S. G. Browne
Brain neurotransmitters and the development and maintenance of experimental hypertension *30*, 127 (1986)	Jerry J. Buccafusco Henry E. Brezenoff
Die Ionenaustauscher und ihre An-wendung in der Pharmazie und Medizin *1*, 11 (1959)	J. Büchi

Wert und Bewertung der Arzneimittel *10*, 90 (1966)	J. Büchi
Cyclopropane compounds of biological interest *15*, 227 (1971) The state of medicinal science *20*, 9 (1976) Isosterism and bioisosterism in drug design *37*, 287 (1991)	A. Burger
Human and veterinary anthelmintics (1965–1971) *17*, 108 (1973)	R. B. Burrows
The antibody basis of local immunity to experimental cholera infection in the rabbit ileal loop *19*, 471 (1975)	W. Burrows J. Kaur
Les dérivés organiques du fluor d'intérêt pharmacologique *3*, 9 (1961)	N. P. Buu-Hoï
Teaching tropical medicine *18*, 35 (1974)	K. M. Cahill
Anabolic steroids *2*, 71 (1960)	B. Camerino G. Sala
Immunosuppression agents, procedures, speculations and prognosis *16*, 67 (1972)	G. W. Camiener W. J. Wechter
Dopamine agonists: Structure-activity relationships *29*, 303 (1985)	Joseph G. Cannon
Therapeutic applications of cytokines for immunostimulation and immuno- suppression: An update *47*, 211 (1996)	Gaetano Cardi Thomas L. Ciardelli Marc S. Ernstoff
Analgesics and their antagonists: Recent developments *22*, 149 (1978)	A. F. Casy
Chemical nature and pharmacological actions of quaternary ammonium salts *2*, 135 (1960)	C. J. Cavallito A. P. Gray
Contributions of medicinal chemistry to medicine – from 1935 *12*, 11 (1968) Changing influences on goals and incentives in drug research and development *20*, 159 (1976) Quaternary ammonium salts – advances in chemistry and pharmacology since 1960 *24*, 267 (1980)	C. J. Cavallito

Über Vorkommen und Bedeutung der Indolstruktur in der Medizin und Biologie *2*, 227 (1960)	A. Cerletti
The new generation of monoamine oxidase inhibitors *38*, 171 (1992)	Andrea M. Cesura Alfred Pletscher
Cholesterol and its relation to atherosclerosis *1*, 127 (1959)	K. K. Chen Tsung-Min Lin
Effect of hookworm disease on the structure and function of small bowel *19*, 44 (1975)	H. K. Chuttani R. C. Misra
Recent developments in antidepressant agents *46*, 183 (1996)	James Claghorn Michael D. Lesem
Generation of new-lead structures in computer-aided drug design *45*, 205 (1995)	Nissim Claude Cohen Vincenzo Tschinke
The psychomimetic agents *15*, 68 (1971)	S. Cohen
The identification and development of antiviral agents for the treatment of hepatitis B virus infection *50*, 259 (1998)	Joseph M. Colacino Kirk A. Staschke
Implementation of disease control in Asia and Africa *18*, 43 (1974)	M. J. Colbourne
Structure-activity relationships in certain anthelmintics *3*, 75 (1961)	J. C. Craig M. E. Tate
Contribution of Haffkine to the concept and practice of controlled field trials of vaccines *19*, 481 (1975)	B. Cvjetanovic
Antifungal agents *22*, 93 (1978)	P. F. D'Arcy E. M. Scott
Carcinogenecity, mutagenecity and cancer preventing activities of flavanoids: A structure-system-activity relationship (SSAR) analysis *42*, 133 (1994)	A. Das J. H. Wang E. J. Lien
Some neuropathologic and cellular aspects of leprosy 18, 53 (1974)	D. K. Dastur Y. Ramamohan A. S. Dabholkar
Autonomic dysfunction as a problem in the treatment of tetanus *19*, 245 (1975)	F. D. Dastur G. J. Bhat K. G. Nair

Studies on *Vibrio parahaemolyticus* infection in Calcutta as compared to cholera infection *19*, 490 (1975)	B. C. Deb
Biochemical effects of drugs acting on the central nervous system *8*, 53 (1965)	L. Decsi
Some reflections on the chemotherapy of tropical diseases: Past, present and future *26*, 343 (1982)	E. W. J. de Maar
Drug research – whence and whither *10*, 11 (1966)	R. G. Denkewalter M. Tishler
Immunization of a village, a new approach to herd immunity *19*, 252 (1975)	N. S. Deodhar
Profiles of tuberculosis in rural areas of Maharashtra *18*, 91 (1974)	M. D. Deshmukh K. G. Kulkarni S. S. Virdi B. B. Yodh
The interface between drug research, marketing, management, and social, political and regulatory forces *20*, 181 (1976) Medicinal research: Retrospectives and perspectives *29*, 97 (1985) Serendipity and structured research in drug discovery *30*, 189 (1986) Medicinal chemistry: A support or a driving force in drug research? *34*, 343 (1990) Heterocyclic diversity: The road to biological activity *44*, 9 (1995)	G. deStevens
Hypolipidemic agents *13*, 217 (1969)	G. deStevens W. L. Bencze R. Hess
Antihypertensive agents *20*, 197 (1976)	G. deStevens M. Wilhelm
RNA virus evolution and the control of viral disease *33*, 93 (1989)	Esteban Domingo

The role of apoptosis in neurodegenerative diseases *48*, 55 (1997)	Iradj Hajimohamadreza J. Mark Treherne
Appetite suppression, pharmacology of *54*, 1 (2000)	Jason C. G. Halford John E. Blundell
Approaches to the rational design of bacterial vaccines *32*, 377 (1988)	Peter Hambleton Stephen D. Prior Andrew Robinson
Clinical field trial of bitoscanate in *Necator americanus* infection, South Thailand *19*, 64 (1975)	T. Harinasuta D. Bunnag
Pharmacological control of reproduction in women *12*, 47 (1968) Contraception – retrospect and prospect *21*, 293 (1977)	M. J. K. Harper
Drug latentiation *4*, 221 (1962)	N. J. Harper
Dopamine receptor diversity: Molecular and pharmacological perspectives *48*, 173 (1997)	Deborah S. Hartman Olivier Civelli
Chemotherapy of filariasis *9*, 191 (1966) Filariasis in India *18*, 173 (1974)	F. Hawking
Production and action of interferons: New insights into molecular mechanisms of gene regulation and expression *43*, 239 (1994)	Mark P. Hayes Kathryn C. Zoon
Recent studies in the field of indole compounds *6*, 75 (1963)	R. V. Heinzelmann J. Szmuszkovicz
Neuere Entwicklungen auf dem Gebiete therapeutisch verwendbarer organischer Schwefelverbindungen *4*, 9 (1962)	H. Herbst
Subclassification and nomenclature of α_1- and α_2-adrenoceptors *47*, 81 (1996)	J. Paul Hieble Robert R. Ruffolo
The management of acute diarrhea in children: An overview *19*, 527 (1975)	N. Hirschhorn
The tetracyclines *17*, 210 (1973)	J. J. Hlavka J. H. Booth
Chemotherapy for systemic mycoses *33*, 317 (1989) Antifungal therapy *44*, 87 (1995)	Paul D. Hoeprich

Biological activity of the terpenoids and their derivatives *6*, 279 (1963)	M. Martin-Smith T. Khatoon
Biological activity of the terpenoids and their derivatives – recent advances *13*, 11 (1969)	M. Martin-Smith W. E. Sneader
Antihypertensive agents 1962–1968 *13*, 101 (1969)	A. Marxer O. Schier
Fundamental structures in drug research – Part I *20*, 385 (1976) Fundamental structures in drug research – Part II *22*, 27 (1978) Antihypertensive agents 1969–1980 *25*, 9 (1981)	A. Marxer O. Schier
Relationships between the chemical structure and pharmacological activity in a series of synthetic quinuclidine derivatives *13*, 293 (1969)	M. D. Mashkovsky L. N. Yakhontov
Further developments in research on the chemistry and pharmacology of synthetic quinuclidine derivatives *27*, 9 (1983)	M. D. Mashkovsky L. N. Yakhontov M. E. Kaminka E. E. Mikhlina S. Ordzhonikidze
Role of neutrotransmitters in the central regulation of the cardiovascular system *35*, 25 (1990) Neurotransmitters involved in the central regulation of the cardiovascular system *46*, 43 (1996)	Robert B. McCall
On the understanding of drug potency *13*, 123 (1971) The chemotherapy of intestinal nematodes *16*, 157 (1972)	J. W. McFarland
Non-steroidal menses-regulating agents: The present status *44*, 159 (1995)	P.K. Mehrotra Sanjay Batra A.P. Bhaduri
Zur Beeinflussung der Strahlen-empfindlichkeit von Säugetieren durch chemische Substanzen *9*, 11 (1966)	H.-J. Melching C. Streffer
Analgesia and addiction *5*, 155 (1963)	L. B. Mellett L. A. Woods
Comparative drug metabolism *13*, 136 (1969)	L. B. Mellett

Effects of NSAIDs on the kidney *49*, 155 (1997)	M. D. Murray D. Craig Brater
A field trial with bitoscanate in India *19*, 81 (1975)	G. S. Mutalik R. B. Gulati A. K. Iqbal
Comparative study of bitoscanate, bephenium hydroxynaphthoate and tetrachlorethylene in hookworm disease *19*, 86 (1975)	G. S. Mutalik R. B. Gulati
Ganglienblocker *2*, 297 (1960)	K. Nádor
Nitroimidazoles as chemotherapeutic agents *27*, 162 (1983)	M. D. Nair K. Nagarajan
Recent advances in cholera pathophysiology and therapeutics *19*, 563 (1975)	D. R. Nalin
Preparing the ground for research: Importance of data *18*, 239 (1974)	A. N. D. Nanavati
Computer-assisted structure – antileukemic activity analysis of purines and their aza and deaza analogs *34*, 319 (1990)	V. L. Narayanan Mohamed Nasr Kenneth D. Paull
Mechanism of drugs action on ion and water transport in renal tubular cells *26*, 87 (1982)	Yu. V. Natochin
Progesterone receptor binding of steroidal and nonsteroidal compounds *30*, 151 (1986)	Neelima M. Seth A. P. Bhaduri
Recent advances in drugs against hypertension *29*, 215 (1985)	Neelima B. K. Bhat A. P. Bhaduri
High resolution nuclear magnetic resonance spectroscopy of biological samples as an aid to drug development *31*, 427 (1987)	J. K. Nicholson Ian D. Wilson
Antibody response to two cholera vaccines in volunteers *19*, 554 (1975)	Y. S. Nimbkar R. S. Karbhari S. Cherian N. G. Chanderkar R. P. Bhamaria P. S. Ranadive B. B. Gaitonde
Surface interaction between bacteria and phagocytic cells *32*, 137 (1988)	L. Öhman G. Maluszynska K. E. Magnusson O. Stendahl

The impact of state and society on medical research *35*, 9 (1990)	C. R. Pfaltz
Transfer factor in malignancy *42*, 401 (1994)	Giancarlo Pizza Caterina De Vinci H. Hugh Fudenberg
Monoaminoxydase-Hemmer *2*, 417 (1960)	A. Pletscher K. F. Gey P. Zeller
Antifungal therapy: Are we winning? *37*, 183 (1991)	A. Polak P. G. Hartman
Antifungal therapy, an everlasting battle *49*, 219 (1997)	A. Polak
Neuropeptides in drug research *54*, 161 (2000)	David Poyner Helen Cox Mark Bushfield J. Mark Treherne Melissa K. Demetrikopoulos
What makes a good pertussis vaccine? *19*, 341 (1975) Vaccine composition in relation to antigenic variation of the microbe: Is pertussis unique? *19*, 347 (1975) Some unsolved problems with vaccines *23*, 9 (1979) Eradication by vaccination: The memorial to smallpox could be surrounded by others *41*, 151 (1993)	N. W. Preston
Peptide drug delivery into the central nervous system *51*, 95 (1998)	Laszlo Prokai
Antibiotics in the chemotherapy of malaria *26*, 167 (1982)	S. K. Puri G. P. Dutta
Potassium channel openers: Airway pharmacology and clinical possibilities in asthma *37*, 161 (1991)	David Raeburn Jan-Anders Karlsson
Isozyme-selective cyclic nucleotide phosphodiesterase inhibitors: Biochemistry, pharmacology and therapeutic potential in asthma *40*, 9 (1993)	David Raeburn John E. Souness Adrian Tomkinson Jan-Anders Karlsson
Clinical study of diphtheria, tetanus and pertussis *19*, 356 (1975)	V. B. Raju V. R. Parvathi
Epidemiology of cholera in Hyderabad *19*, 578 (1975)	K. Rajyalakshmi P. V. Ramana Rao
Present status of hepatoprotectants *52*, 53 (1999)	Vishnu Ji Ram Atul Goel

Tetrahydroisoquinolines and β-carbolines: Putative natural substances in plants and animals *29*, 415 (1985)	H. Rommelspacher R. Susilo
Functional significance of the various components of the influenza virus 18, 253 (1974)	R. Rott
Drug receptors and control of the cardiovascular system: Recent advances *36*, 117 (1991)	Robert R. Ruffolo Jr J. Paul Hieble David P. Brooks Giora Z. Feuerstein Andrew J. Nichols
Behavioral correlates of presynaptic events in the cholinergic neurotransmitter system *32*, 43 (1988)	Roger W. Russell
Epidemiology of pertussis *19*, 257 (1975)	J. A. Sa
Surgical amoebiasis *18*, 77 (1974)	A. E. de Sa
Role of beta-adrenergic blocking drug propranolol in severe tetanus *19*, 361 (1975)	G. S. Sainani K. L. Jain V. R. D. Deshpande A. B. Balsara S. A. Iyer
Studies on *Vibrio parahaemolyticus* in Bombay *19*, 586 (1975)	F. L. Saldanha A. K. Patil M. V. Sant
Leukotriene antagonists and inhibitors of leukotriene biosynthesis as potential therapeutic agents *37*, 9 (1991)	John A. Salmon Lawrence G. Garland
Pharmacology and toxicology of axoplasmic transport *28*, 53 (1984)	Fred Samson Ralph L. Smith J. Alejandro Donoso
Clinical experience with bitoscanate *19*, 96 (1975)	M. R. Samuel
Tetanus: Situational clinical trials and therapeutics *19*, 367 (1975)	R. K. M. Sanders M. L. Peacock B. Martyn B. D. Shende
Epidemiological studies on cholera in non-endemic regions with special reference to the problem of carrier state during epidemic and non-epidemic period *19*, 594 (1975)	M. V. Sant W. N. Gatlewar S. K. Bhindey

Endogenous digitalis-like factors *41*, 249 (1993)	Wilhelm Schoner
Die Anwendung radioaktiver Isotope in der pharmazeutischen Forschung *7*, 59 (1964)	K. E. Schulte
Natürliche und synthetische Acetylen-Verbindungen als Arzneistoffe *14*, 387 (1970)	K. E. Schulte G. Rücker
The role of cytokines in macrophage activation *35*, 105 (1990) The potential role of cytokines in cancer therapy *39*, 219 (1992) Newer antifolates in cancer therapy *44*, 129 (1995)	Richard M. Schultz
Central control of aterial pressure by drugs *26*, 353 (1982)	A. Scriabine D. G. Taylor E. Hong
Pharmacological properties of the natural polyamines and their depletion by biosyn- thesis inhibitors as a therapeutic approach *37*, 107 (1991)	Nikolaus Seiler
The natural polyamines and the immune system *43*, 87 (1994)	Nikolaus Seiler C. L. Atanassov
Aminoglycosides and polyamines: Targets and effects in the mammalian organism of two important groups of natural ali- phatic polycations *46*, 183 (1996)	N. Seiler A. Hardy J. P. Moulinoux
Chemistry and pharmacology of cannabis *36*, 71 (1991)	Renu Seth Shradha Sinha
The structure and biogenesis of certain antibiotics *2*, 591 (1960)	W. A. Sexton
Quinolones *31*, 243 (1987)	P. M. Shah
Role of periodic deworming of pre-school community in national nutrition programmes *19*, 136 (1975)	P. M. Shah A. E. Junnarkar R. D. Khare
Advances in the treatment and control of tissue-dwelling helminth parasites *30*, 473 (1986) The benzimidazole anthelmitics chemistry and biological activity *27*, 85 (1983)	Satyavan Sharma

Treatment of helminth diseases, challenges and achievements *31*, 9 (1987) Vector-borne diseases *35*, 365 (1990)	Satyavan Sharma
Chemotherapy of cestode infections *24*, 217 (1980)	Satyavan Sharma S. K. Dubey R. N. Iyer
Chemotherapy of hookworm infections *26*, 9 (1982)	Satyavan Sharma Elizabeth S. Charles
Ayurvedic medicine – past and present *15*, 11 (1971)	Shiv Sharma
Mechanisms of anthelmintic action *19*, 147 (1975)	U. K. Sheth
Aspirin as an antithrombotic agent *33*, 43 (1989)	Melvin J. Silver Giovanni Di Minno
Immunopharmacological approach to the study of chronic brain disorders *30*, 345 (1986) Implications of immunomodulant therapy in Alzheimer's disease *32*, 21 (1988)	Vijendra K. Singh H. Hugh Fudenberg
Neuroimmune axis as a basis of therapy in Alzheimer's disease *34*, 383 (1990) Immunoregulatory role of neuropeptides *38*, 149 (1992) Neuropeptides as native immune modulators *45*, 9 (1995) Immunotherapy for brain diseases and mental illnesses *48*, 129 (1997)	Vijendra K. Singh
Natural products as anticancer agents *42*, 53 (1994)	Shradha Sinha Sudha Jain
Biologically active quinazolones *43*, 143 (1994)	Shradha Sinha Mukta Srivastava
Some often neglected factors in the control and prevention of communicable diseases *18*, 277 (1974)	C. E. G. Smith
Tetanus and its prevention *19*, 391 (1975)	J. W. G. Smith
Growth of *Clostridium tetani in vivo* *19*, 384 (1975)	J. W. G. Smith A. G. MacIver
The biliary excretion and enterohepatic circulation of drugs and other organic compounds *9*, 299 (1966)	R. L. Smith

Aspects of social pharmacology *22*, 9 (1978)	J. Venulet
The current status of cholera toxoid research in the United States *19*, 602 (1975)	W. F. Verwey J. C. Guckian J. Craig N. Pierce J. Peterson H. Williams Jr
Systemic cancer therapy: Four decades of progress and some personal perspectives *34*, 76 (1990)	Charles L. Vogel
Abnormalities of protein kinases in neurodegenerative diseases *51*, 133 (1998)	Ravenska T. E. Wagey Charles Krieger
The problem of diphtheria as seen in Bombay *19*, 452 (1975)	M. M. Wagle R. R. Sanzgiri Y. K. Amdekar
Drug nephrotoxicity – The significance of cellular mechanisms *41*, 51 (1993)	Robert J. Walker J. Paul Fawcett
Protease inhibitors as potential antiviral agents for the treatment of picornaviral infections *52*, 197 (1999)	Q. May Wang
Recent advances in prevention and treatment of hepatitis C virus infection *55*, 1 (2000)	Q. May Wang Beverly A. Heinz
Nicotine: An addictive substance or a therapeutic agent? *33*, 9 (1989)	David M. Warburton
Cell-wall antigens of *Vibrio cholerae* and their implication in cholera immunity *19*, 612 (1975)	Y. Watanabe R. Ganguly
Steroidogenic capacity in the adrenal cortex and its regulation *34*, 359 (1990)	Michael R. Watermann Evan R. Simpson
Antigen-specific T-cell factors and drug research *32*, 9 (1988)	David R. Webb
Where is immunology taking us? *20*, 573 (1976) Immunology in drug research *28*, 233 (1984)	W. J. Wechter Barbara E. Loughman
Natriuretic hormones *34*, 231 (1990)	W. J. Wechter Elaine J. Benaksas
The effects of NSAIDs and E-prosta- glandins on bone: A two signal hypothesis for the maintenance of skeletal bone *39*, 351 (1992)	William J. Wechter

Backlist

Vol. 1–46 available

Vol. 47, 1996, 346 pp. ISBN 3-7643-5299-X
Kurt R. H. Repke, Kathleen J. Sweadner,
Jürgen Weiland, Rudolf Megges and
Rudolf Schön: In search of ideal inotropic
steroids: Recent progress
Silvano Sozzani, Paola Allavena, Paul Proost,
Jo Van Damme and Alberto Mantovani:
Chemokines as targets for pharmacologi-
cal intervention
J. Paul Hieble and Robert R. Ruffolo, Jr: Sub-
classification and nomenclature of α_1-
and α_2-adrenoceptors
E. Leong Way, Yong Qing Liu and Chieh-Fu
Chen: Perspective and overview of Chi-
nese traditional medicine and contempo-
rary pharmacology
Jeanne Fürst Jucker and Gary P. Anderson:
Emerging drug targets in the molecular
pathogenesis of asthma
Gaetano Cardi, Thomas L. Ciardelli and
Marc S. Ernstoff: Therapeutic applications
of cytokines for immunostimulation and
immunosuppression: An update
Pushkar N. Kaul: Alternative therapeutic
modalities. Alternative medicine
Leo E. Hollister and Enrique S. Garza-
Trevino: Calcium channel blockers in
psychiatry

Vol. 48, 1997, 288 pp. ISBN 3-7643-5671-5
Eric J. Lien, Arima Das, Partha Nandy and
Shijun Ren: Physicochemical basis of the
universal genetic codes – quantitative
analysis
Horst Kleinkauf and Hans von Döhren:
Enzymatic generation of complex pep-
tides
Iradj Hajimohamadreza and J. Mark Tre-
herne: The role of apoptosis in neurode-
generative diseases
Esteban Domingo, Luis Menéndez-Arias,
Miguel E. Quiñones-Mateu, Africa Hol-
guín, Mónica Gutiérrez-Rivas, Miguel A.
Martínez, Josep Quer, Isabel S. Novella
and John J. Holland: Viral quasispecies

and the problem of vaccine-escape and
drug-resistant mutants
Vijendra K. Singh: Immunotherapy for
brain diseases and mental illnesses
Shijun Ren and Eric J. Lien: Natural products and their derivatives as cancer
chemopreventive agents
Deborah S. Hartman and Olivier Civelli:
Dopamine receptor diversity: Molecular
and pharmacological perspectives
Vera M. Kolb: Novel and unusual nucleo-
sides as drugs

Vol. 49, 1997, 373 pp. ISBN 3-7643-5672-3
Richard M. Eglen: 5-Hydroxytryptamine (5-
HT)4 receptors and central nervous
system function: An update
Mont R. Juchau: Chemical teratogenesis in
humans: Biochemical and molecular
mechanisms
Gillian Edwards and Arthur H. Weston:
Recent advances in potassium channel
modulation
Helen Wise: Neuronal prostacyclin receptors
M.D. Murray and D. Craig Brater: Effects of
NSAIDs on the kidney
Olivier Valdenaire and Philippe Vernier: G
protein coupled receptors as modules of
interacting proteins: A family meeting
Annemarie Polak: Antifungal therapy, an
everlasting battle

Vol. 50, 1998, 373 pp. ISBN 3-7643-5821-1
P.N. Kaul: Drug discovery: Past, present and
future
G. Edwards and A.H. Weston: Endothelium-
derived hyperpolarizing factor – a critical
appraisal
M. Rohmer: Isoprenoid biosynthesis via the
mevalonate-independent route, a novel
target for antibacterial drugs
R.W. Rockhold: Glutamatergic involvement
in psychomotor stimulant action
T.D. Johnson: Polyamines and cerebral
ischemia
J.M. Colacino and K.A. Staschke: The identification and development of antiviral
agents for the treatment of chronic
hepatitis B virus infection